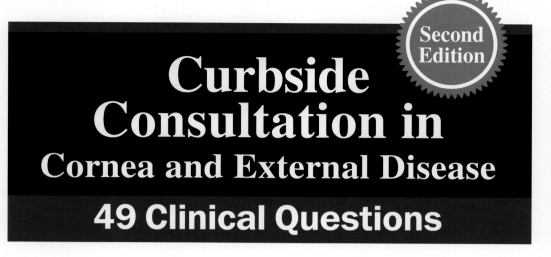

Curbside Consultation in
Cornea and External Disease

Second Edition

49 Clinical Questions

Curbside Consultation in Ophthalmology
Series

SERIES EDITOR, DAVID F. CHANG, MD

Second Edition

Curbside Consultation in
Cornea and External Disease

49 Clinical Questions

EDITORS

David R. Hardten, MD
Minnesota Eye Consultants
Minnetonka, Minnesota
University of Minnesota
Minneapolis, Minnesota

Mark S. Hansen, MD
Attending Surgeon
Minnesota Eye Consultants
Minnetonka, Minnesota

ASSOCIATE EDITOR

Celine E. Satija, MD
Sight MD
Brooklyn and Hewlett, New York
Department of Ophthalmology and Visual Neurosciences
University of Minnesota
Minneapolis, Minnesota

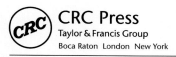

CRC Press
Taylor & Francis Group
Boca Raton London New York

CRC Press is an imprint of the
Taylor & Francis Group, an **informa** business

First published 2022 by SLACK Incorporated

Published 2024 by CRC Press
2385 NW Executive Center Drive, Suite 320, Boca Raton FL 33431

and by CRC Press
4 Park Square, Milton Park, Abingdon, Oxon, OX14 4RN

CRC Press is an imprint of Taylor & Francis Group, LLC

Cover Artist: Donna Trapani

Library of Congress Cataloging-in-Publication Data

Names: Hardten, David R., 1961- editor. | Hansen, Mark S, editor. | Satija,
  Celine E., editor.
Title: Curbside consultation in cornea and external diseases : 49 clinical
  questions / editors, David R Hardten, Mark S Hansen ; associate editor,
  Celine E. Satija
Other titles: Curbside consultation in cornea and external disease. |
  Curbside consultation in ophthalmology series.
Description: Second edition. | Thorofare, NJ : SLACK Incorporated, [2022] |
  Series: Curbside consultation in ophthalmology | Preceded by Curbside
  consultation in cornea and external disease / editor, Francis W. Price
  Jr ; associate editors, Marianne O. Price, Erik Letko. c2010. | Includes
  bibliographical references and index.
Identifiers: LCCN 2022002653 (print) | ISBN 9781630917746 (paperback) |
Subjects: MESH: Corneal Diseases--complications | Corneal Diseases--therapy
  | Corneal Injuries--therapy | BISAC: MEDICAL / Ophthalmology
Classification: LCC RE336 (print) | NLM WW 220 | DDC
  617.7/19--dc23/eng/20220131
LC record available at https://lccn.loc.gov/2022002653

ISBN: 9781630917746 (pbk)
ISBN: 9781003523499 (ebk)

DOI: 10.1201/9781003523499

Dedication

We dedicate this book to all ophthalmologists and optometrists around the globe who are treating patients who may benefit from a curbside consultation with the cornea specialists who contributed to this effort.

Contents

Acknowledgments

We would like to acknowledge the work that Francis W. Price Jr, MD; Marianne Price, PhD; and Erik Letko, MD, put forth in creating the first edition of this text. While we attempted to update this book to reflect the rapidly changing field of cornea, many of the prompts from the first edition still remain relevant in this edition. Their foundation demonstrated that there is a high need for a text such as this one, and we are happy to continue to meet the needs of the eye care providers who review this text.

About the Editors

David R. Hardten, MD is a cornea, refractive, and anterior surgery subspecialist in Minnesota. He teaches at many national and international meetings, and he highly values his involvement in resident and fellow teaching. He has served in leadership positions in many national ophthalmology organizations.

Mark S. Hansen, MD is an anterior segment surgeon at Minnesota Eye Consultants. He is the fellowship director of the cornea and glaucoma fellowship program and enjoys teaching. He also participates in international ophthalmology trips and works to train local residents and surgeons in Central America. He is on the board of directors for a nonprofit organization, Central American Eye Clinics.

About the Associate Editor

Celine E. Satija, MD is a clinical cornea fellow at Tufts University New England Eye Center and Ophthalmic Consultants of Boston. She graduated from Princeton University with her undergraduate degree, after which she attended Tulane University School of Medicine. She completed her ophthalmology residency at the University of Minnesota.

Contributing Authors

Natalie A. Afshari, MD (Question 16)
Shiley Eye Institute
Viterbi Family Department of Ophthalmology
University of California San Diego
San Diego, California

Zaina Al-Mohtaseb, MD (Question 47)
Baylor College of Medicine
Houston, Texas

Brian D. Alder, MD (Question 24)
Shepherd Eye Center
Las Vegas, Nevada

Shelby Anderson, OD (Question 34)
Sanford Health
Sioux Falls, South Dakota

Penny Asbell, MD, MBA (Question 33)
Barrett G. Haik Endowed Chair
Professor of Ophthalmology
Department of Ophthalmology
The University of Tennessee
    Health Science Center
Hamilton Eye Institute
Memphis, Tennessee

Brandon Baartman, MD (Question 10)
Vance Thompson Vision
Omaha, Nebraska

James R. Barnes, BS (Question 39)
Virginia Commonwealth University
    School of Medicine
Richmond, Virginia

Melissa Barnett, OD (Question 12)
University of California
Davis Eye Center
Sacramento, California

John Berdahl, MD (Question 49)
Vance Thompson Vision
Sioux Falls, South Dakota

Benjamin B. Bert, MD (Question 23)
Health Sciences Assistant Professor
Doheny and Stein Eye Institutes
David Geffen School of Medicine
University of California, Los Angeles
Los Angeles, California

Andrea Blitzer, MD (Question 36)
University of Iowa
Iowa City, Iowa

Daniel Brocks, MD (Question 33)
BostonSight
Needham, Massachusetts

Jessica Chow, MD (Question 22)
Yale University School of Medicine
Department of Ophthalmology and
    Visual Science
New Haven, Connecticut

Reza Dana, MD, MSc, MPH (Question 15)
Cornea Service, Massachusetts Eye & Ear
Harvard Medical School
Boston, Massachusetts

Derek W. DelMonte, MD (Question 29)
Carolina Eye Associates, P.A.
Cornea, Cataract and Refractive Surgery
Greensboro/Winston-Salem, North Carolina

Deepinder K. Dhaliwal, MD, L.Ac (Question 35)
UPMC Eye Center
Pittsburgh, Pennsylvania

Ali R. Djalilian, MD (Question 21)
Illinois Eye and Ear Infirmary
University of Illinois at Chicago
Chicago, Illinois

Ahmad Fahmy, OD (Question 34)
Co-Founder, Eyes On Dry Eye
Founder, Twin Cities Ocular Surface Disease
    Symposium
Consultative Optometry, Minnesota Eye
    Consultants
Adjunct Clinical Professor
Optometric Externship Director
Illinois College of Optometry
Chicago, Illinois

Brad H. Feldman, MD (Question 16)
Philadelphia Eye Associates
Wills Eye Hospital
Sidney Kimmel Medical College of
    Thomas Jefferson University Hospital
Philadelphia, Pennsylvania

C. Stephen Foster, MD (Question 19)
Harvard Medical School
Boston, Massachusetts

Martin L. Fox, MD (Question 6)
Medical Director
Cornea and Refractive Surgery Practice
    of New York
New York, New York
Surgeon Consultant
Kismet New Vision Holdings
Cincinnati, Ohio

Frederick (Rick) W. Fraunfelder, MD (Question 25)
Mason Eye Institute
Department of Ophthalmology
University of Missouri
Columbia, Missouri

Prashant Garg, MD (Question 28)
LV Prasad Eye Institute
Hyderabad, India

Mark S. Gorovoy, MD (Question 1)
Gorovoy MD Eye Specialists
Fort Myers, Florida

Preeya K. Gupta, MD (Question 4)
Triangle Eye Consultants
Cary, North Carolina

Ramon Joaquim Hallal Jr, MD (Question 41)
Cornea and Refractive Surgery Specialist
Cascavel, Paraná, Brazil

Sadeer B. Hannush, MD (Question 2)
Professor of Ophthalmology
Sidney Kimmel Medical College of
    Thomas Jefferson University
Wills Eye Hospital
Philadelphia, Pennsylvania

Grant C. Hopping, MD (Question 39)
McGovern Medical School
University of Texas Health Science Center
    at Houston
Houston, Texas
Hoopes Durrie Rivera Research Center
Hoopes Vision
Draper, Utah
Utah Lions Eye Bank
Murray, Utah
John A. Moran Eye Center
Department of Ophthalmology and
    Visual Sciences
University of Utah School of Medicine
Salt Lake City, Utah

Mitch Ibach, OD (Question 37)
Vance Thompson Vision
Sioux Falls, South Dakota

Bennie H. Jeng, MD (Question 42)
Department of Ophthalmology and
    Visual Sciences
University of Maryland School of Medicine
Baltimore, Maryland

Kyle Jones, MD (Question 22)
John A. Moran Eye Center
University of Utah
Salt Lake City, Utah

Sumitra S. Khandelwal, MD (Question 9)
Associate Professor of Ophthalmology
Baylor College of Medicine
Houston, Texas

Terry Kim, MD (Question 38)
Professor of Ophthalmology
Duke University School of Medicine
Chief, Cornea Division
Director, Refractive Surgery Service
Duke University Eye Center
Durham, North Carolina

Thomas Kohnen, MD, PhD (Question 8)
Professor and Chair
Department of Ophthalmology
University Clinic Frankfurt
Goethe University
Frankfurt am Main, Germany

Brent Kramer, MD (Question 37)
Duke Eye Center
Durham, North Carolina

Bryan S. Lee, MD, JD (Question 48)
Altos Eye Physicians
Los Altos, California

Gary Legault, MD (Question 46)
Brooke Army Medical Center
San Antonio, Texas
Uniformed Services University of the
    Health Sciences
Bethesda, Maryland

Erik Letko, MD (Question 31)
Kaiser Permanente
Lafayette, Colorado

Wendy Liu, MD (Question 27)
Department of Anesthesiology
University of Miami
Miller School of Medicine
Miami, Florida

Marian Macsai, MD (Question 36)
Northshore University Health System
Glenview, Illinois

Yuri McKee, MD, MS (Question 44)
East Valley Ophthalmology
Mesa, Arizona

Jill S. Melicher, MD (Question 26)
Ophthalmic Plastics, Orbit and
    Reconstructive Surgery
Minnesota Eye Consultants
Minnetonka, Minnesota

Mark S. Milner, MD (Question 13)
Precision Lasik Group
Cheshire, Connecticut

Majid Moshirfar, MD (Question 39)
Director of Clinical Research
Hoopes Vision Research Center
Draper, Utah
Adjunct Professor of Ophthalmology
Department of Ophthalmology and
    Visual Sciences
John Moran Eye Center
University of Utah
Salt Lake City, Utah
Co-Director, Utah Lions Eye Bank
Murray, Utah

Muanploy Niparugs, MD (Question 21)
Department of Ophthalmology
Faculty of Medicine, Chiang Mai University
Chiang Mai, Thailand

Manachai Nonpassopon, MD (Question 21)
Cornea and Refractive Surgery Unit
Department of Ophthalmology
Faculty of Medicine, Ramathibodi Hospital
Mahidol University
Bangkok, Thailand

Walter T. Parker, MD (Question 43)
Alabama Ophthalmology Associates, P.C.
Birmingham, Alabama

Samuel Passi, MD (Question 5)
Cornea Specialist
The Eye Institute of Utah
Salt Lake City, Utah

Stephen C. Pflugfelder, MD (Question 11)
Baylor College of Medicine
Houston, Texas

Roberto Pineda, MD (Question 41)
Massachusetts Eye and Ear
Harvard Medical School
Boston, Massachusetts

Christopher J. Rapuano, MD (Question 3)
Chief, Cornea Service
Wills Eye Hospital
Professor of Ophthalmology
Sidney Kimmel Medical College at
    Thomas Jefferson University
Philadelphia, Pennsylvania

Nikolas Raufi, MD (Question 38)
Rhode Island Eye Institute
Cataract and Refractive Surgery
Providence, Rhode Island

Sherman W. Reeves, MD, MPH (Question 5)
Minnesota Eye Consultants
Minnetonka, Minnesota

Yasmyne C. Ronquillo, MD, MSc, JD (Question 39)
Hoopes Vision Research Center
Draper, Utah

Cullen D. Ryburn, MD (Question 29)
Eye Center of Northern Colorado
Cornea, Cataract and Refractive Surgery
Fort Collins, Colorado

*Konstantinos D. Sarantopoulos, MD, PhD
    (Question 27)*
Professor of Anesthesiology
Department of Anesthesiology
Perioperative Medicine and Pain Management
Professor of Ophthalmology
Bascom Palmer Eye Institute
University of Miami
    Miller School of Medicine
Miami, Florida

Mohamed Abou Shousha, MD, PhD (Question 18)
Bascom Palmer Eye Institute
University of Miami
    Miller School of Medicine
Miami, Florida

Krishna Surapaneni, MD (Question 45)
SuraVision
Houston, Texas

Daniel Terveen, MD (Question 49)
Vance Thompson Vision
Sioux Falls, South Dakota

Tarika Thareja, MD (Question 35)
Geisinger Eye Institute
Danville, Pennsylvania

Vance Thompson, MD (Question 49)
Director of Refractive Surgery
Vance Thompson Vision
Sioux Falls, South Dakota
Professor of Ophthalmology
University of South Dakota
    Sanford School of Medicine
Vermillion, South Dakota

Kevin R. Tozer, MD (Question 7)
Tozer Eye Center
Scottsdale, Arizona

Elmer Y. Tu, MD (Question 30)
Eye and Ear Infirmary
Chicago, Illinois

Nandini Venkateswaran, MD (Question 4)
Massachusetts Eye and Ear Infirmary
Harvard Medical School
Boston, Massachusetts

David D. Verdier, MD (Question 20)
Clinical Professor
Michigan State University
    College of Human Medicine
Director, Verdier Eye Center PLC
Grand Rapids, Michigan

Jesse M. Vislisel, MD (Question 17)
Associated Eye Care
Stillwater, Minnesota

Laura Voicu, MD (Question 45)
Ophthalmic Consultants of Boston
Boston, Massachusetts

Michael Wallace, MD (Question 33)
Mobile Infirmary Diagnostic and
　　Medical Clinic
Mobile, Alabama

Yvonne Wang, MD (Question 9)
Assistant Professor of Ophthalmology
Yale School of Medicine
New Haven, Connecticut

Steven E. Wilson, MD (Question 14)
Cole Eye Institute, Cleveland Clinic
Cleveland, Ohio

Sonia H. Yoo, MD (Question 18)
Bascom Palmer Eye Institute
University of Miami
　　Miller School of Medicine
Miami, Florida

Zachary Zavodni, MD (Question 40)
The Eye Institute of Utah
Jon A. Moran Eye Center
University of Utah
Salt Lake City, Utah

Elaine Zhou, MD (Question 47)
Baylor College of Medicine
Houston, Texas
Bascom Palmer Eye Institute
Miami, Florida

Preface

The *Curbside Consultation in Cornea and External Disease: 49 Clinical Questions, Second Edition* is an updated collection of clinical questions that comprehensive ophthalmologists, optometrists, and ophthalmology residents are most likely to encounter in the area of cornea. Experts in the field of cornea provide their clinical approach to the difficult questions they come across in their day-to-day practices. We hope this text will help to guide your clinical decisions in these difficult topics, creating better outcomes for your patients.

SECTION I

CORNEAL DYSTROPHY

I HAVE A PATIENT WITH FUCHS' ENDOTHELIAL CORNEAL DYSTROPHY. IS THERE ANYTHING NEW TO IMPROVE THEIR VISION?

Mark S. Gorovoy, MD

Fuchs' endothelial corneal dystrophy (FECD), defined by the presence of dark spots (guttae) on corneal endothelium (Figure 1-1), is the leading indication for corneal transplant in the Western world. This hereditary condition is rarely symptomatic before the sixth decade of life when gradual reduction in visual acuity sets in (Figure 1-2). First guttae and then corneal edema due to endothelial cell insufficiency contribute to reduction of visual acuity. The quality of vision also becomes affected by halos and glare from bright light or while driving at night. Diurnal fluctuation of visual acuity—worse in the morning—is pathognomonic for this condition. In later stages, epithelial edema and progressive stromal fibrosis may develop, resulting in further decrease of vision. At that point, patients may also experience eye irritation and foreign body sensations from an irregular ocular surface and ruptured epithelial bullae.

Diagnosis

Early diagnosis of FECD is important because this condition, even in the beginning stages, may increase the risk for corneal decompensation with intraocular surgery or corneal procedures such as laser in situ keratomileusis (LASIK). The diagnosis is relatively easy to make once guttae can be visualized bilaterally on slit-lamp examination. Ancillary testing, including specular or confocal microscopy and pachymetry, is typically not necessary for the purpose of diagnosis but becomes helpful when monitoring progression of the disease. In contrast, confocal or specular microscopy in the early stages of FECD might play a crucial role in diagnosis, particularly during preoperative evaluation for intraocular or corneal surgery in cases where the degree of suspicion is high and the slit-lamp exam is inconclusive.

Hardten DR, Hansen MS.
Curbside Consultation in Cornea and External Disease:
49 Clinical Questions, Second Edition (pp 3-6).
© 2022 Taylor & Francis Group.

Figure 1-1. Confluent guttae in a patient with Fuchs' corneal endothelial dystrophy.

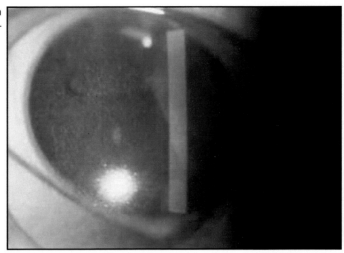

Figure 1-2. Focal corneal edema in a patient with Fuchs' corneal endothelial dystrophy.

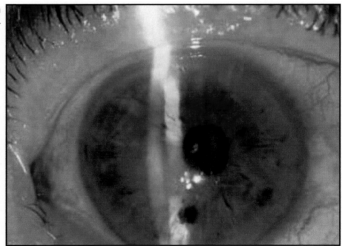

Treatment

Essentially, there is no medical treatment for FECD. Hypertonic saline solution has been used to reduce corneal edema, but its efficacy is limited and is temporary at best. Treatment is typically indicated when the patient becomes symptomatic. Corneal transplantation offers a definitive solution for a symptomatic patient. Penetrating keratoplasty was the standard of treatment for corneal decompensation secondary to FECD. Due to a long vision rehabilitation period and a high risk of vision-threatening complications during and after surgery, penetrating keratoplasty was typically indicated in advanced stages of FECD, when a patient's vision became very poor. Treatment of corneal decompensation secondary to endothelial failure was revolutionized in the late 1990s[1] and was gradually replaced by posterior lamellar endothelial keratoplasty (most recently referred to as *Descemet's stripping [automated] endothelial keratoplasty* [DSEK or DSAEK]).[2] In 2007, 85% of patients in the United States who underwent a corneal transplant for corneal decompensation from endothelial failure also underwent DSAEK. This procedure removes the diseased patient's corneal endothelium with Descemet's membrane and replaces it with a layer of donor cornea,

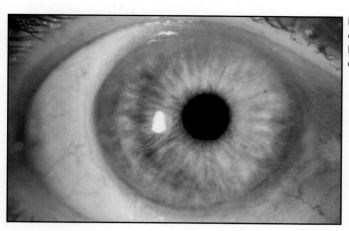

Figure 1-3. A patient with Fuchs' corneal endothelial dystrophy after Descemet's stripping automated endothelial keratoplasty.

consisting of posterior corneal stroma, Descemet's membrane, and healthy endothelial cells. There are numerous advantages of DSAEK when compared to penetrating keratoplasty. Unlike penetrating keratoplasty, the surgery is performed through a small incision, which reduces the chance for catastrophic intraoperative subchoroidal hemorrhage during the surgery that can result in permanent loss of vision or the eye. The likelihood of such catastrophic bleeding with incidental ocular trauma after surgery is small compared to penetrating keratoplasty. Furthermore, vision recovery after DSAEK is faster and superior to the vision recovery after penetrating keratoplasty. Patients typically reach near full recovery of vision within 1 month after DSAEK (Figure 1-3). The best-corrected visual acuity ranges between 20/20 and 20/40 in most patients and the amount of surgically induced postoperative astigmatism is minimal compared to penetrating keratoplasty. Moreover, unlike penetrating keratoplasty, DSAEK does not lead to ocular surface disturbance, which typically contributes to a decrease in vision and prolonged vision recovery. On the other hand, the long-term data on endothelial cell count after DSAEK compare favorably to those seen after penetrating keratoplasty.[3]

Most recently, attempts to further improve vision after DSAEK have been made by Descemet's membrane endothelial keratoplasty (DMEK). The donor tissue in DMEK, unlike in DSAEK, has no corneal stroma adhering to the Descemet's membrane. Visual acuity after DMEK is superior to that seen after DSAEK, with 26% of patients achieving 20/20 and 63% achieving 20/25 or better. The rejection rate is reduced to 1% to 2% vs 5% to 9% found in DSAEK. However, the trade-off is a new surgeon learning curve innate to any new novel procedure as well as increased donor harvesting failure, primary graft failure, and increased donor dislocations.[4] Eye bank donor acquisition has eliminated the donor harvesting issue. The rapid acceptance of DMEK has made it the most common procedure for uncomplicated Fuchs' dystrophy.

The evolution of surgical treatment for Fuchs' dystrophy has further been advanced with a procedure named *Descemet stripping only* (DSO).[5] This novel procedure eliminates the guttae by stripping away the central Descemet's membrane and allowing the mid-peripheral endothelial cells to migrate centrally and fill in this stripped area, totally eliminating any donor. The best candidates are those Fuchs' patients whose symptomatic guttae clustered centrally. The time to clear can be as long as 8 weeks, and the benefit of adding a Rho kinase inhibitor class drop (a glaucoma eye drop) is currently under investigation. Those patients who do not clear can still undergo a DMEK without any adverse sequela from the failed DSO surgery.

Currently, studies are investigating the use of cultured human corneal endothelial cells that can be injected directly into the anterior chamber to increase endothelial cell density.[6] These cells may also be aided by a Rho kinase class drop. This method does not rely on donor tissue and requires very little surgical manipulation. Studies are ongoing, but initial reports appear promising.

References

1. Melles GRJ, Eggink FAGJ, Lander F, et al. A surgical technique for posterior lamellar keratoplasty. *Cornea*. 1998;17(6):618-626.
2. Gorovoy MS. Descemet-stripping automated endothelial keratoplasty. *Cornea*. 2006;25(8):886-889.
3. Price MO, Price FW. Endothelial cell density after Descemet's stripping endothelial keratoplasty: influencing factors and 2-year trend. *Ophthalmology*. 2008;115(5):857-865.
4. Gorovoy MS. DMEK complications. *Cornea*. 2014;33(1):101-104.
5. Moloney G, Petsoglou C, Ball M, et al. Descemetorhexis without grafting for Fuchs' endothelial dystrophy–supplementation with topical ripasudil. *Cornea*. 2017;36(6):642-648.
6. Kinoshita S, Koizumi N, Ueno M, et al. Injection of cultured cells with a ROCK inhibitor for bullous keratopathy. *N Engl J Med*. 2018;378(11):995-1003.

QUESTION

2

I AM SEEING A 64-YEAR-OLD WOMAN FOR CATARACT EVALUATION. THE SLIT-LAMP EXAMINATION IS SIGNIFICANT FOR ANTERIOR BASEMENT MEMBRANE DYSTROPHY AFFECTING THE VISUAL AXIS AND 3+ NUCLEAR SCLEROSIS OF THE LENS IN BOTH EYES. HOW SHOULD I MANAGE THIS PATIENT?

Sadeer B. Hannush, MD

It is important for the clinician to determine the contribution of both the corneal dystrophy and the cataract to the patient's visual compromise.

Anterior basement membrane dystrophy (ABMD), or epithelial basement membrane dystrophy, is the most common corneal dystrophy, with a predilection for women over men. The clinical appearance may vary, and it has been extensively described in the ophthalmic literature over the past century. *Map-dot, fingerprint, mare's tail* (Figure 2-1), and *Cogan's dystrophy* are terms used to describe this entity. Histopathologically, a thickened layer of epithelium is recognized, together with reduplication of the epithelial basement membrane and entrapment of debris in cyst-like structures. Many corneal specialists, especially after the publication of the 2015 update to the International Classification of Corneal Dystrophies,[1] no longer consider ABMD a dystrophy but rather as a degenerative change frequently associated with chronic blepharitis. In clinical practice, we encounter 2 presentations of ABMD: (1) pain, photophobia, and tearing, usually associated with a recurrent erosion syndrome[2-4] (discussed in a different chapter of this book) and (2) decreased visual acuity, associated with an irregular corneal surface overlying the pupillary aperture.

Workup and Treatment

ABMD is often easily observable on slit-lamp examination alone. Characteristic findings include *maps*, which appear as clear zones within gray amorphous or geographic areas; *dots*, which consist of gray putty-like lesions; and *fingerprints*, or parallel curved lines. Even if not easily visible,

Hardten DR, Hansen MS.
Curbside Consultation in Cornea and External Disease:
49 Clinical Questions, Second Edition (pp 7-11).
© 2022 Taylor & Francis Group.

Figure 2-1. Cornea with ABMD, manifesting as "mare's tail."

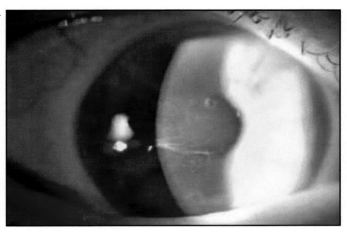

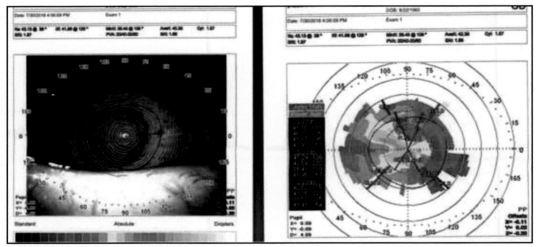

Figure 2-2. Placido disc–based topography of a patient with ABMD showing irregular mires (left) and a high surface regularity index of 1.97 (right).

the negative staining pattern can identify ABMD when fluorescein is added. Also, irregularity on any keratometry readings or topography can clue the clinician to look for this condition.

In this case, when trying to determine how visually significant the central ABMD changes may be to the patient's blurred vision, Placido disc–based corneal topography may be an invaluable tool (Figure 2-2). Irregular mires and an increased surface regularity index usually imply that the surface is a significant contributor to the visual compromise. This may be further confirmed with a rigid gas permeable (RGP) contact lens diagnostic evaluation. If the patient's vision improves significantly with an RGP lens, the cataract may not be the main factor in the patient's poor vision, and cataract surgery should not be rushed into. Moreover, intraocular lens (IOL) implant power calculations are likely to be inaccurate in the setting of inaccurate keratometry measurements. This has become very important in modern cataract surgery, with patients investing in toric and/ or presbyopia-correcting IOL implants to hopefully achieve spectacle-free vision at distance, near, or both.

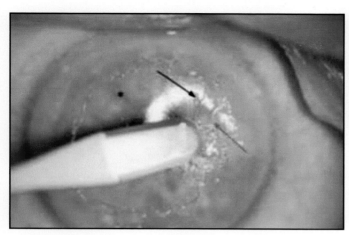

Figure 2-3. Superficial keratectomy, removing the epithelium and basement membrane, baring Bowman's layer. Asterisk: Bowman's layer. Black arrow: edge of epithelial basement membrane, which must also be removed. Blue arrow: edge of the debrided epithelium.

In the preceding scenario, consideration should be given to treating the basement membrane changes prior to cataract surgery.[5] The patient is counseled that treatment of the basement membrane dystrophy may improve her vision enough to delay or obviate the need for cataract surgery. Moreover, treatment will likely create a smooth corneal surface, allowing more accurate calculation of IOL implant power. Should the resultant vision after treatment of the basement membrane changes be inadequate, it may be decided to proceed with cataract surgery. With an irregular surface, any IOL implant power calculation is an estimate at best. After the irregularity is corrected and the surface is smooth, lens power calculations may be made more predictably and the choice of the IOL can be more confidently discussed with the patient.

If, on the other hand, the computerized corneal topography mires are relatively smooth from the outset, and there is minimal improvement in vision with an RGP contact lens, the surgeon may determine that the contribution of the basement membrane changes to the patient's vision is minimal and may decide to proceed with cataract surgery alone. IOL implant power calculation may be carried out using the surgeon's technique of choice. The patient should still be counseled that vision after cataract surgery, with or without spectacle correction, might not be as crisp as desired because of the corneal dystrophy, albeit mild.

When ABMD is visually significant, treatment usually consists of a superficial keratectomy. We favor a dull, rounded or crescent knife to remove the central 5 to 6 mm of corneal epithelium overlying the pupillary aperture (Figure 2-3). The epithelial layer usually cleaves easily off of the basement membrane. It is very important to then deliberately remove the irregular and frequently redundant (duplicated) basement membrane until Bowman's layer is recognized, with its characteristic sheen (Figure 2-4). The same keratectomy/epitheliectomy may be accomplished with 20% ethanol, provided that meticulous attention is given to removal of the abnormal basement membrane. Importantly, a diamond-dusted burr is not required in this setting. Because eliminating recurrent erosions is not the focus of treatment, roughening up Bowman's layer to improve epithelial adherence is not required (unnecessary diamond-dusted burr polishing of Bowman's layer may result in some fibrosis and visually significant haze). Similarly, antifibrosis treatment with mitomycin is not necessary. Moreover, there is no real role for excimer laser phototherapeutic keratectomy in the treatment of ABMD in the absence of recurrent erosions. A therapeutic bandage contact lens is placed instead. I start my patients on a topical steroid, a nonsteroidal anti-inflammatory agent, and a fluoroquinolone antibiotic, which is the custom with most of my ocular surface procedures. Re-epithelialization usually takes place over the next 3 to 7 days. The bandage contact lens is then removed, the topical nonsteroidal anti-inflammatory agent and antibiotic discontinued, and the steroid tapered rapidly. A couple of weeks later, the patient is re-evaluated,

Figure 2-4. Peeling off basement membrane with forceps after epithelial removal. This photo demonstrates the sheen of Bowman's layer after the keratectomy.

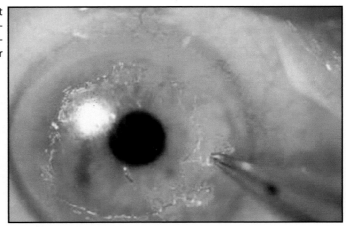

visual acuity is measured again, and computerized corneal topography is repeated. If the patient is pleased with the resultant vision, the endpoint of treatment is achieved. Otherwise, consideration may be given to proceeding with cataract surgery. IOL implant power calculation may be carried out using the technique preferred by the surgeon, usually optical biometry.

The availability of new technology IOLs and the heightened expectations among patients and surgeons of excellent postoperative vision, unaided by spectacle or contact lens correction, necessitate paying extra attention to detail, specifically the identification of contributors to visual compromise other than the cataract. Optimization of the ocular surface, including the preoperative treatment of visually significant ABMD, becomes very important.

Conclusion

Corneal ABMD is most commonly responsible for 2 clinical presentations:

1. Painful corneal erosions

2. Visual compromise

The ophthalmic literature is replete with articles describing techniques for the treatment and prevention of painful recurrent corneal erosions. These techniques most commonly employ a diamond-dusted burr[2-4] or excimer laser phototherapeutic keratectomy[3] to improve epithelial adherence after keratectomy, presumably by creating a mild inflammatory response and subclinical fibrosis of the anterior aspect of Bowman's layer. When ABMD manifests as visual compromise alone, without painful erosions, only removal of the corneal epithelium and underlying basement membrane is necessary. This may be achieved with a blade or with diluted ethanol. No adjuvant therapy with a diamond-dusted burr or laser is required. If there is any doubt regarding the corneal surface's contribution to visual compromise, cataract surgery should be delayed until the surface is optimized.[5] After the surface is made pristine, if the vision remains compromised, presumably secondary to the nuclear sclerotic cataract, the surgeon may proceed with cataract surgery and depend on optical biometry in choosing an IOL, including the new technology IOL varieties.

References

1. Weiss JS, Møller HU, Aldave AJ, et al. IC3D classification of corneal dystrophies—edition 2. *Cornea*. 2015;34(2):117-159. doi:10.1097/ICO.0000000000000307
2. Buxton JN, Constad WH. Superficial epithelial keratectomy in the treatment of epithelial basement membrane dystrophy. *Cornea*. 1987;6(4):292-297.
3. Sridhar MS, Rapuano CJ, Cosar CB, Cohen EJ, Laibson PR. Phototherapeutic keratectomy versus diamond burr polishing of Bowman's membrane in the treatment of recurrent corneal erosions associated with anterior basement membrane dystrophy. *Ophthalmology*. 2002;109(4):674-679.
4. Wong VWY, Chi SCC, Lam DSC. Diamond burr polishing for recurrent corneal erosions: results from a prospective randomized controlled trial. *Cornea*. 2009;28(2):152-156.
5. Goerlitz-Jessen MF, Gupta PK, Kim T. Impact of epithelial basement membrane dystrophy and Salzmann nodular degeneration on biometry measurements. *J Cataract Refract Surg*. 2019;45(8):1119-1123.

I Have a Patient With Bilateral Granular Corneal Dystrophy Who Is Struggling With Their Vision. What Can I Do to Help Them, Short of a Penetrating Keratoplasty?

Christopher J. Rapuano, MD

Granular dystrophy is an autosomal dominant condition, where hyaline material is progressively deposited in the corneas. The opacities are generally first noted in the first to second decades of life and usually become visually significant in the third to fourth decades of life. Initially, the deposits tend to be in the anterior to mid stroma but are discreet, with clear intervening spaces through which the patient can usually see fairly well. These opacities may cause some irregular astigmatism, which can be treated with rigid contact lenses. Additionally, very superficial opacities may cause painful episodes, known as *recurrent erosions*, which can be managed with medications and sometimes a bandage soft contact lens. As patients age, new deposits tend to be rather superficial but much more confluent—it is these confluent opacities that can significantly affect the vision. As the opacities worsen, medications, glasses, and contact lenses are no longer effective and surgery is considered. Depending on the degree and depth of the opacities, a stepwise approach to surgery is usually recommended, starting with a lamellar keratectomy, then a partial-thickness corneal transplant, then a deep anterior lamellar transplant or a full-thickness corneal transplant. Patients need to understand that the granular opacities will recur over months to years.

Lamellar Keratectomy

A lamellar keratectomy is a procedure that removes a superficial layer of cornea. Preoperatively, it is important to determine whether the bulk of the opacities are located in the superficial cornea and are thereby treatable with a lamellar keratectomy or not. As mentioned previously, the deep scattered granules are not usually that visually significant, but as the disease progresses and the

Hardten DR, Hansen MS.
Curbside Consultation in Cornea and External Disease:
49 Clinical Questions, Second Edition (pp 13-17).
© 2022 Taylor & Francis Group.

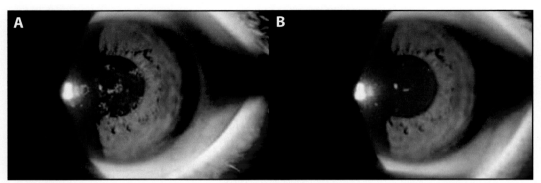

Figure 3-1. (A) Moderate granular corneal dystrophy involving the central cornea. Fortunately, most of the opacities are fairly superficial, making this eye a good candidate for excimer laser PTK. (B) Five weeks after excimer laser PTK, the central cornea is much clearer, and the vision much better, although a few deeper granular opacities remain.

opacities become more confluent, vision can deteriorate significantly. Fortunately, these confluent opacities are usually rather superficial and amenable to treatment with a lamellar keratectomy. Lamellar keratectomy can be performed freehand with a blade, but that typically results in a very irregular surface and poor vison. It can also be performed using a mechanical microkeratome or femtosecond laser to create a "free cap" that is then discarded.[1] The disadvantage of these 2 procedures is that you need to set the depth prior to surgery and cannot modify it during the procedure. An advantage is that tissue can be sent for pathologic examination if desired. Excimer laser phototherapeutic keratectomy (PTK) is a procedure where an excimer laser is used to shave off opacities in the superficial cornea to make the cornea clearer and more regular, ideally improving vision. The primary advantage of PTK over the other lamellar keratectomy procedures is that it is titratable during the procedure.

Phototherapeutic Keratectomy

A wide variety of techniques can be used for the PTK procedure.[2-4] When the epithelium is smooth, as in most eyes with granular dystrophy, I prefer a transepithelial approach, where I set the laser to a large-diameter spot size (eg, 6.5 mm), center the laser on the pupil, and ablate through the epithelium into the stroma. I initially ablate about 66% to 75% of the depth of the opacity, as predicted by a combination of the preoperative slit-lamp examination, pachymetry, and anterior segment optical coherence tomography (when available). I then stop and check the corneal clarity. If the bulk of the opacity has been removed and the cornea is fairly clear, then I stop. Otherwise, I continue ablating small amounts at a time until the cornea is fairly clear. Sometimes, a thin layer of a masking agent (eg, saline) is helpful to achieve the smoothest surface. The general goal is to remove as little tissue as possible to clear most of the opacity. The cornea does not have to be crystal clear for the patient's vision to improve considerably (Figure 3-1). Deeper ablations result in greater scarring and larger hyperopic shifts in refraction.[5] If a deep ablation is required, an anti-hyperopia PTK can be performed by ablating the periphery of the central ablation or a hyperopic PTK card can be used to mitigate some of the expected induction of hyperopia.[6] Mitomycin C 0.02% on an 8-mm sponge for approximately 60 seconds, then irrigated with saline, can also be used to prevent post-PTK haze/scar when deep ablations are necessary. Postoperatively, these eyes are usually treated with a bandage soft contact lens and antibiotic drops and followed closely until the epithelium heals.

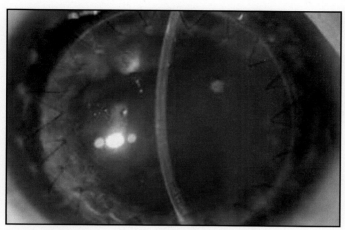

Figure 3-2. This eye underwent a fairly deep anterior lamellar graft for granular dystrophy with posterior involvement. The slit-beam demonstrates an approximately two-thirds–depth graft, with some mild residual granular opacities in the patient's own deep stroma.

In eyes with significant corneal opacities that reach into the mid-stroma, PTK is not a great choice, and a corneal transplant should be considered. Because the endothelium is generally healthy in these eyes, a partial-thickness graft is often a good alternative. A "half-thickness" graft is a good option for some of these eyes, as the risk of perforation and the need to convert to a full-thickness corneal transplant is low (Figure 3-2). There are a variety of techniques for this type of transplant, but the general idea is to remove approximately one-half of the patient's anterior cornea and replace it with a half-thickness corneal transplant. The patient's anterior cornea can be removed with a microkeratome, a femtosecond laser, or by using a manual blade dissection technique. The donor cornea can also be prepared with a microkeratome, femtosecond laser, or, much less common, by using a manual blade dissection technique on an artificial anterior chamber. The hemi-automated lamellar keratoplasty technique uses a partial-thickness trephination of the patient's cornea, which is then manually removed with a semisharp dissector blade. A microkeratome is used to fashion the donor corneal button, which is then trephined to the same (or 0.25 mm larger) diameter as the recipient trephination and then sutured into place.[7]

Deep Anterior Lamellar Keratoplasty

When the opacities reach into the deep cornea, then a deep anterior lamellar keratoplasty (DALK) may be indicated. This technique removes most or all of the stroma, leaving Descemet's membrane and endothelium in place. The primary advantage of DALK over a full-thickness penetrating keratoplasty is the elimination of endothelial rejection. Here too, a variety of DALK techniques are available. The most popular is the "big bubble" technique, where the cornea is trephined and an air bubble is injected into the deep stroma to separate Descemet's membrane from the stroma. The stroma is carefully removed, taking great care not to puncture Descemet's membrane. Descemet's membrane and endothelium are stripped from a full-thickness cornea donor button, which is then sutured into place; again, taking great care not to rupture Descemet's membrane. If a large tear in Descemet's membrane occurs during the DALK procedure, or if the endothelium is abnormal in a patient with granular dystrophy, a full-thickness corneal transplant (penetrating keratoplasty) can be performed.

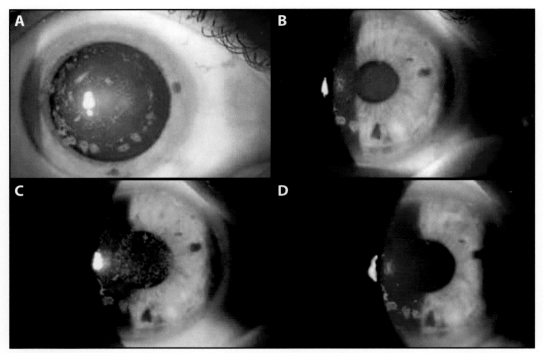

Figure 3-3. (A) Right eye has recurrent granular dystrophy opacities centrally 5 years after excimer laser PTK. (B) Four days after repeat excimer laser PTK of the patient's right eye, the central cornea is much clearer, and the vision greatly improved. (C) Four years later, there is significant recurrent granular dystrophy opacities in the patient's right eye. As is common with recurrent granular dystrophy, these opacities were rather superficial, so were treatable with repeat excimer laser PTK. (D) One day after repeat excimer laser PTK of the patient's right eye, the central cornea is again much clearer, with improved vision.

Other Corneal Dystrophies

The same stepwise approach is used for many other corneal dystrophies, including lattice and Reis-Bücklers' corneal dystrophies, with the caveats that the opacities in lattice corneal dystrophy tend to be deeper and less amenable to PTK, whereas those in Reis-Bücklers' corneal dystrophy tend to be more superficial and more likely to be treatable with PTK. Macular corneal dystrophy involves the full-thickness cornea. PTK can be used to treat the superficial macules, which may help some patients. DALK is somewhat controversial in eyes with macular corneal dystrophy because the endothelium in these eyes is often abnormal. Schnyder corneal dystrophy is another full-thickness corneal dystrophy where PTK may be helpful to remove the superficial crystalline opacities but does not result in crystal-clear cornea. Finally, patients with granular corneal dystrophy type 2 (combined granular-lattice dystrophy, Avellino dystrophy), should avoid LASIK, as it can cause severe exacerbation of the opacities and significantly affect vision.[8]

Using this general treatment algorithm, most patients with granular dystrophy can achieve very good visual outcomes. The granules will recur over time, but the same stepwise approach can used to treat patients with recurrent granular dystrophy[9,10] (Figures 3-3 and 3-4).

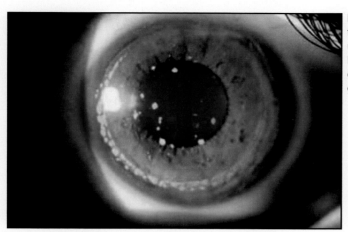

Figure 3-4. This eye underwent a full-thickness corneal graft for granular dystrophy many years before. Note the many recurrent granular dystrophy opacities throughout the graft.

References

1. Steger B, Romano V, Biddolph S, Willoughby CE, Batterbury M, Kaye SB. Femtosecond laser-assisted lamellar keratectomy for corneal opacities secondary to anterior corneal dystrophies: an interventional case series. *Cornea.* 2016;35(1):6-13.
2. Ayres BD, Rapuano CJ. Excimer laser phototherapeutic keratectomy. *Ocul Surf.* 2006;4(4):196-206.
3. Rapuano CJ. Phototherapeutic keratectomy: who are the best candidates and how do you treat them? *Curr Opin Ophthalmol.* 2010;21(4):280-282.
4. Reddy JC, Rapuano CJ, Nagra PK, Hammersmith KM. Excimer laser phototherapeutic keratectomy in eyes with corneal stromal dystrophies with and without a corneal graft. *Am J Ophthalmol.* 2013;155(6):1111-1118.e2.
5. Nakamura T, Kataoka T, Kojima T, Yoshida Y, Sugiyama Y. Refractive outcomes after phototherapeutic refractive keratectomy for granular corneal dystrophy. *Cornea.* 2018;37(5):548-553.
6. Amano S, Kashiwabuchi K, Sakisaka T, Inoue K, Toda I, Tsubota K. Efficacy of hyperopic photorefractive keratectomy simultaneously performed with phototherapeutic keratectomy for decreasing hyperopic shift. *Cornea.* 2016;35(8):1069-1072.
7. Yuen LH, Mehta JS, Shilbayeh R, Lim L, Tan DT. Hemi-automated lamellar keratoplasty (HALK). *Br J Ophthalmol.* 2011;95(11):1513-1518.
8. Woreta FA, Davis GW, Bower KS. LASIK and surface ablation in corneal dystrophies. *Surv Ophthalmol.* 2015;60(2):115-122.
9. Dinh R, Rapuano CJ, Cohen EJ, Laibson PR. Recurrence of corneal dystrophy after excimer laser phototherapeutic keratectomy. *Ophthalmology.* 1999;106(8):1490-1497.
10. Lewis DR, Price MO, Feng MT, Price FW Jr. Recurrence of granular corneal dystrophy type 1 after phototherapeutic keratectomy, lamellar keratoplasty, and penetrating keratoplasty in a single population. *Cornea.* 2017;36(10):1227-1232.

SECTION II

CORNEAL DEGENERATION

WHAT SHOULD I DO FOR A YOUNG PATIENT WITH MILD KERATOCONUS?

Nandini Venkateswaran, MD and Preeya K. Gupta, MD

Keratoconus is a progressive, noninflammatory corneal ectatic disorder that typically affects individuals starting in the adolescent years and progresses throughout the second and third decades of life. In adults, the prevalence of the condition has been reported to be 0.05%, whereas in the pediatric population, the incidence has been reported to be 0.16%.[1] Although keratoconus initially manifests as corneal steepening and apical corneal thinning, subsequent vision loss can ensue secondary to worsening irregular corneal astigmatism, corneal hydrops, and irreversible corneal scarring.[2,3]

Diagnosis

Although a definitive pattern of inheritance has not been established for keratoconus, there can be a positive family history. Most cases of keratoconus are bilateral, but they can at times be asymmetric. Despite extensive research, the etiology of keratoconus has not yet been clearly elucidated. Several systemic syndromes that can be associated with keratoconus include Down syndrome, Leber congenital amaurosis, Ehlers-Danlos syndrome or other connective tissue disorders, atopy (often associated with eye rubbing), sleep apnea, and floppy eyelid syndrome. A thorough examination should include a review of the patient's prior ocular and medical history (ie, history of any associated syndromes), visual acuity with and without correction, refractive error (ie, asymmetric refractive error or high degrees of myopic astigmatism), external examination (eg, for floppy lids, signs of atopy), and slit-lamp biomicroscopy of the anterior segment (eg, scissoring of the red

Hardten DR, Hansen MS.
Curbside Consultation in Cornea and External Disease:
49 Clinical Questions, Second Edition (pp 21-27).
© 2022 Taylor & Francis Group.

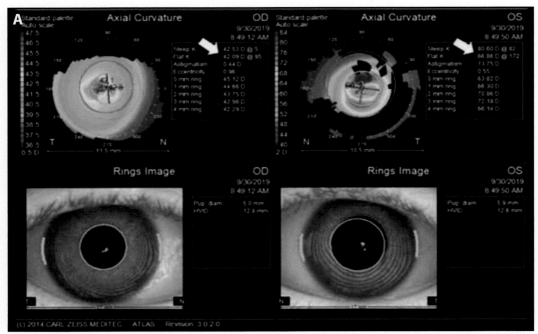

Figure 4-1. Topographic evaluation of a 23-year-old man with asymmetric keratoconus. His keratoconus is mild in the right eye but is advanced in the left eye, with marked corneal thinning, scarring, and ectatic changes. This patient will need to be monitored closely for progression of ectasia in the right eye (ie, every 4 to 6 months). He deferred any surgical intervention at this time in the left eye. (A) Placido-based topography images demonstrating steep keratometry values of 42.53 diopters in the right eye and 80.60 diopters in the left eye. Central steepening can be seen in both eyes. *(continued)*

reflex, Rizutti's sign, Vogt's striae, Kayser–Fleisher rings, Munson's sign and/or apical corneal thinning, signs of hydrops or stromal scarring). In addition, use of Placido-disc–based topography and Scheimpflug tomography elevation–based maps can be used to evaluate for irregularities of the anterior and posterior corneal surfaces that can help to detect early changes that are characteristic for keratoconus (ie, steepening of keratometry [K] values, particularly inferiorly; skewed axes of astigmatism; posterior elevation; corneal thinning, often with inferotemporal displacement of thinnest corneal point)[2,4] (Figure 4-1).

Recently, a genetic test to diagnose keratoconus and corneal dystrophies was US Food and Drug Administration (FDA) approved. The AvaGen genetic test by Avellino allows physicians to perform a simple cheek swab and submit specimens to test for 75 genes and over 2000 gene variants that are associated with keratoconus, as well as gene variants for TGFB1 gene related corneal dystrophies. Particularly for keratoconus, a polygenic risk stratification score is provided, categorized as low, medium, or high risk of keratoconus, along with genetic variant analysis. Access is also given to a genetic counseling to assist patients and physicians in interpretation of tests. This genetic test is a valuable tool for the early and accurate detection of keratoconus, especially in patients in whom clinical or topographic signs may be subtle or early (Figure 4-2).

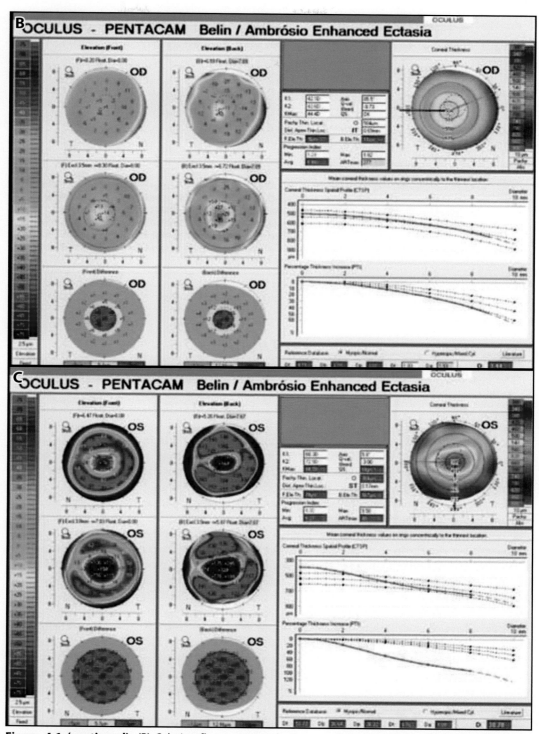

Figure 4-1 (continued). (B) Scheimpflug tomography images demonstrating mild posterior corneal elevation in the right eye and (C) marked posterior corneal elevation in the left eye. The Belin/Ambrosio Enhanced Ectasia display is abnormal in both eyes. The central corneal thickness in the left eye is 385 microns, rendering the patient a suboptimal candidate for corneal cross-linking.

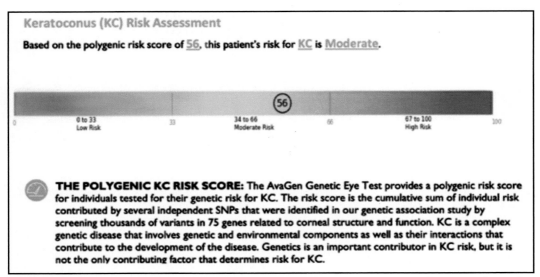

Figure 4-2. Sample genetic test report for a patient with suspected keratoconus. The report shows that based on genetic analysis, this patient had a moderate polygenic risk score.

Treatment

The key to the treatment of keratoconus is prompt recognition of risk factors and early diagnosis. Particularly in the pediatric and adolescent patient population, early detection can allow for more timely intervention and ultimately prevent amblyopia and facilitate visual rehabilitation and preservation.

Progression of keratoconus, especially in younger patients, is a topic of paramount concern.[5] However, the criteria and guidelines used to determine progression are not clearly defined in the literature. Generally, parameters used to define progression include consistent steepening of the anterior and posterior corneal surfaces (often a 1 diopter or more increase in the K max or sim K values on topography), changes in the manifest refraction (ie, myopic shift of 0.5 diopters or more and/or increase of more than 1 diopter of astigmatism), and/or continued corneal thinning on pachymetry.[6] Corneal cross-linking is a technique that employs ultraviolet light and the photosensitizer riboflavin to strengthen the chemical bonds of corneal collagen fibrils and halt progressive and irregular changes of the cornea. Cross-linking is typically pursued when there is evidence of ectasia progression. It is the only FDA-approved treatment that has been shown to halt the progression of keratoconus. Patients are often followed for serial visits—often at 4- to 6-month intervals—to establish definitive progression prior to undergoing cross-linking. Two primary methods of corneal cross-linking are currently available in the United States. The epithelium-off method was approved by the FDA in 2016, which applies ultraviolet light to a cornea soaked with riboflavin, with or without dextran (riboflavin with dextran is used when the corneal stromal bed thickness is less than 400 microns), using the Dresden protocol, after removal of the central 8 to 10 mm of corneal epithelium. Several studies have shown beneficial results of epithelium-off

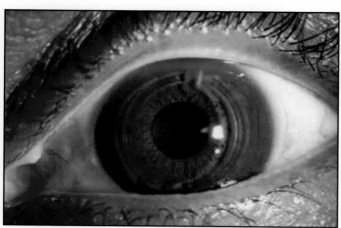

Figure 4-3. Slit-lamp photography of intracorneal ring segments in a middle-aged Hispanic patient with stable keratoconus who was experiencing contact lens intolerance in the left eye. The patient experienced improved comfort with contact lenses after her intracorneal ring segments procedure.

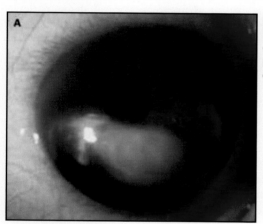

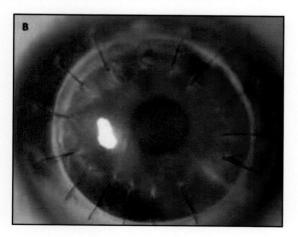

Figure 4-4. (A) Slit-lamp photograph of a young Black patient with inferior corneal scarring after an episode of acute hydrops. (B) Slit-lamp photograph of the same patient 3 months post–penetrating keratoplasty for corneal scarring in his fellow eye.

cross-linking treatment in visual acuity and topographic indices.[7] The epithelium-on method is currently under FDA clinical trials and utilizes a similar cross-linking procedure but without the removal of the epithelium. The epithelium-on protocol may permit cross-linking in thinner corneas and cause less pain and risk of infection for patients. Internationally, corneal cross-linking has been widely used for the treatment of progressive keratoconus and has been shown to stabilize disease progression in pediatric patients.[8,9] Rarely, corneal cross-linking can be associated with infectious keratitis or corneal scarring.

When considering therapeutic options, it is first important to determine whether the patient can achieve good vision with spectacles and/or contact lenses. In many mild cases, patients can often tolerate soft spherical or toric contact lenses without complications. However, in advancing cases, with higher amounts of astigmatism or corneal scarring, hard, rigid gas permeable, hybrid (central rigid gas permeable lenses with soft peripheral lens skirts), piggyback (rigid gas permeable lenses over soft silicone hydrogel lenses), or scleral contact lenses are often necessary. Collaboration with a skilled contact lens specialist is critical in helping these patients become educated about their vision correction options that can help them achieve excellent best-corrected visual acuity.

With progressive astigmatism or corneal ectasia causing an irregular corneal shape, patients may begin to grow intolerant of contact lenses. In such cases, the corneal specialist can consider implantation of intracorneal ring segments. These segments are polymethylmethacrylate implants that are surgically inserted at a 70% to 80% depth of the peripheral corneal stroma through a small radial incision (Figure 4-3). These implants help flatten the patient's ectatic cone and normalize the asymmetry of the corneal tissue, allowing for better tolerance and fitting of contact lenses and/or spectacles. Severe corneal thinning (typically < 450 microns in the 7-mm optical zone) or central corneal scarring can preclude implantation of intracorneal ring segments, and patients must be chosen judiciously for this treatment option. In rare circumstances, these segments can be explanted if they are not tolerated or if there are signs of ring extrusion or corneal infection.[10]

In advanced cases of keratoconus with apical or diffuse corneal scarring or hydrops, anterior lamellar keratoplasty or penetrating keratoplasty can be pursued to help achieve visual rehabilitation (Figure 4-4). In most of these cases, patients still need to wear spectacles and/or contact lenses after surgical intervention; however, tolerance of correction and quality of vision in the long term will be improved.

In summary, the treatment of keratoconus should utilize a stepwise approach that must take into consideration the patient who is affected by the condition, their preferences for visual recovery, and the degree and speed of progression. Prompt treatment is employed in cases detected later to facilitate rapid stabilization, whereas other individuals who are keratoconus suspects can be monitored every 6 months. Ultimately, with all the powerful technologies available in our armamentarium for the treatment of keratoconus, fewer patients will need to undergo keratoplasty if we implement the available tools to halt the progression of this condition.

References

1. Moshirfar M, Heiland MB, Rosen DB, Ronquillo YC, Hoopes PC. Keratoconus screening in elementary school children. *Ophthalmol Ther.* 2019;8(3):367-371.
2. Rabinowitz YS. Keratoconus. *Surv Ophthalmol.* 1998;42(4):297-319.
3. Davidson AE, Hayes S, Hardcastle AJ, Tuft SJ. The pathogenesis of keratoconus. *Eye (Lond).* 2014;28(2):189-195.
4. Mas Tur V, MacGregor C, Jayaswal R, O'Brart D, Maycock N. A review of keratoconus: diagnosis, pathophysiology, and genetics. *Surv Ophthalmol.* 2017;62(6):770-783.
5. Barbisan PRT, Pinto RDP, Gusmao CC, de Castro RS, Arieta CEL. Corneal collagen cross-linking in young patients for Progressive keratoconus. *Cornea.* 2019;39(2):186-191.
6. Duncan JK, Belin MW, Borgstrom M. Assessing progression of keratoconus: novel tomographic determinants. *Eye Vis (Lond).* 2016;3:6.
7. Belin MW, Lim L, Rajpal RK, Hafezi F, Gomes JAP, Cochener B. Corneal cross-linking: current USA status: report from the Cornea Society. *Cornea.* 2018;37(10):1218-1225.
8. Godefrooij DA, Soeters N, Imhof SM, Wisse RP. Corneal cross-linking for pediatric keratoconus: long-term results. *Cornea.* 2016;35(7):954-958.
9. Sarac O, Caglayan M, Uysal BS, Uzel AGT, Tanriverdi B, Cagil N. Accelerated versus standard corneal collagen cross-linking in pediatric keratoconus patients: 24 months follow-up results. *Cont Lens Anterior Eye.* 2018;41(5):442-447.
10. Vega-Estrada A, Alio JL. The use of intracorneal ring segments in keratoconus. *Eye Vis (Lond).* 2016;3:8.

I Have a Patient Who Is 25 Years Old With Progressive Keratoconus. Would It Be More Effective to Do Cross-Linking With the Epithelium On or Off in This Patient?

Samuel Passi, MD and Sherman W. Reeves, MD, MPH

Keratoconus is a subtype of corneal ectasias that is defined by noninflammatory progressive apical thinning with steepening. It is the most common corneal ectasia, affecting more than 1 in 1000 people worldwide, based on a recent meta-analysis of more than 7 million people.[1] Since 2007, keratoconus has remained the most common indication for penetrating keratoplasty in the United States, despite a dramatic decrease in the overall number of penetrating keratoplasties from more than 42,000 in 2007 to fewer than 20,000 in 2014.[2] The disease commonly presents in early puberty and progresses throughout adulthood, often not stabilizing until the fourth or fifth decade of life. It is a bilateral disease but is often asymmetric. Although a genetic component exists, environmental factors seem to play an equal if not greater role in the manifestation of the disease. Initially, visual symptoms are the result of progressive changes in refractive error and increasing irregular astigmatism, which are both treatable with scleral or hard contact lenses. However, later in the disease, the corneal ectasia may become so severe that patients are unable to fit into a scleral or hard contact lens. In its most severe stages, the cornea develops significant apical scarring and is prone to episodes of hydrops.

Diagnosis

Early diagnosis of keratoconus is challenging, based solely on refractive change and slit-lamp examination. Refractive change is exceedingly common in the adolescent age group, and the corneal thinning and steeping on examination can be very subtle and challenging to identify apart from topographic and Scheimpflug imaging. As the disease progresses, the clinical manifestations

Hardten DR, Hansen MS.
Curbside Consultation in Cornea and External Disease:
49 Clinical Questions, Second Edition (pp 29-33).
© 2022 Taylor & Francis Group.

Figure 5-1. Fleischer ring of iron deposition around the base of the cone in a patient with keratoconus.

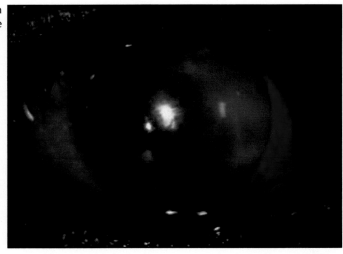

Figure 5-2. Corneal topography showing inferior steepening in a patient with keratoconus.

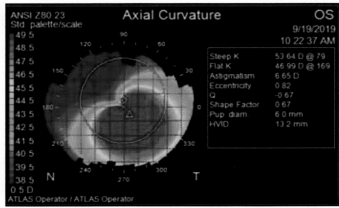

become more apparent, with notable scissoring of the red reflex on retinoscopy, iron deposition around the base of the cone (Fleischer ring; Figure 5-1), conical depression of the lower eyelid on downgaze (Munson's sign), central vertical striae (Vogt striae), and a conical reflection on the nasal cornea when a penlight is shone temporally (Rizzutti sign). Excessive change to refractive error or higher than average astigmatism in any adolescent patient should prompt the eye care provider to obtain further baseline testing. With modern diagnostic imaging devices, including topography (Figure 5-2) and Scheimpflug imaging (Figure 5-3), the diagnosis can be readily made. Further, in cases of questionable keratoconus or in older patients with potentially stable keratoconus, serial imaging with subtraction maps can be of great utility for monitoring progression.

Treatment

The treatment of keratoconus can be separated into 2 groups—visual rehabilitation and halting progression. With regard to visual rehabilitation, it is important to educate the patient on the unique optics of the cornea with keratoconus. While keratoconus makes them poor candidates for soft contact lenses or spectacles, it still allows them to be good candidates for scleral and hard

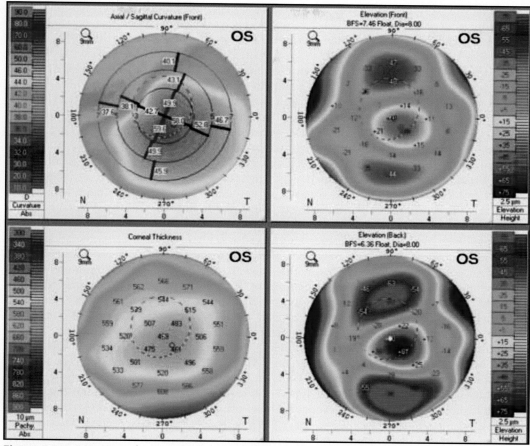

Figure 5-3. Scheimpflug imaging showing apical steepening, with anterior and posterior elevation, in a patient with keratoconus.

contact lenses. Especially in more advanced states of ectasia, contact lens fitting can become extremely challenging. It is recommended to work closely with contact lens specialists who have experience with complex scleral and hard contact lens fittings. For those patients unable to fit or tolerate a scleral or hard contact lens due to the severity of their corneal steepening, corneal ring segments can be of benefit. Although these ring segments have no effect on halting disease progression, they can permit the use of specialty contact lenses and help to avoid the need for a corneal transplant. Additionally, due to the atypical corneal curvature, normal ocular wetting and tear film stability are compromised and require special attention and treatment.

Regarding halting the disease progression, the focus should always begin with identifying modifiable risk factors, including eye rubbing and stomach sleeping (often with 1 hand resting underneath the worst eye). Ocular allergies are aggressively treated with topical therapy when indicated. Finally, for those patients without excessive apical scarring or thinning, corneal cross-linking (CXL) should be explored.

Prior to the US Food and Drug Administration (FDA) approval of CXL in 2016, there was no existing treatment available for patients in the United States with keratoconus except for a corneal transplant. As a testament to its efficacy, the number of penetrating keratoplasties has dramatically decreased in countries where CXL has been approved for a longer period of time. For example, one study in the Netherlands showed a decrease in corneal transplantation by approximately 25%.[3] In a similar study in Norway, greater than a 50% reduction in corneal transplantation rates for patients with keratoconus was found.[4] As CXL has evolved internationally over the past decade, numerous protocols and variations have been developed. However, in all variations, the key ingredients remain: riboflavin, ultraviolet A light (UVA), oxygen, and corneal collagen. The riboflavin serves to both absorb UVA and protect the corneal endothelium. The UVA, together with riboflavin and oxygen, causes photooxidation. This results in the desired collagen CXL, which ultimately strengthens and stabilizes the cornea. Although currently the Dresden epithelial-off CXL (epi-off CXL) protocol is the only FDA-approved method, epithelium-on CXL (epi-on CXL), also known as *transepithelial CXL*, has been utilized for years outside of the United States and is currently being evaluated in the United States through several active FDA trials.

With regard to efficacy, both epi-on CXL and epi-off CXL have been shown to halt progression and stabilize the cornea in patients with progressive keratoconus.[5] However, when using standard protocols, epi-off CXL has shown a greater ability to decrease maximum keratometry over time.[6-8] The reasons for the discrepancy in efficacy have been researched heavily; consequently, several modulations to the protocol have been explored. First, it is known that an intact epithelium limits corneal riboflavin absorption as well as UVA absorption. Thus, alterations to the riboflavin formulation have been developed, which allow for sustained release and better epithelial penetration, enhancing its efficacy.[8] Second, we know that an intact epithelium limits atmospheric oxygen. Researchers have found that by pulsing the UV light, oxygen levels can partially recover during the off cycle.[9] Further, specialty goggles have been developed that deliver continuous supplemental oxygen throughout the UVA light treatment.[8] Currently, these modifications are being tested in both nonhuman and human studies.

Finally, with regard to the efficacy of visual improvement, in a meta-analysis by Li and Wang,[5] they found that patients who underwent epi-on CXL gained more improvement in corrected distance visual acuity compared with epi-off CXL patients.

Although both epi-off and epi-on CXL protocols have good safety profiles, several studies have shown a higher incidence of complications with epi-off CXL protocols, including corneal haze, stromal edema, microbial keratitis, and scar.[6,10] While most of these complications are transient, some can persist and lead to permanent degradation of vision.[10] In addition to the increased incidence of complications, patients who undergo epi-off CXL experience prolonged visual recovery and increased pain compared with epi-on CXL, due to the induced large epithelial defect.

Conclusion

Keratoconus is by definition a progressive condition, and all adolescents/young adults should be considered for corneal CXL. Given its proven efficacy and FDA approval, epi-off CXL is the currently the most widely used protocol in the United States. However, given international trends and ongoing FDA trials, future epi-on CXL options may exist with equivalent efficacy and improved safety profiles over epi-off CXL.

References

1. Hashemi H, Heydarian S, Hooshmand E, et al. The prevalence and risk factors for keratoconus: a systematic review and meta-analysis. *Cornea*. 2020;39(2):263-270.
2. Park CY, Lee JK, Gore PK, Lim CY, Chuck RS. Keratoplasty in the United States: A 10-year review from 2005 through 2014. *Ophthalmology*. 2015;122(12):2432-2442.
3. Godefrooij DA, Gans R, Imhof SM, Wisse RP. Nationwide reduction in the number of corneal transplantations for keratoconus following the implementation of cross-linking. *Acta Ophthalmol*. 2016;94(7):675-678.

4. Sandvik GF, Thorsrud A, Råen M, Østern AE, Sæthre M, Drolsum L. Does corneal collagen cross-linking reduce the need for keratoplasties in patients with keratoconus? *Cornea.* 2015;34(9):991-995.
5. Li W, Wang B. Efficacy and safety of transepithelial corneal collagen crosslinking surgery versus standard corneal collagen crosslinking surgery for keratoconus: a meta-analysis of randomized controlled trials. *BMC Ophthalmol.* 2017;17(1):262.
6. Shalchi Z, Wang X, Nanavaty MA. Safety and efficacy of epithelium removal and transepithelial corneal collagen crosslinking for keratoconus. *Eye (Lond).* 2015;29(1):15-29.
7. Soeters N, Wisse RPL, Godefrooij DA, Imhof SM, Tahzib NG. Transepithelial versus epithelium-off corneal cross-linking for the treatment of progressive keratoconus: a randomized controlled trial. *Am J Ophthalmol.* 2015;159(5):821-828.e3.
8. Raizman, M. The science behind epi-on: clinical trials evaluate the safety and efficacy of epithelium-off corneal collagen cross-linking treatment protocols with supplemental oxygen. *The Ophthalmologist.* 2019;37(1):18-19.
9. Sun L, Li M, Zhang X, et al. Transepithelial accelerated corneal collagen cross-linking with higher oxygen availability for keratoconus: 1-year results. *Int Ophthalmol.* 2018;38(6):2509-2517.
10. Hersh PS, Stulting RD, Muller D, Durrie DS, Rajpal RK, US Crosslinking Study Group. U.S. multicenter clinical trial of corneal collagen crosslinking for treatment of corneal ectasia after refractive surgery. *Ophthalmology.* 2017;124(10):1475-1484.

I HAVE A 38-YEAR-OLD PATIENT WITH FAIRLY ADVANCED KERATOCONUS. IS THERE ANYTHING I CAN DO FOR THEM?

Martin L. Fox, MD

Keratoconus is a bilateral noninflammatory corneal disease that is characterized by a progressive loss of corneal structural integrity due to loss of collagen, eventually producing irregularity in corneal shape, scarring, and severe ocular morbidity. The disease usually presents in late adolescence and can progress in severity into the fifth decade of life, with varying morphological presentations and rates of progression. Until very recently, therapeutic options were extremely limited for patients with the condition—many of whom were destined to experience progressive corneal weakening and irregular astigmatism—making it impossible to achieve adequate spectacle-corrected visual acuity and eventually requiring a variety of rigid lenses as the only modality for providing adequate functional vision. For many with advanced disease and contact lens intolerance, penetrating keratoplasty was the only means of reversing the inevitable corneal blindness.

New technologies have provided increased hope for affected patients, including corneal collagen cross-linking (CXL), Intacs intrastromal rings (Addition Technology), and topography-driven excimer laser treatments, improving the prognosis for limiting disease progression and achieving considerably better visual function. There has never been a better time for the successful management of our patients with keratoconus, and there is much that can be offered to improve the clinical status of our patient in question.

Hardten DR, Hansen MS.
Curbside Consultation in Cornea and External Disease:
49 Clinical Questions, Second Edition (pp 35-40).
© 2022 Taylor & Francis Group.

Corneal Collagen Cross-Linking

In 2003, Wollensak et al[1] reported the first clinical study on riboflavin—an ultraviolet A–induced corneal collagen CXL procedure for the treatment of progressive keratoconus in adults. Iseli et al[2] developed the primary animal models and performed the first clinical trials of corneal CXL, hoping to provide a treatment for keratoconus that could actually halt progression of the disease. They reasoned that combining CXL with a refractive treatment would be the ultimate goal by both preventing progression and rehabilitating vision. Since its first description, corneal CXL has grown in acceptance and has been widely used for the treatment of progressive keratoconus as well as other conditions, including post-LASIK ectasia.[2]

Combined Cross-Linking and Excimer Laser Treatments

Treatments designed to regularize the keratoconic cornea at the time of CXL have also been the subject of recent studies as a natural evolution of this technology. In one variant demonstrating great promise—transepithelial phototherapeutic keratectomy with CXL—the corneal epithelium is removed with phototherapeutic keratectomy designed to not only remove the epithelium, but also to ablate the superficial corneal stroma to regularize the superficial corneal surface. Studies on the so-called *Cretan protocol* have indicated benefits of such an approach.[3] Additionally, recent interest in combined topography-linked photorefractive keratectomy treatments limited to 40 to 50 microns at the time of CXL are also attracting great interest in reporting excellent results internationally and appear to hold great promise in carefully selected individuals presenting before significant disease progression.[4]

Combining Intacs With Corneal Cross-Linking

Although collagen corneal CXL is effective in stabilizing the cornea in keratoconus and providing some element of corneal flattening, many treated patients are unable to find satisfactory improvement in visual function and still may have issues achieving adequate spectacle-corrected visual acuity or improved contact lens tolerance.

In seminal reports by Colin et al[5] and others,[6,7] the long-term beneficial effects of stromal polymethylmethacrylate ring (Intacs) implantation on enhanced morphology and stability in keratoconus has been well documented. Further, combining Intacs implantation with simultaneous CXL has been shown to provide additive effects on visual outcomes.[8-10] Treated patients can often achieve improved "walking around" vision, enhanced spectacle correction, and better contact lens tolerance, often allowing patients to find success with soft toric lenses rather than rigid modalities. Our reported results also indicated that the simultaneous approach, making use of ring placement with CXL, provide superior outcomes over either procedure alone (Figure 6-1).[8]

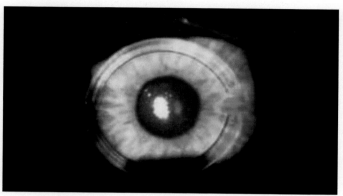

Figure 6-1. Symmetrical Intacs rings.

Approach for Matching Keratoconus Patients to Intacs Procedures

In planning our treatment approach using Intacs, we evaluate each patient from 2 distinct standpoints: risk of progression and degree of visual impairment. Patients early in the disease course are best addressed with CXL alone, but we advise those with significant visual function issues to consider Intacs ring placement in concert with CXL. In general, patients with mean keratometry values well above 60 diopters are usually not good candidates for Intacs surgery. Those with corneas steeper than this do not usually respond as well but remain viable candidates if expectations are limited to achieving better contact lens tolerance. Such patients may benefit from specialty Intacs, manufactured with a severe keratoconus modification, which are placed at a 6-mm optical zone and can allow for an enhanced flattening effect. Unfortunately, the severe keratoconus ring is not currently available in the United States and is awaiting FDA approval. Individuals with significant scarring are not good candidates for Intacs surgery. For those patients outside of the Intacs treatment range or with significant scarring, we consider femtosecond laser–assisted keratoplasty as the best logical alternative for visual rehabilitation.

Intacs surgical planning consists of a complete examination, combined with Pentacam tomography (OCULUS Optikgeräte GmbH), to better delineate the pattern of ectasia and corneal thinning to allow the most effective positioning and placement of rings in a symmetrical (double ring) or asymmetrical (single ring) approach.[8] In our hands, evaluation of the corneal shape against the red reflex (Charleaux's sign) using a direct ophthalmoscope allows for the characterization of ectasia patterns as being central symmetric (round type) or asymmetric (oval sagging type). Such findings are essential in planning the appropriate custom surgical approach. Symmetrical surgery, consisting of insertion of 2 rings on the steep meridian, is used with round central cases, and asymmetric single-ring placement is typically used in the approach to oval sagging pathology. In our clinic, we use 0.45-mm standard thickness rings in all cases.

We use the IntraLase femtosecond laser (Johnson & Johnson Vision) to create ring channels at a depth of 75% of the thinnest corneal pachymetry at a radius of 7 mm around the visual axis. The entrance incision is placed at the steepest corneal axis, determined by Pentacam tomography and confirmed with manual Placido ring topography. Following ring placement, CXL is added in the classic epithelium-off approach, allowing for an enhanced flattening effect of ring placement. Patients can expect to experience an evolution of visual improvement over a period of 2 to 3 months.

Femtosecond Laser–Assisted Keratoplasty

Keratoconus patients with advanced disease can benefit greatly from the addition of femtosecond laser technology in keratoplasty. The use of the femtosecond laser has completely altered the landscape of laser vision correction, allowing surgeons to create predictable LASIK flaps that can be customized to the architecture of each eye. The resulting planar flaps, when used in combination with custom excimer laser ablations, have allowed for superior safety, stability, and visual outcomes. In the same way, femtosecond laser–assisted keratoplasty has allowed for a beneficial improvement in predictability and biomechanical stability.

Prior to the advent of laser-assisted keratoplasty, patients having corneal transplant surgery with standard mechanical trephine or mechanical punch transplant surgery could expect a lengthy period of visual rehabilitation of upwards to 1 year. Outcomes notoriously included high levels of irregular astigmatism and wound instability. With femtosecond technology, patients can expect improved recovery speed and outcomes (Figures 6-2 and 6-3).

In femtosecond laser keratoplasty, the corneal surgeon can either calculate a unique pattern of corneal cuts or work off a set group of precalculated templates that best fit the patient.[11] Participating eye banks will make use of the same corneal cut parameters to prepare laser-cut donor tissue. In the operating room, the recipient's pathology is removed and the custom corneal replacement is sutured in place.

A series of 14 consecutive keratoconus cases performed over a 1-year period with the IntraLase femtosecond laser zigzag patterning was evaluated in our clinic. We documented visual rehabilitation during a 3-to 6-month follow-up period. The series consisted of patients ranging in age from 22 to 62 years with a best spectacle-corrected visual acuity range of counting fingers to 20/100. The 3-month postoperative data revealed that 100% of patients had spectacle-corrected visual acuity of 20/40 or better, with 64% achieving correctable vision of 20/25 or better. In laser-assisted keratoplasty, precise matching of complex donor and recipient tissue planes has allowed for accelerated healing, enabling the removal of sutures as early as 6 weeks postoperative, with more than 75% of patients manifesting very acceptable levels of regular astigmatism (2.5 diopters or less).[11]

Femtosecond laser technology can also allow for safe astigmatism "touch-ups" for patients with higher levels of postoperative astigmatism. Making use of the anterior side-cut setting of the IntraLase, we can place safe, accurate, paired astigmatic keratotomy arcuate incisions inside of the graft/host interface to address any astigmatism concerns.[12]

Conclusion

Surgical management of keratoconus has clearly reached a point where we can offer new hope to this population of patients. Timely CXL has been demonstrated to provide the opportunity to halt disease progression in young patients who might otherwise be passed over. For those patients with keratoconus who are unable to tolerate contact lens correction, precise placement of Intacs intrastromal rings can reshape corneal morphology, allowing for improvement in best-corrected visual acuity as well as contact lens tolerance. Topography-assisted photorefractive keratectomy combined with CXL can also allow for significant improvement of vision in selected individuals. Patients presenting with advanced disease should be considered for laser-assisted keratoplasty, which offers the prospect of rapid recovery of quality vision and corneal stability.

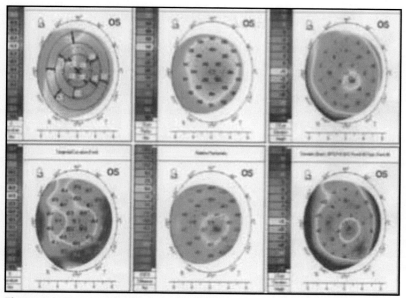

Figure 6-2. Topography showing central symmetrical keratoconus pattern.

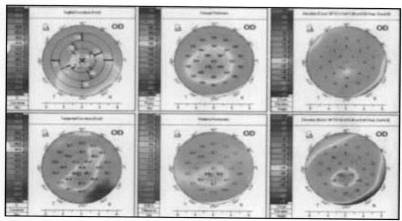

Figure 6-3. Topography showing sagging asymmetric pattern.

References

1. Wollensak G, Spoerl E, Seiler T. Riboflavin/ultraviolet-a–induced collagen crosslinking for the treatment of keratoconus. *Am J Ophthalmol*. 2003;135(5):620-627.
2. Iseli HP, Thiel MA, Hafezi F, Kampmeier J, Seiler T. Ultraviolet A/riboflavin corneal cross-linking for infectious keratitis associated with corneal melts. *Cornea*. 2008;27(5):590-594.
3. Kymionis GD1, Grentzelos MA, Kounis GA, Diakonis VF, Limnopoulou AN, Panagopoulou SI. Combined transepithelial phototherapeutic keratectomy and corneal collagen cross-linking for progressive keratoconus. *Ophthalmology*. 2012;119(9):1777-1784.
4. Shetty R, D'Souza S, Srivastava S, Ashwini R. Topography-guided custom ablation treatment for treatment of keratoconus. *Indian J Ophthalmol*. 2013;61(8):445-450. doi:10.4103/0301-4738.116067
5. Colin J, Cochener B, Savary G, Malet F. Correcting keratoconus with intracorneal rings. *J Cataract Refract Surg*. 2000;26(8):1117-1122.
6. Bethke WC. Corralling keratoconus with Intacs. *Review of Ophthalmology*. September 15, 2005. Accessed October 1, 2021. https://www.reviewofophthalmology.com/article/corralling-keratoconus-with-intacs
7. Kymionis GD, Siganos CS, Tsiklis NS, et al. Long-term follow-up of Intacs in keratoconus, *Am J Ophthalmol*. 2007;144(2):236-244.
8. Fox ML. Intrastromal rings for keratoconus. *Ophthalmology Times*. May 1, 2015.
9. Chan CCK, Sharma M, Boxer Wachler BS. Effect of inferior segment Intacs with and without C3-R on keratoconus. *J Cataract Refract Surg*. 2007;33(1):75-80.
10. Coskunseven E, Jankov MR II, Hafezi F, Atun S, Arslan E, Kymionis G. Effect of treatment sequence in combined intrastromal corneal rings and corneal collagen crosslinking for keratoconus. *J Cataract Refract Surgery*. 2009;35(12):2084-2091.
11. Fox ML. Laser assisted keratoplasty–the changing paradigm. *Eye World News*. October 2014.
12. Fox ML. Femtosecond astigmatic keratotomy before LASIK can be beneficial. *Ocular Surgery News, US Edition*. August 25, 2014. Accessed October 1, 2021. https://www.healio.com/news/ophthalmology/20140822/femtosecond-astigmatic-keratotomy-before-lasik-can-be-beneficial

A Patient With High Cylinder Has Sudden Onset of Pain, Blurry Vision, and Corneal Edema. How Do I Manage This Patient?

Kevin R. Tozer, MD

This clinical scenario is a common presentation for acute corneal hydrops secondary to advanced keratoconus. Keratoconus is a bilateral noninflammatory corneal ectatic disease. Some estimates place its prevalence at 1 in 2000 within the general population. However, others estimate a much higher rate, approaching 1 in 500[1] in certain populations, such as those with atopic keratoconjunctivitis or those living in hot, dry environments. The natural history of keratoconus is a progressive increase in corneal astigmatism that becomes more irregular over time, associated with posterior corneal elevation and corneal thinning. One of the most potentially devastating complications of keratoconus is acute corneal decompensation, referred to as *corneal hydrops*. Hydrops occurs when a tear develops in Descemet's membrane secondary to mechanical stretching associated with the abnormal posterior corneal curvature. The normal pump function of the endothelium is disrupted, creating a pathway for fluid to enter the stroma. This results in sudden, often painful, corneal swelling. Hydrops occurs only in advanced cases of keratoconus, affecting approximately 3% of these patients.[2] Although hydrops is commonly associated with keratoconus, it can also be less frequently seen in pellucid marginal degeneration, post-refractive ectasia, Terrien marginal degeneration, and keratoglobus.

Diagnosis

If the patient has no previous diagnosis of keratoconus, it can be difficult to determine whether the cornea was ectatic before the hydrops developed. The swelling can be so severe that the normal corneal anatomy is distorted, which makes topography or tomography less helpful in establishing the diagnosis of keratoconus. In this situation, it is helpful to look for the pathognomonic sign

Hardten DR, Hansen MS.
Curbside Consultation in Cornea and External Disease:
49 Clinical Questions, Second Edition (pp 41-45).
© 2022 Taylor & Francis Group.

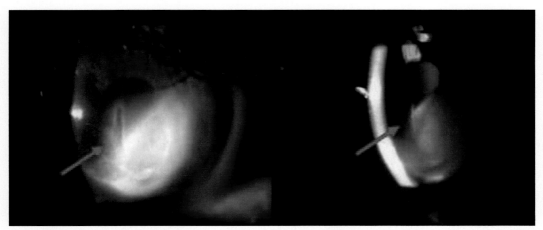

Figure 7-1. Wide-beam and slit-beam photos of a cornea with hydrops. The red line (red arrow) identifies a Descemet's membrane tear.

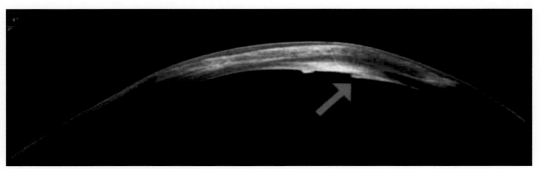

Figure 7-2. Anterior-segment optical coherence tomography identifying a break in Descemet's membrane (blue arrow) with associated cornea edema. (Reproduced with permission from Dr. Josh Duncan.)

of hydrops—a tear in Descemet's membrane (Figure 7-1). This may be visualized under higher magnification at the slit-lamp biomicroscope. However, if the edema obscures the view, then ultrasound biomicroscopy or anterior-segment optical coherence tomography (Figure 7-2) can be helpful. Both of these imaging modalities are useful in identifying and measuring tears in Descemet's membrane and associated stromal clefts. Additionally, examining the contralateral eye is important, as keratoconus is rarely unilateral. If the fellow eye shows any signs of keratoconus on examination (Table 7-1) or with topography/tomography (Table 7-2), the diagnosis of hydrops in the affected eye is likely confirmed. Also, it is important to consider the entire clinical scenario. Keratoconus is typically a disease of the young. Its natural history is a gradual progression from the teenage years through the fifth decade of life. When a person reaches the sixth decade of life, the disease naturally stabilizes in most patients. Furthermore, the prevalence of keratoconus appears to decrease with age. Keratoconus in the Medicare-age population is quite low, decreasing to approximately 18 per 100,000.[3] Even within a population of keratoconus patients, younger persons who develop hydrops tend to have more severe episodes and sequelae.[4] Therefore, if a 75-year-old patient presents with corneal edema, it would less likely be due to hydrops and more likely due to another cause of the painful swelling, such as ruptured bullae from pseudophakic bullous keratopathy.

Table 7-1

Clinical Signs of Keratoconus

External Examination	
Munson's sign	V-shaped displacement of lower lid on downgaze
Rizutti phenomenon	Focusing on light from penlight onto the nasal limbus when light is held temporal to the cornea
Retinoscopy	
Scissoring	Splitting of retinoscopy beam
Slit-Lamp	
Vogt's striae	Vertical endothelial striae that disappear with corneal compression
Charleaux oil drop sign	Distortion of red reflex seen in retroillumination
Stromal thinning	Most commonly seen apically or slightly inferiorly
Fleischer ring	Iron deposition at base of or around corneal cone
Scarring	Typically a late finding after an episode of hydrops

Treatment

It is important to understand that corneal hydrops is self-limiting. The natural history of hydrops is a gradual resolution over 2 to 4 months. Typically, the Descemet's detachment resolves as the endothelial cells develop polymegathism while migrating over the exposed areas. Although this invariably leaves a scar, it can also lead to significant flattening of the corneal curvature. If the scar is peripheral and not visually significant, some patients experience an improvement in contact lens tolerance after a hydrops episode due to this flattening effect.

The conventional treatment for hydrops consists of topical hypertonic, steroid, and cycloplegic agents and bandage contact lenses. To promote deturgescence of the cornea while the steroids help to control inflammation and prevent subsequent neovascularization, 5% sodium chloride solutions are used. Cycloplegic drugs are used to help with photosensitivity and pain. Bandage contact lenses may also be used for comfort and may assist in managing swelling. Additionally, topical antibiotics are important if any epithelial defects develop.

In the last several years, numerous studies have explored using intracameral air or gas to promote Descemet's reattachment. These also act as a mechanical tamponade, preventing aqueous from entering the stroma, which enhances healing. Sterile air, 14% perfluoropropane (C_3F_8), and 20% sulfur hexafluoride (SF_6), have been used with some success. Volumes between 0.1 and 0.2 mL at isoexpansile concentrations are recommended to minimize post-injection intraocular pressure spikes. Although air or gas injections have been shown to decrease the time to edema resolution by approximately 1 month,[5] most studies show no improvement in final visual acuity outcomes over conventional therapy.[6] Additionally, any injections carry risks, including infection, intrastromal gas migration, and pupillary block glaucoma. In one study using C_3F_8 in 90 patients, 10 (16%) eyes developed pupillary block glaucoma.[6] In addition to the risk of complications, compliance is

Table 7-2
Topography and Tomography Signs of Keratoconus

Topography	
Focal area of increased corneal power	Typically will have a maximum keratometry > 48 diopters; usually inferiorly but may also be superiorly
Inferior to superior power asymmetry	Average dioptric power of inferior hemisphere vs superior
Skewed steep axis	Can give "lazy bow-tie" configuration/irregular astigmatism
Tomography	
Anterior elevation	Elevation in anterior surface of cornea, corresponds to the area cone formation
Posterior elevation	Often seen prior to anterior corneal changes
Corneal thinning	Typically worse inferotemporally or centrally
Decreased posterior radius of curvature	Measured at 3-mm zone; normal would be > 7.25 mm
Decreased anterior radius of curvature	Measured at 3-mm zone; normal would be > 5.9 mm

difficult because patients are required to be supine from several days up to 2 weeks, depending on the type of injection used. These factors, combined with the need for frequent reinjections, have led to a decrease in popularity of intracameral injections among some cornea specialists.

When the acute episode resolves, either naturally or augmented by intracameral air, the next step is visual rehabilitation. As mentioned previously, if the scar is peripheral and not visually significant, the patient may do well with a simple update to their scleral or rigid gas permeable lens. Unfortunately, frequent scarring or subsequent neovascularization will prevent adequate vision. In these cases, corneal transplant is usually necessary. Traditionally, full-thickness penetrating keratoplasty (PKP) has been the preferred transplant procedure. Although patients with keratoconus often have among the best outcomes with PKP, evidence suggests that PKP performed following acute hydrops have a higher incidence of endothelial rejection.[2] Therefore, some have proposed attempting to perform deep anterior lamellar keratoplasty in these patients. Although intraoperative focal Descemet's perforations are common in these cases, conversion rates to PKP can be kept low with surgical experience.[7]

One final consideration for treating acute hydrops is corneal cross-linking (CXL). CXL, which has been used internationally for more than a decade, was approved by the US Food and Drug Administration in 2016. It is known to stabilize the shape of the cornea and prevent further progression of both keratoconus and post-refractive ectasia. There does not appear to be a role for CXL in the acute stage of hydrops. However, if the patient heals with acceptable visual acuity and does not require a transplant, CXL is reasonable. Additionally, because keratoconus is nearly always bilateral, the fellow eye should be considered for CXL to prevent a similar outcome.

References

1. Jonas JB, Nangia V, Matin A, Kulkarni M, Bhojwani K. Prevalence and associations of keratoconus in rural Maharashtra in central India: the central India eye and medical study. *Am J Ophthalmol.* 2009;148(5):760-765.
2. Tuft SJ, Gregory WM, Buckley RJ. Acute corneal hydrops in keratoconus. *Ophthalmology.* 1994;101(10):1738-1744.
3. Reeves SW, Ellwein LB, Kim T, Constantine R, Lee PP. Keratoconus in the Medicare population. *Cornea.* 2009;28(1):40-42.
4. Al Suhaibani AH, Al-Rajhi AA, Al-Motowa S, Wagoner MD. Inverse relationship between age and severity and sequelae of acute corneal hydrops associated with keratoconus. *Br J Ophthalmol.* 2007;91(7):984-985.
5. Miyata K, Tsuji H, Tanabe T, Mimura Y, Amano S, Oshika T. Intracameral air injection for acute hydrops in keratoconus. *Am J Ophthalmol.* 2002;133(6):750-752.
6. Basu S, Vaddavalli PK, Ramappa M, Shah S, Murthy SI, Sangwan VS. Intracameral perfluoropropane gas in the treatment of acute corneal hydrops. *Ophthalmology.* 2011;118(5):934-939.
7. Nanavaty MA, Daya SM. Outcomes of deep anterior lamellar keratoplasty in keratoconic eyes with previous hydrops. *Br J Ophthalmol.* 2012;96(10):1304-1309.

A Patient With Eye Irritation While Wearing Soft Contact Lenses Is Noted to Have White Elevated Nodules at the Limbus. Do They Need Surgery?

Thomas Kohnen, MD, PhD

Salzmann's nodular degeneration (SND) is a noninflammatory, slowly progressive degenerative disorder. It is characterized by bluish-gray (or white) nodules that usually vary in number and are elevated above the corneal surface; sometimes they are confluent. The nodules occur in either the scarred cornea or at the edge of the transparent cornea, with or without the presence of vascularization. When they start to cause vision loss by enlarging into the visual axis or if they are causing substantial astigmatism, they can be excised. Many years can elapse before SND causes loss of vision or change in astigmatism, requiring surgery. The disease may be unilateral or bilateral, which suggests a careful examination of the fellow eye if SND is diagnosed in 1 eye. SND affects patients of various ages and races. The disease displays a predilection for the female sex, so this case is very typical. SND can be associated with a history of ocular surface diseases (eg, phlyctenular keratitis, interstitial keratitis, vernal keratitis, trachoma, Thygeson's superficial punctate keratitis, scarlet fever, measles, and keratoconjunctivitis). In other cases, however, there is no history of previous eye disease.

Diagnosis

SND will not be very frequent in general practice; more often, it will be seen by cornea specialists. Therefore, you should consider every case very carefully. The first diagnostic instrument should always be an evaluation of the anterior segment with the slit lamp (Figure 8-1). Tomography of the cornea can reveal a typical pattern of circular peripheral elevations. Further, in

Hardten DR, Hansen MS.
Curbside Consultation in Cornea and External Disease:
49 Clinical Questions, Second Edition (pp 47-49).
© 2022 Taylor & Francis Group.

Figure 8-1. Slit-lamp examination of SND prior to treatment.

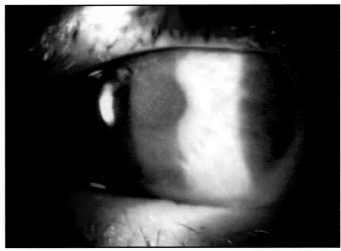

Figure 8-2. Slit-lamp examination after PTK.

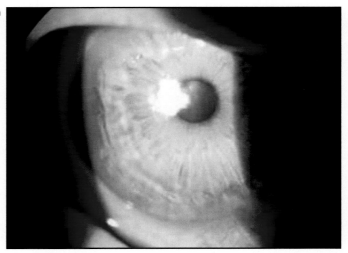

vivo confocal microscopy has shown its applicability for the diagnosis of SND by being correlated to histopathological findings.[1] Using in vivo confocal microscopy will give you important information about the degree of your patient's SND and thus the required treatment.

Treatment

The etiology of SND is unknown, and a spontaneous cure or remission has not been reported. Therefore, surgical treatment is the only option for improving the vision of patients with SND. Nodules can be successfully removed manually by superficial keratectomy, provided the opacity is confined to the superficial layers of the cornea, with or without subsequent phototherapeutic keratectomy (PTK) using an excimer laser.[2] In most instances, healing is rapid and visual disturbances decrease. Even without performance of PTK, rehabilitation and healing give a good result, but PTK may provide a more regular surface and therefore could be added to the surgical treatment.

If the SND recurs, one should consider PTK as a possible treatment as well (Figure 8-2). Large nodules can extend deeply into the stroma. Such cases may require PTK or, in severe cases, lamellar or penetrating keratoplasty. Severin and Kirchhof[3] reported the superficial opacity of grafts 2.5 and 9 years after penetrating keratoplasty due to recurring SND. Recurrence can also occur after surgical treatments such as keratoplasty or PTK.

Postoperative Protocol

The usual postoperative medical therapy consists of artificial tears and antibiotic eye drops. Both should be applied until total healing of epithelium is achieved, followed by steroid eye drops up to 4 weeks after surgery. To prevent such recurrence, Bowers et al[4] applied mitomycin-C (MMC) after superficial keratectomy. None of the patients treated in this manner suffered a recurrence of SND during a follow-up period of up to 4 years. However, MMC for prophylaxis of SND is an off-label use. I do not typically use MMC. However, if SND recurs, one should consider it as an option for retreatment.

Correction of Ametropia

One female patient with SND had +6.00 diopters of ametropia prior to surgery. After epithelial removal and performance of PTK, the patient was emmetropic.[1] Because of the change in corneal refractive power induced by the nodules, refractive surgery should not be combined with SND treatment. It seems to me that SND causes poor predictability in refractive surgery and thus should not be performed to avoid any risk of large under- or overcorrections.

Due to the irregular corneal surface, contact lens fitting will be difficult in patients still suffering from SND. One should not consider contact lens fitting prior to the treatment. However, after the treatment and complete wound healing, contact lenses may be fit. It is important to schedule regular visits to control the contact lens fitting and the possible recurrence of SND afterward. If there is any sign of contact lens intolerance, their use should be discontinued. One has to instruct patients very carefully to take out their contact lenses if they have any discomfort.

Similarly, if considering SND removal and cataract surgery, intraocular lens biometry will be more accurate after removal of SND. It may take several months to achieve a stable corneal topography. I would confirm a stable topography before proceeding with intraocular lens measurements for cataract surgery.

References

1. Meltendorf C, Bühren J, Bug R, Ohrloff C, Kohnen T. Correlation between clinical in vivo confocal microscopic and ex vivo histopathologic findings of Salzmann nodular degeneration. *Cornea.* 2006;25(6):734-738.
2. Das S, Langenbucher A, Pogorelov P, Link B, Seitz B. Long-term outcome of excimer laser phototherapeutic keratectomy for treatment of Salzmann's nodular degeneration. *J Cataract Refract Surg.* 2005;31(7):1386-1391.
3. Severin M, Kirchhof B. Recurrent Salzmann's corneal degeneration. *Graefes Arch Clin Exp Ophthalmol.* 1990;228(2):101-104.
4. Bowers PJ Jr, Price MO, Zeldes SS, Price FW Jr. Superficial keratectomy with mitomycin-C for the treatment of Salzmann's nodules. *J Cataract Refract Surg.* 2003;29(7):1302-1313.

SECTION III

EXTERNAL DISEASE

I Have a Patient With Significant Facial Rosacea With Chronic, Red, Irritated Eyes. They Have Some Peripheral Corneal Neovascularization and Are Struggling With Contact Lens Wear. How Can I Manage This Patient?

Yvonne Wang, MD and Sumitra S. Khandelwal, MD

Ocular rosacea is an overlooked cause of chronic eye irritation and contact lens intolerance. Rosacea is an inflammatory dermatologic condition characterized by facial erythema, papules, pustules, and telangiectasias on the cheek, chin, nose, and forehead. It has an estimated prevalence of a little over 20% in fair-skinned patients, and more than 50% of the patients have ocular symptoms. In fact, the presence of ocular rosacea is a major feature, with >50% agreement for the diagnosis of rosacea.[1] Ocular rosacea presents as blepharitis and keratitis (Figure 9-1). The symptoms of rosacea blepharitis range from mild irritation to severe ocular surface disease, causing significant vision loss. Patients experience dryness, irritation, photophobia, discharge, crusting, and blurry vision. Ocular symptoms may not correlate with dermatological findings and can even precede skin involvement.[2]

The pathophysiology of rosacea blepharitis is unknown. Studies have suggested a correlation of increased inflammatory markers caused by *Staphylococcus epidermidis* and *Demodex*. These microorganisms are hypothesized to release proteins that increase the levels of the inflammatory markers interleukin-1β and matrix metalloproteinase-9.[3]

Determining the underlying etiology for a patient's blepharitis can help direct the management. If ocular rosacea is established as the etiology, treatment can be guided to address the inflammation related to this type of blepharitis.

Hardten DR, Hansen MS.
Curbside Consultation in Cornea and External Disease:
49 Clinical Questions, Second Edition (pp 53-57).
© 2022 Taylor & Francis Group.

Figure 9-1. Facial erythema and rhinophyma are noted, which are characteristic of rosacea.

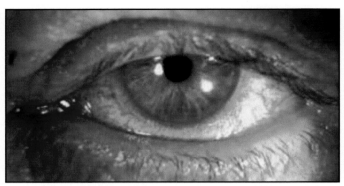

Figure 9-2. Conjunctival injection caused by rosacea blepharitis.

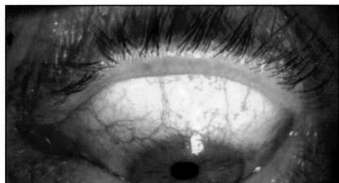

Diagnosis

The vision care provider should conduct a careful slit-lamp examination focused on the eyelashes and eyelid margin. Crusting of the eyelashes is a hallmark of anterior blepharitis. Eyelash misdirection can cause trichiasis and epithelial erosions. Collarettes, or sleeves, on the eyelashes may be a sign of *Demodex* infection. Chronic inflammation leads to telangectasias and eyelid margin thickening (Figure 9-2). Oily, inspissated meibomian glands that are difficult to express are seen in posterior blepharitis. Meibomian gland disease can cause recurrent chalazia and lead to eyelid margin ulceration and scarring. A disruption of the oily secretions of the meibomian glands lead to tear instability, a rapid tear break-up time, and ocular surface staining using fluorescein.

Examination of the ocular surface may show chronic conjunctival injection, pannus formation, punctate epithelial erosions, and, in severe cases, corneal scarring and neovascularization. Meibography is a relatively new technique that uses infrared imaging of the meibomian glands. With meibography, we can now quantify the degree of gland destruction, which helps to score the severity of disease.[4]

It also is important to examine the face for signs of rosacea, specifically telangiectasias of the nose and cheek. Often, these are chronic changes that patients have noted but not addressed. If facial rosacea is a concern, it can tailor treatment to a more systemic approach.

Treatment

Treatment of rosacea blepharitis is directed toward symptom alleviation and decreasing inflammation. There is no cure for the disease, and patients should be counseled that long-term management is needed.

EYELID HYGIENE

Warm compresses and eyelid scrubs have been shown to improve symptoms and are simple, noninvasive treatments to start for patients. Warming of the meibomian glands encourages the flow of meibum. However, compliance can be an issue because patients should apply the heat via a warmed washcloth or eye mask for at least 5 to 10 minutes, followed by a gentle massage of the eyelid margins. In-office procedures to assist with lid warming can also be utilized. A variety of devices are available that will warm the eyelid margin either internally or externally, followed by lid expression by the device or the provider.

In cases of suspected *Demodex*, eyelid scrubs with 50% tea tree oil has been shown to decrease the parasite load. Eyelid scrubs help to clean the meibomian gland orifices, which can have a buildup of biofilm that causes inflammation. Commercial scrubs with hypochlorous acid 0.01% can be obtained via over-the-counter purchase and have been shown to be bactericidal for organisms at the eyelid margin that are commonly associated with blepharitis.[5]

DIETARY SUPPLEMENTATION

Dietary supplementation with essential fatty acids is hypothesized to change the composition of the meibum secretions to improve tear film stability and may also have anti-inflammatory properties. Omega-3 fatty acids from fish oil or flaxseed oil and omega-6 gamma linoleic fatty acids from black currant seed have shown improvements in symptoms. These supplements are readily available over the counter and can be given as 500 mg of eicosapentaenoic acid/docosahexaenoic acid from fish oil per day and 1000 mg of gamma linoleic acid.[6]

TOPICAL TREATMENT

Topical steroids can be used to control episodes of acute inflammation. Short courses with loteprednol or fluorometholone, either as drops or ointment, is typically well tolerated. If the patient has cornea neovascularization and/or keratitis, it becomes important to use topical anti-inflammatory agents initially to control the inflammation. Treatment should be tapered to the lowest effective dose and discontinued when symptoms are improved. The risk of elevated intraocular pressure and cataract formation should be weighed when considering use of topical steroids. Topical cyclosporine A is a nonsteroidal immune-suppressive medication that has been used for ocular surface disease and avoids the side effects of steroids. It also has been shown to improve the ocular surface and symptoms of blepharitis associated with rosacea.[7-9] Dapsone gel is a topical treatment for facial rosacea that has been shown to be effective for decreasing skin lesions in papulopustular rosacea, although its effect on ocular manifestations are yet to be evaluated.[10]

ANTIBIOTICS

Topical antibiotics help to decrease the bacterial load at the eyelid margin and in the tear film. Topical azithromycin 1% is administered twice daily for 2 days, then once nightly for 28 days. Several studies have shown that topical azithromycin improves symptoms and signs of inflammation associated with blepharitis.[8] Topical fluoroquinolones have been shown to decrease the bacterial load of the conjunctiva, but clinical improvement in blepharitis is not well established, and there is concern for increasing drug resistance.[8] Topical tobramycin, administered by itself or in combination with a steroid, has been shown to improve symptoms.[7-9]

ORAL ANTIBIOTICS

Doxycycline, azithromycin, and minocycline have been well studied in their use for meibomian gland dysfunction. At low doses, they have an anti-inflammatory effect by decreasing the levels of metalloproteinases in the tear film. Doxycycline can be prescribed as 100 mg twice daily for 1 month, then 100 mg daily for several months thereafter. A lower dose of 20 mg twice daily can be used for a longer term if needed. Minocycline is prescribed as 50 mg twice daily for 3 months. The prescriber should warn patients about sun sensitivity while taking tetracyclines, and their use in children and pregnant women is contraindicated. Azithromycin is an alternative to tetracyclines, and is given as a pulse dose course, and 500 mg once daily given for 3 days every 7 days has been shown to improve symptoms and tear break-up time.[7-9]

INTENSE PULSED LIGHT THERAPY

Intense pulsed light therapy (IPL) is an in-office–based procedure that uses lights of specific wavelengths to penetrate through the skin and is absorbed by oxyhemoglobin in the blood vessels, which is converted into heat. This heat ablates the dilated telangiectasias seen in the eyelid margins of patients with rosacea and decreases inflammatory markers. Additionally, this therapy may also decrease the bacterial load at the meibomian gland orifices and warms the glands to promote better secretion. IPL has been shown to improve tear film function and patient-reported symptoms in those with meibomian gland dysfunction associated with rosacea.[11] Following treatment, manual expression of the glands by a provider can assist in improving gland function. The main limitation of IPL therapy is that it can be used only for patients with a Fitzpatrick skin type of 4 or less, which means light to fair skin. It is important to note that it is not US Food and Drug Administration (FDA)-approved for periorbital use and its off-label use is not covered by insurance.

THERMAL PULSATION SYSTEMS

Various in-office devices are available for meibomian gland expression, involving applications of heat and pressure to express meibum. At the time of this publication, 2 devices are FDA-cleared. LipiFlow thermal pulsation system was the first of these such devices to receive FDA clearance. It was shown to improve both meibomian gland secretion and tear beak-up time after one 12-minute procedure.[12] The second, iLux, which uses light-based heat and pulsation to achieve meibomian gland expression, has received FDA clearance as well. These devices have good safety profiles. However, they have not been studied in ocular rosacea specifically. Further, they may exacerbate severe lid inflammation and may not be appropriate for first-line therapy in patients with severe inflammation but rather as an adjunct therapy when inflammation is under control.

BLEPHEX

BlephEx is a handheld device that targets the bacterial biofilm of eyelids and lashes. It uses a patented microsponge to clean the base of the eyelashes and lids. It may need to be repeated at regular intervals of 4 to 6 months. It has been cleared by the FDA for treatment of blepharitis, but it has not been studied in the setting of ocular rosacea.

Scleral Contact Lens Options

For a patient who is intolerant to soft contact lenses, scleral lenses can provide improved vision, without issues with marginal keratitis or cornea neovascularization if fit correctly. In addition, these lenses protect the cornea from the eyelid margin, leading to improved inflammation on the surface. However, the challenge of scleral lenses is the fogging that can occur with initial wear. Initiation of the previously described treatments can minimize the tear film debris that leads to fogging initially.

Conclusion

Blepharitis is a broad diagnosis, but it is important to understand its etiology. In a patient with rosacea causing contact lens intolerance, addressing the facial and eyelid rosacea is important. With the proper diagnosis and treatment for both chronic inflammation as well as flare-ups, patients can continue to wear contact lenses or change to alternate options, such as scleral contact lenses.

References

1. Tan J, Almeida LMC, Bewley A, et al. Updating the diagnosis, classification and assessment of rosacea: recommendations from the global ROSacea COnsensus (ROSCO) panel. *Br J Dermatol.* 2017;176(2):431-438.
2. Vieira AC, Mannis MJ. Ocular rosacea: common and commonly missed. *J Am Acad Dermatol.* 2013;69(6 Suppl 1):S36-S41.
3. Stone DU, Chodosh J. Ocular rosacea: an update on pathogenesis and therapy. *Curr Opin Ophthalmol.* 2004;15(6):499-502.
4. Palamar M, Degirmenci C, Ertam I, Yagci A. Evaluation of dry eye and meibomian gland dysfunction with meibography in patients with rosacea. *Cornea.* 2015;34(5):497-499.
5. Lindsley K, Matsumura S, Hatef E, Akpek EK. Interventions for chronic blepharitis. *Cochrane Database Syst Rev.* 2012;2012(5):CD005556.
6. Bhargava R, Kumar P, Kumar M, Mehra N, Mishra A. A randomized controlled trial of omega-3 fatty acids in dry eye syndrome. *Int J Ophthalmol.* 2013;6(6):811-816.
7. Wladis EJ, Adam AP. Treatment of ocular rosacea. *Surv Ophthalmol.* 2018;63(3):340-346.
8. Pflugfelder SC, Karpecki PM, Perez VL. Treatment of blepharitis: recent clinical trials. *Ocul Surface.* 2014;12(4):273-284.
9. Jackson WB. Blepharitis: current strategies for diagnosis and management. *Can J Ophthalmol.* 2008;43(2):170-179.
10. Faghihi G, Khosravani P, Nilforoushzadeh MA, et al. Dapsone gel in the treatment of papulopustular rosacea: a double-blind randomized clinical trial. *J Drugs Dermatol.* 2015;14(6):602-606.
11. Seo KY, Kang SM, Ha DY, Chin HS, Jung JW. Long-term effects of intense pulsed light treatment on the ocular surface in patients with rosacea-associated meibomian gland dysfunction. *Cont Lens Anterior Eye.* 2018;41(5):430-435.
12. Lane SS, DuBiner HB, Epstein RJ, et al. A new system, the LipiFlow, for the treatment of meibomian gland dysfunction. *Cornea.* 2012;31(4):396-404. doi:10.1097/ICO.0b013e318239aaea

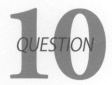

An 18-Year-Old Man Complaining of Severe Itchy Eyes and Redness Has Diffuse Eyelid Erythema With Dry Scaly Skin, Meibomian Gland Dysfunction, 2+ Conjunctival Bulbar and Palpebral Injection, and 3+ Papillae. Does He Need Steroid Drops?

Brandon Baartman, MD

The clinical picture painted here is certainly suggestive of an atopic ocular condition. Atopic conditions of the eye and ocular adnexa include vernal keratoconjunctivitis (VKC), atopic keratoconjunctivitis (AKC), and giant papillary conjunctivitis. Although all have certain unique, disease-defining characteristics, a shared pathophysiology of hypersensitivity exists in each case, which can lead to some overlap in signs and symptoms. While giant papillary conjunctivitis could be included in the differential diagnosis, in the absence of obvious contact lens history, VKC and AKC are the 2 most likely causative culprits in this 18-year old young man. We will discuss some of the clinical features of atopic ocular conditions and return to our case to discuss the management plan.

Diagnosis

Atopy as a systemic disease, including hay fever, eczema or atopic dermatitis, and allergic rhinitis, exists in about 10% to 20% of people of Western populations.[1] In the course of evaluation for atopic ocular disease, such as VKC or AKC, it is important to ask the patient about these systemic symptoms and any prior management. Additionally, discussing aggravating and alleviating environmental factors can be helpful, as this is a tenet of successful management, which we will discuss later. It is often simple to arrive at the diagnosis of atopic or allergic ocular

Hardten DR, Hansen MS.
*Curbside Consultation in Cornea and External Disease:
49 Clinical Questions, Second Edition* (pp 59-63).
© 2022 Taylor & Francis Group.

Figure 10-1. Periocular dermatitis with resultant medial ectropion, keratinization of the lid margin, and mild symblepharon in this patient with chronic, steroid-dependent AKC.

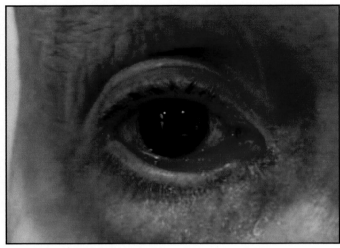

disease, but it can be more difficult to distinguish between VKC and AKC. Both conditions typically present with any combination of symptoms, including ocular irritation, itching, photophobia, and blurred vision. Signs of the diseases are also similar, including conjunctival injection, mucous discharge, and varying degrees of corneal involvement, but with a few defining features in each case that can help lead to the correct diagnosis. Age at presentation is commonly considered a diagnostic clue, with VKC classically presenting in young men, while AKC generally manifests later in life.[2] Periocular findings can be seen in both entities but are generally mild in VKC, with the most common manifestation being mild mechanical ptosis. In AKC, periocular findings are often diagnostic and classically include dermatitis, which can result in a rough, leather-like skin quality. Additional lid findings can include ectropion, entropion, anterior and posterior blepharitis, and keratinization of the lid margins, as seen in Figure 10-1.[2] The conjunctival involvement can appear similar in both VKC and AKC on cursory inspection, with injection of the perilimbal zones and Horner-Trantas dots, which are distinct elevations of hyperplastic epithelial cells and eosinophils.[3] Further evaluation of the conjunctiva can reveal differences among the diseases. While VKC will typically present with large papillae of the upper tarsus, the conjunctival papillary reaction of AKC is often greatest in the inferior conjunctiva and fornix and may produce symblepharon.[2] Both VKC and AKC can result in vision loss from corneal disease. In VKC, the classic "shield ulcer" can be seen in the superior cornea and may result in scarring and irregular astigmatism, while in AKC, chronic punctate keratitis early in the disease can lead to chronic epithelial erosion and corneal neovascularization. In severe cases of AKC, symblepharon and limbal stem cell deficiency may develop.[4]

Management

Now that we have shared the characteristics of the top 2 conditions on our differential diagnosis, let us reconsider the characteristics of the patient at hand. We have an 18-year old man with itching and redness of both eyes, with conjunctival injection and papillae, which, taken alone, could be either AKC or VKC. However, we also know that there are erythematous skin changes, dry and scaly skin (suggestive of eczema; Figure 10-2), and meibomitis—all which more strongly suggest AKC, which is the most likely diagnosis for this patient. A careful history should be taken to determine the patient's atopic history and use of antihistamine or steroid medications. Asthma and allergic rhinitis can be present in up to 65% of patients with AKC.[5] Patients will often report a family history of atopic disease as well. Examination should include inspection of the fornices for symblepharon and careful evaluation of the cornea for scarring, neovascularization, and inferior steepening, as keratoconus may develop from chronic eye rubbing (see Figure 10-2). A dilated examination of the lens evaluating for cataract is also important, as this can be seen secondary to AKC as well as from chronic steroid use.

The management of this patient should be comprehensive, with the goal of quieting inflammation and reducing the risks of sequelae and chronic vision loss. Deliberate evaluation for and avoidance of environmental irritants is critical and may be best facilitated by a primary care physician or allergy specialist. Because atopy, at its root, is a systemic condition, treatment with oral antihistamine agents is critical to reducing the systemic inflammatory response to allergens. Topical steroids are often required to reduce the ocular surface inflammation and should be started in this patient. Typical practice will employ prednisolone acetate 1% or difluprednate 0.05% up to 8 times daily for a period of 2 weeks, and it is critical that the patient be educated about the temporary intent of the medication and the side effects with chronic use. Topical steroids should be started in conjunction with topical mast cell stabilizers, such as cromolyn, nedocromil, or lodoxamide, which can be continued with less risk of chronic complications.[6] Newer formulations, with antihistamines such as olapatadine or ketotifen, may also be employed this way. Other topical immunomodulatory medications have shown benefit in the chronic management of inflammation in AKC as well, such as cyclosporine and tacrolimus, and may be a beneficial addition to medication regimens for patients who are either steroid-dependent or those with refractory inflammation.[7,8]

Although the control of inflammation is paramount to the management of AKC, optimizing the ocular surface health is a mainstay of treatment as well. Preservative-free artificial tears and ointments are critical to provide adequate lubrication in the setting of poor tear film quality and should be used frequently in patients with AKC. Meibomian gland dysfunction (MGD) in AKC is also thought to be more severe than in simple obstructive MGD,[9] and while meibomian clearance therapies such as LipiFlow, iLux, or TearCare have not been formally studied in the setting of AKC, these may be employed as well. Newer treatment modalities, such as intense pulsed light therapy, have been shown to be effective in obstructive MGD as well and can be considered.[10]

In short, this patient does likely require topical steroid therapy, but it should be used judiciously in this young patient and in conjunction with other environmental modifications, systemic antihistamine medications, and topical immunomodulator therapy for the best possible management of this chronic disease.

Figure 10-2. (A) A patient with severe facial eczema, with leathery periocular skin wrinkling. (B) Corneal topography of the same patient, demonstrating inferior steepening from chronic eye rubbing, suggestive of early keratoconus.

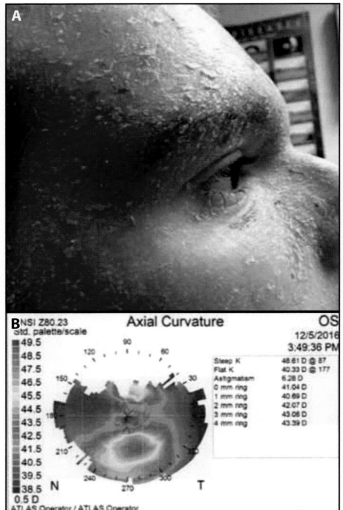

References

1. Thomsen SF. Epidemiology and natural history of atopic diseases. *Eur Clin Respir J.* 2015;2. doi:10.3402/ecrj. v2.24642
2. Foster CS, Calonge M. Atopic keratoconjunctivitis. *Ophthalmology.* 1990;97(8):992-1000.
3. Barney NP. Vernal and atopic keratoconjunctivitis. In: Mannis MJ, Holland EJ, eds. *Cornea. Fundamentals, Diagnosis and Management.* 4th ed. Elsevier; 2017:533-541.
4. Jabbehdari S, Stames TW, Kurji KH, et al. Management of advanced ocular surface disease in patients with severe atopic keratoconjunctivitis. *Ocul Surf.* 2019;17(2):303-309.
5. Power WJ, Tugal-Tutkun I, Foster CS. Long-term follow-up of patients with atopic keratoconjunctivitis. *Ophthalmology.* 1998;105(4):637-642.
6. Chen JJ, Applebaum DS, Sun GS, Pflugfelder SC. Atopic keratoconjunctivitis: a review. *J Am Acad Dermatol.* 2014;70(3):569-575.
7. Utine CA, Stern M, Akpek EK. Immunopathological features of severe chronic atopic keratoconjunctivitis and effects of topical cyclosporine treatment. *Ocul Immunol Inflamm.* 2019;27(7):1184-1193.
8. Al-Amri AM. Long-term follow-up of tacrolimus ointment for treatment of atopic keratoconjunctivitis. *Am J Ophthalmol.* 2014;157(2):280-286.
9. Ibrahim OMA, Matsumoto Y, Dogru M, et al. In vivo confocal microscopy evaluation of meibomian gland dysfunction in atopic-keratoconjunctivitis patients. *Ophthalmology.* 2012;119(10):1961-1968.
10. Toyos R, McGill W, Briscoe D. Intense pulsed light treatment for dry eye disease due to meibomian gland dysfunction; a 3-year retrospective study. *Photomed Laser Surg.* 2015;33(1):41-46.

HOW CAN I HELP A 47-YEAR-OLD WOMAN WHO USES ARTIFICIAL TEARS 6 TIMES DAILY AND CONTINUES TO COMPLAIN OF DRY EYES?

Stephen C. Pflugfelder, MD

This patient's history suggests that she has a chronic and severe dry eye condition. Evaluation should begin with a thorough systemic and ocular history, with attention to symptoms of a systemic autoimmune condition, such as Sjögren's syndrome (SS) or rheumatoid arthritis. These would include symptoms of dry mouth; difficulty chewing and swallowing dry food; or painful, tender, or stiff joints. The systemic medications currently being taken should be reviewed to identify any with anticholinergic effects that could be causing dry eye. Most commonly, these include antihistamine, antispasmodic, and antidepressant medications. The patient should be questioned about the severity and nature of the ocular discomfort, with attention to exacerbating factors (eg, low humidity or computer use) and symptoms of blurred vision. The patient should be asked about their ability to reflex tear in response to emotional or environmental stimuli.

A detailed ocular surface and tear evaluation should be performed. The components of this examination should include visual acuity and evaluation of lid closure, blink rate, the presence of anterior or posterior blepharitis, and punctal position and patency. Conjunctival (scarring, chalasis, pinguecula, or pterygium) and corneal epithelial (punctate erosions, filaments, or epithelial defects) signs should be noted (Figure 11-1). If the patient is complaining of blurred vision, corneal topography should be performed to assess corneal smoothness. Irregularity or poor reflectivity of Placido rings or elevated surface regularity indices (eg, the surface regularity index) may be noted (Figure 11-2).[1] Fluorescein should be instilled using a fluorescein strip that is wet with preservative-free saline, and tear break-up time and presence, location, and severity of the corneal staining should be measured. Lissamine green staining should be performed to evaluate the conjunctiva, with attention to the exposure zone (Figure 11-3) and superior bulbar conjunctiva. Staining in the latter area is a sign of superior limbic keratoconjunctivitis. Tear production should be evaluated with a Schirmer test. In my hands, the Schirmer-I test performed without anesthesia provides the

Hardten DR, Hansen MS.
Curbside Consultation in Cornea and External Disease:
49 Clinical Questions, Second Edition (pp 65-68).
© 2022 Taylor & Francis Group.

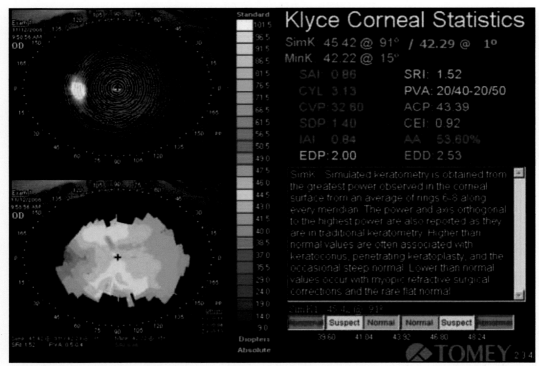

Figure 11-1. Corneal topography showing marked irregularity of Placido rings and elevated surface regularity index.

Figure 11-2. Corneal epithelial filaments stained with fluorescein.

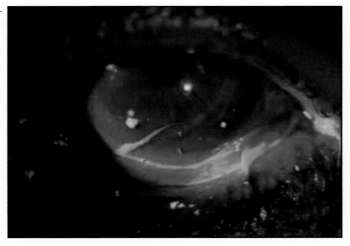

most valuable information because it tests one's ability to reflex tear in response to sensory stimulation. If the patient has a Schirmer test less than 5 mm and moderate-to-severe exposure zone corneal and conjunctival staining, I recommend that the patient have serological testing to look for the presence of circulating autoantibodies associated with SS, including rheumatoid factor, antinuclear antibody, and SS-associated antibodies A and B. Consultation with a rheumatologist is suggested if autoantibodies are detected. Corneal sensitivity should be evaluated in selected cases, particularly when an exposure zone corneal epithelial defect is present.

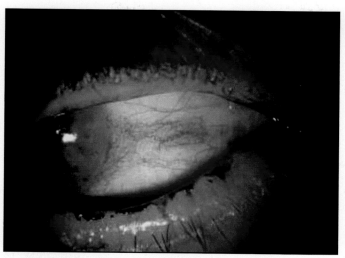

Figure 11-3. Conjunctival lissamine green staining in the exposure zone.

Table 11-1
Dry Eye Management

Severity Level	Treatment
1	Education; environmental/dietary modification; eliminate offending systemic medications; artificial tear substitutes, gels/ointments; lid therapy
2	Anti-inflammatory medications[a]; tetracyclines, AZM for meibomianitis, rosacea; plugs, secretagogues; moisture chamber specs
3	Serum/plasma; contact lenses; permanent punctal occlusion
4	Systemic IS therapy; surgery (AMT lid surgery tarsorrhaphy, MM and SG transplant)

[a]Corticosteroids, cyclosporine, lifitegrast.

AMT = amniotic membrane transplant; AZM = azithromycin; IS = immunosuppression; MM = mucous membrane; Pl = plasma; SG = salivary gland.

Treatment Options

My treatment regimen is grounded on the severity-based algorithm proposed by the Tear Film and Ocular Surface Society Dry Eye WorkShop (Table 11-1).[2] Generally, chronic dry eye that is not adequately treated with artificial tears will require 1 or more therapeutic agents. If tear production is 5 mm or less in the presence of moderate-to-severe ocular surface dye staining, punctal occlusion is performed.

Figure 11-4. Cornea with severe epitheliopathy and previous sterile ulcers is fit with the PROSE, a sclera-bearing lens with a fluid-filled reservoir, over the cornea.

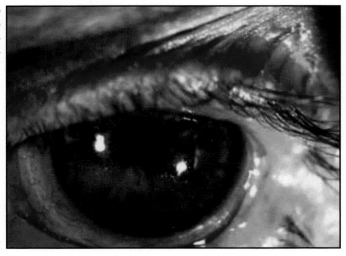

I recommend thermal cautery for patients who have lost the ability to reflex tear, whereas extended-duration intracanalicular punctal plugs are used for patients who maintain the ability to reflex tear. Patients with reduced vision due to corneal epithelial disease require the most aggressive therapy, which typically would include artificial tears with preservatives, pulsed topical corticosteroid steroid (eg, loteprednol, etabonate 0.5% 4 times daily for 2 weeks, followed by twice daily for 2 weeks), cyclosporine A 0.05% emulsion 2 to 4 times daily, oral doxycycline 40 mg per day (given in 1 or 2 doses), and topical autologous serum or plasma. If vision remains decreased or if the patient continues to complain of moderate-to-severe irritation or photophobia, a scleral lens, such as the Prosthetic Replacement of the Ocular Surface Ecosystem (PROSE; Boston Sight), is recommended (Figure 11-4).[3]

References

1. de Paiva CS, Lindsey JL, Pflugfelder SC. Assessing the severity of keratitis sicca with videokeratoscopic indices. *Ophthalmology.* 2003;110(6):1102-1109.
2. Jones L, Downie LE, Korb D, et al. TFOS DEWS II management and therapy report. *Ocul Surf.* 2017;15(3):575-628.
3. Romero-Rangel T, Stavrou P, Cotter J, Rosenthal P, Baltatzis S, Foster CS. Gas-permeable scleral contact lens therapy in ocular surface disease. *Am J Ophthalmol.* 2000;130(1):25-32.

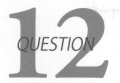

A 43-YEAR-OLD WOMAN IS COMPLAINING OF DRY EYES.
THE EXAM SHOWS PUNCTATE KERATOPATHY IN THE
INFERIOR THIRD OF HER CORNEAS. WHAT IS THE
OPTIMAL MANAGEMENT?

Melissa Barnett, OD

Dry eye disease is the primary reason that patients see their eye care practitioners.[1] There is an increasing awareness for both practitioners and the public of the magnitude of this condition. More than 30 million Americans have symptoms of dry eye disease; however, only 16 million are diagnosed and only 1 million are treated.[2] Needless to say, there is massive potential and opportunity to address this highly prevalent condition.

Dry eye disease can negatively affect one's quality of life,[3] with symptoms such as grittiness, foreign body sensation, debilitating ocular pain, and photophobia. Visual fluctuations and distortion may also occur. It is well established that the signs and symptoms of dry eye do not correlate, which may be attributed to the neurosensory component of dry eye disease, as emphasized by the Tear Film and Ocular Surface Society Dry Eye WorkShop II (DEWS II).

Diagnosis

In a 43-year-old patient who presents with dry eye signs and symptoms, a dry eye questionnaire is a helpful place to start the evaluation. Myriad questionnaires, such as the Standard Patient Evaluation of Eye Dryness Questionnaire (SPEED), Ocular Surface Disease Index (OSDI), Dry Eye Questionnaire (DEQ), Canadian Dry Eye Epidemiology Study (CANDEES), and the Contact Lens Dry Eye Questionnaire (CLDEQ) are available.

Hardten DR, Hansen MS.
Curbside Consultation in Cornea and External Disease:
49 Clinical Questions, Second Edition (pp 69-74).
© 2022 Taylor & Francis Group.

In addition to asking standard dry eye questions, it is important to ask whether dry mouth or arthritis symptoms exist to investigate the presence of autoimmune disease, including Sjögren's disease, rheumatoid arthritis, and systemic lupus erythematosus. Sjögren's disease is a chronic, autoimmune, systemic disease characterized by lymphocytic infiltration and malfunction of the exocrine glands, resulting in predominant symptoms of dry eye and dry mouth.[4] Sjögren's disease is a highly prevalent condition and is one of the most common systemic, rheumatic, autoimmune diseases, affecting up to 1.4% of adults in the United States—second only to rheumatoid arthritis in its prevalence in North America.[5] Prompt diagnosis and management is imperative due to the predominance of diffuse large B-cell lymphoma in patients with Sjögren's disease.[6]

Ocular Surface Evaluation

Meibomian gland dysfunction is the most frequent cause of dry eye and is present in as many as 86 of 100 cases of dry eye.[7] The precise etiology of meibomian gland dysfunction is unknown. However, is it clear that there are 2 pathologies that contribute to meibomian gland dysfunction— a decrease in the lipid layer due to keratinization of the terminal duct anatomy and an accumulation of cellular and lipid material within the duct lamina.[8] In addition to traditional management strategies for meibomian gland dysfunction, including warm compresses, eyelid massage, and eyelid scrubs, there are many promising in-office manual and mechanical treatments that may provide symptomatic relief for patients with meibomian gland dysfunction. In this case, in addition to evaluating and imaging the meibomian glands, it is pertinent to evaluate for nonobvious obstructive meibomian gland dysfunction, which is perhaps the most common form of obstructive meibomian gland dysfunction.[9] Nonobvious obstructive meibomian gland dysfunction appears to be the precursor to obvious obstructive meibomian gland dysfunction, is highly underdiagnosed, and is the most common cause of evaporative dry eye.[9] Meibomian gland evaluation and expression, even if nonobvious obstructive meibomian gland dysfunction is suspected, is valuable to determine whether the meibomian gland dysfunction is contributing to a patient's dry eye.

In this patient case example with inferior punctate keratopathy, it is important to consider nighttime evaporative stress. Nighttime evaporative stress may have various dynamic, often overlapping causes, such as incomplete eyelid seal, nocturnal lagophthalmos, sleep apnea, floppy eyelid syndrome, and aqueous deficient dry eye.[10,11] A recent study demonstrated that incomplete eyelid seal correlated well with the presence of moderate-to-severe dry eye signs and symptoms, moderate incomplete lid seal was common in the general patient population, and lid seal problems were extremely common in patients older than 50 years, with 50% of patients aged 61 to 80 years showing signs of poor seal.[10] That study reinforces the belief that every patient with dry eye should be evaluated for incomplete eyelid seal, especially those with morning dry eye symptoms and those with meibomian gland dysfunction, which greatly exacerbate the problem.

To evaluate for incomplete eyelid seal, in a dark room, place a fully illuminated transilluminator gently against the closed relaxed upper eyelid at the superior junction of the tarsal plate. The amount of light escaping between the upper and lower lid margins indicates a lack of closure. Sodium fluorescein corneal staining and lissamine green staining are used to supplement this technique (Figure 12-1). Management options for nighttime evaporative stress include nighttime lubricant ointment, eyelid taping and/or a high-quality sleep mask to seal in moisture, improve eye lubrication, and provide eye protection.

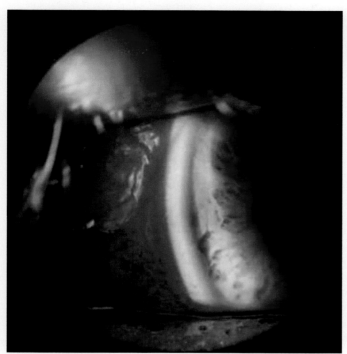

Figure 12-1. An eye with ocular surface disease demonstrating lissamine green staining on the cornea and conjunctiva.

Contact Lenses

Asking the patient about a history of contact lens wear or discontinuation of contact lens wear is also important. A 43-year-old person may be approaching or entering presbyopia and desires to wear contact lenses. In the global market, contact lens dropout is estimated to be approximately equal to the number of new lens wearers each year.[12] Numerous publications have established that the rate of contact lens dropout ranges from 15% to more than 20%.[13-15] Contact lens dropout increases around age 40 years and significantly increases around age 42 years. Comfort issues are the key reason for contact lens dropout for patients younger than age 45 years.[16] After age 45, vision and comfort are almost equally stated as the reason for contact lens dropout.[17] Of interest, in the soft contact lens population, 93% of patients were not wearing multifocal contact lenses at the time of dropout. If ocular surface disease is present, the quality of the tear film is diminished, increasing contact lens discomfort. Dry eye significantly increases the chance of contact lens drop out.[12]

The main indications for use of scleral lenses are visual rehabilitation in irregular corneas and the therapeutic treatment of ocular surface disease.[18] The scleral lens' post-lens fluid reservoir provides continuous corneal lubrication and ocular protection (Figure 12-2). Scleral lenses prevent mechanical damage, prevent tissue desiccation, promote healing, and disrupt the pain cycle. Large-diameter scleral lenses cover most of the ocular surface and protect corneal and conjunctival tissue from potential aggravation due to friction between the ocular surface and the palpebral surface of the lids.

Figure 12-2. Scleral lens for a normal cornea compared with a dime.

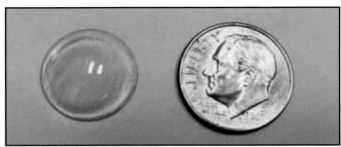

When conventional treatments are insufficient, scleral lenses are a viable management option for patients with dry eye.[18] Therapeutic scleral lens indications for ocular surface disease include neurotrophic keratitis, exposure keratitis, dry eye syndrome, graft vs host disease, Stevens-Johnson syndrome, ocular cicatricial pemphigoid, chemical burns, limbal stem cell deficiency, Sjögren's disease, and persistent epithelial defects.[18] Additionally, scleral lenses have been indicated for the treatment of conditions that are associated with neuropathic ocular pain.[18]

Scleral lens designs are also available for patients with normal, healthy eyes. Scleral lenses can be used for corneas with a regular, normal, prolate shape, without disease, ectasia, or irregularities, and can significantly improve the lens-wearing experience for patients with normal eyes (Figure 12-3). Scleral lenses for normal eyes are beneficial for a patient who is not satisfied with their current soft, corneal gas permeable, or hybrid contact lenses. Perhaps the vision is not clear enough nor consistent or lens awareness and discomfort are present. Consider patients with refractive errors, such as myopia, regular astigmatism, hyperopia, and presbyopia, for scleral lenses. Transitioning a patient from other contact lens modalities to scleral lenses is easily attainable and improves the contact lens experience of patients. If vision, comfort, or both are not optimal with the current contact lens modality, consider a scleral lens option. It is still critical to discuss realistic expectations with the patient, including scleral lens risks, benefits, handling, solutions, and the scleral lens fitting process.

In patients with mild to moderate dry eye without systemic comorbidities, scleral lenses should not be the primary therapy. Other conventional treatment options should be tried first, including environment modifications, preservative-free eye drops, prescription dry eye medications, eyelid hygiene, nighttime lubrication or goggles, and punctal occlusion. When conventional treatments are insufficient, scleral lenses are a viable management option for patients with dry eye.

According to DEWS II, scleral lenses are tertiary therapy, after prescription medications and overnight treatments, such as ointment or moisture goggles, and before the long-term use of steroids, amniotic membrane grafts, surgical punctal occlusion, or other surgical procedures such as tarsorrhaphy or salivary gland transplantation.[19] Other step 3 therapy options for dry eye, along with scleral lenses, include oral secretagogues, autologous/allogenic serum eye drops, and soft bandage contact lenses.

Scleral lenses are ideal for presbyopic patients who often have concomitant dry eye. Numerous multifocal scleral lens options are available that provide exceptional vision at all distances. Because scleral lenses protect and bathe the ocular surface, scleral lenses are fantastic for patients with dry eye. Of note, multifocal scleral lens optics may be used in patients with corneal irregularities, as a scleral lens neutralizes the irregularities. In this case example, a multifocal scleral lens is a reasonable option.

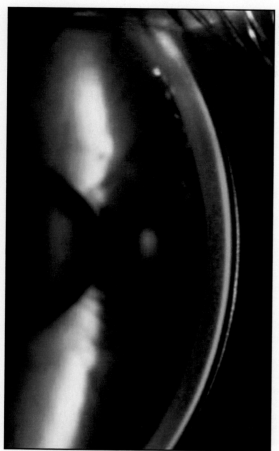

Figure 12-3. A cross-sectional view of a scleral lens with sodium fluorescein. (Reproduced with permission from Tom Arnold, OD.)

A study published in *Contact Lens Anterior Eye* assessed the performance of scleral lenses for a wide range of clinical indications.[20] That prospective, cross-sectional study evaluated 281 existing contact lens patients who were fit with lenses based on a lens selection algorithm. The authors determined that wearing contact lenses significantly improved corrected distance visual acuity compared with wearing spectacles. In addition, there was an improvement in satisfactory wearing time. Both the scleral lens and soft lens groups were generally effective and had high subjective scores with similar results. Additionally, wearers reported that scleral lenses were as comfortable as soft lenses, and 75% of wearers preferred their vision with a scleral lens.[20]

Conclusion

When evaluating a patient for ocular surface disease, many factors are essential to be considered. The evaluation of dry eye symptoms, lifestyle factors, and systemic disease are all pertinent. In addition, evaluating corneal and conjunctival staining, tear break-up time, osmolarity, and incomplete eyelid seal are all critical factors to consider. It is also valuable to determine whether the patient has an interest in contact lens wear and to provide scleral lenses as an option. The popularity of scleral lenses is immense and continues to grow. Multifocal scleral lens options may be considered, especially in a patient with symptomatic dry eye.

References

1. Gayton JL. Etiology, prevalence, and treatment of dry eye disease. *Clin Ophthalmol*. 2009;3:405-412.
2. Farrand KF, Fridman M, Stillman IO, Schaumberg DA. Prevalence of diagnosed dry eye disease in the United States among adults aged 18 years and older. *Am J Ophthalmol*. 2017;182:90-98. doi:10.1016/j.ajo.2017.06.033
3. Paulsen AJ, Cruickshanks KJ, Fischer ME, et al. Dry eye in the beaver dam offspring study: prevalence, risk factors, and health-related quality of life. *Am J Ophthalmol*. 2014;157(4):799-806.
4. Bloch KJ, Buchanan WW, Wohl MJ, Bunim JJ. Sjogren's syndrome: a clinical, pathological and serological study of 62 cases. *Medicine (Baltimore)*. 1965;44:187-231.
5. Helmick CG, Felson DT, Lawrence RC, et al. Estimates of the prevalence of arthritis and other rheumatic conditions in the United States. Part 1. *Arthritis Rheum*. 2008;58(1):15-25.
6. Navazesh M, Christensen C, Brightman V. Clinical criteria for the diagnosis of salivary gland hypofunction. *J Dent Res*. 1992;71(7):1363-1369.
7. Lemp MA, Crews LA, Bron AJ, Foulks GN, Sullivan BD. Distribution of aqueous deficient and evaporative dry eye in a clinic-based patient population: a retrospective study. *Cornea*. 2012;31(5):472-478.
8. Tomlinson A, Bron AJ, Korb D, et al. The International Workshop on Meibomian Gland Dysfunction: report of the diagnosis subcommittee. *Invest Ophthalmol Vis Sci*. 2011;52(4):2006-2049.
9. Blackie CA, Korb DR, Knop E, Bedi R, Knop N, Holland EJ. Nonobvious obstructive meibomian gland dysfunction. *Cornea*. 2010;29(12):1333-1345. doi:10.1097/ICO.0b013e3181d4f366
10. Korb DR, Blackie CA, Nau AC. Prevalence of compromised lid seal in symptomatic refractory dry eye patients and asymptomatic patients. *Invest Ophthalmol Vis Sci*. 2017;58(8):2696.
11. Liu DTS, Di Pascuale MA, Sawai J, Gao YY, Tseng SCG. Tear film dynamics in floppy eyelid syndrome. *Invest Ophthalmol Vis Sci*. 2005;46(4):1188-1194. doi:10.1167/iovs.04-0913
12. Pucker AD, Jones-Jordan LA, Marx S, et al. Clinical factors associated with contact lens dropout. *Cont Lens Anterior Eye*. 2019;42(3):318-324. doi:10.1016/j.clae.2018.12.002
13. Pritchard N, Fonn D, Brazeau D. Discontinuation of contact lens wear: a survey. *Int Contact Lens Clin*. 1999;26(6):157-162.
14. Young G, Veys J, Pritchard N, Coleman S. A multi-centre study of lapsed contact lens wearers. *Ophthalmic Physiol Opt*. 2002;22(6):516-527.
15. Richdale K, Sinnott LT, Skadahl E, Nichols JJ. Frequency of and factors associated with contact lens dissatisfaction and discontinuation. *Cornea*. 2007;26(2):168-174.
16. Nichols JJ, Willcox MDP, Bron AJ, et al. The TFOS International Workshop on Contact Lens Discomfort: executive summary. *Invest Ophthalmol Vis Sci*. 2013;54(11):TFOS7-TFOS13.
17. Brujic M, Miller, J. Minimizing dropouts: what you can do. *Rev Cornea Contact Lens*. March 17, 2011. Accessed October 4, 2021. https://www.reviewofcontactlenses.com/article/minimizing-dropouts-what-you-can-do
18. Barnett M, Johns LK, eds. Ophthalmology current and future developments. Vol 4. *Contemporary scleral lenses: theory and application*. Bentham Books; 2017.
19. Jones L, Downie LE, Korb D, et al. TFOS DEWS II management and therapy report. *Ocul Surf*. 2017;15(3):575-628. doi:10.1016/j.jtos.2017.05.006
20. Michaud L, Bennett ES, Woo SL, et al. Clinical evaluation of large diameter rigid-gas permeable versus soft toric contact lenses for the correction of refractive astigmatism. A multicenter study. *Eye Contact Lens*. 2018;44(3):164-169.

13

I Have a Patient With Significant Dry Eye. Is There Anything I Can Do in the Office to Help This Patient With Their Eye Problems?

Mark S. Milner, MD

Dry eye may be the most common disease an optometrist or ophthalmologist sees in their office, and, unfortunately, most eye care professionals dread seeing these patients on their schedules. Although cornea specialists see most patients with significant dry eye, the impact on the ocular surface affects every subspecialty—from cataract and refractive surgery to glaucoma and retina. Based on the Tear Film and Ocular Surface Society (TFOS) Dry Eye WorkShop (DEWS) II definition, "Dry eye disease is a multifactorial disease of the ocular surface characterized by a loss of homeostasis of the tear film and accompanied by ocular surface symptoms, in which tear film instability and hyperosmolarity, ocular surface inflammation and damage, and neurosensory abnormalities play etiological roles."[1]

Our understanding of dry eye has changed over the past 20 years in several ways. We now know that dry eye is an inflammatory process of the lacrimal gland, ocular surface, and tear film, even if it is not clinically apparent. We also believe that dry eye may be a chronic, progressive disease, and that if left untreated, may result in damage to the ocular surface. There are now approved treatments to address dry eye disease and the surface inflammation, as opposed to just palliative therapies. Finally, dry eye is now thought of as not just a problem with tear quantity but tear quality as well.

Hardten DR, Hansen MS.
*Curbside Consultation in Cornea and External Disease:
49 Clinical Questions, Second Edition* (pp 75-85).
© 2022 Taylor & Francis Group.

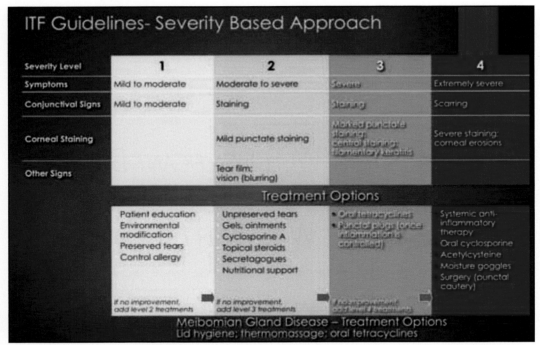

Figure 13-1. International Task Force Delphi panel guidelines for a severity-based treatment algorithm. (Reproduced with permission from Behrens A, Doyle JJ, Stern L, et al. Dysfunctional tear syndrome: a Delphi approach to treatment recommendations. *Cornea.* 2006;25[8]:900-907.)

Diagnosis

What makes this disease so complex is that both the diagnosis and treatment are difficult because there are multiple triggers, signs, and symptoms that do not always correlate, and, until several years ago, treatment options were limited. There have been numerous algorithms developed to simplify or clarify the process of diagnosis and treatment. One of the earliest was the International Task Force Delphi panel guidelines,[2] which separated dry eye into 4 categories of severity based on symptoms and signs (both conjunctival and corneal), with treatment options suggested for each severity level (Figure 13-1). Three new algorithms have been published to help clinicians diagnose and treat this complex disease, including the TFOS DEWS II,[1] the American Society of Cataract and Refractive Surgery (ASCRS) Preoperative Ocular Surface Disease algorithm,[3] and the Cornea External Disease and Refractive Surgery Society (CEDARS) Dysfunctional Tear Syndrome (DTS) algorithm.[4] The ASCRS algorithm is a specific guideline to help surgeons address the ocular surface prior to cataract and refractive surgery. The DEWS II comprises 11 separate reports, totaling approximately 400 pages, and is extremely comprehensive. This algorithm is extensive and detailed, with road maps (Figures 13-2 and 13-3) available to help clinicians diagnose dry eye as aqueous deficient, evaporative, or both.[1] The CEDARS DTS algorithm was developed with 3 goals in mind.[4] First, was to design a diagnostic-based approach to treatment. Many of the prior algorithms are severity-based approaches, meaning that treatment is based on separating patients into mild, moderate, or severe dry eye. The second goal was to provide innovative treatment options (compounded and off-label), in addition to the commercially available drugs, to address this complex disease. The third goal was to create a facile algorithm that clinicians can use in their offices to simplify the process of diagnosis and treatment.

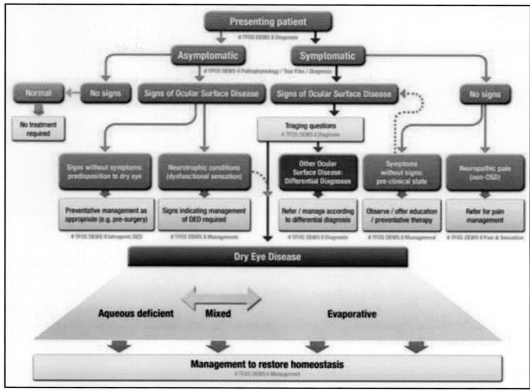

Figure 13-2. TFOS DEWS II algorithm. DED = dry eye disease; OSD = ocular surface disease. (Reprinted from *Ocul Surf,* 15[3], Craig JP, Nichols KK, Akpek EK, et al, TFOS DEWS II definition and classification report, 276-283, Copyright 2017, with permission from Elsevier.)

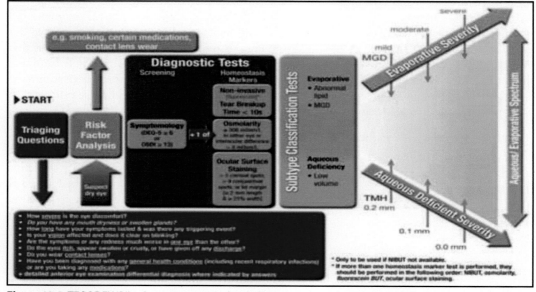

Figure 13-3. TFOS DEWS II—Process associated with diagnosis of dry eye disease. DEQ-5 = Dry Eye Questionnaire 5; MGD = meibomian gland dysfunction; NIBUT = noninvasive tear breakup time; OSDI = Ocular Surface Disease Index; TMH = tear meniscus height. (Reprinted from *Ocul Surf,* 15[3], Wolffsohn JS, Arita R, Chalmers R, et al, TFOS DEWS II Diagnostic Methodology report, 539-574, Copyright 2017, with permission from Elsevier.)

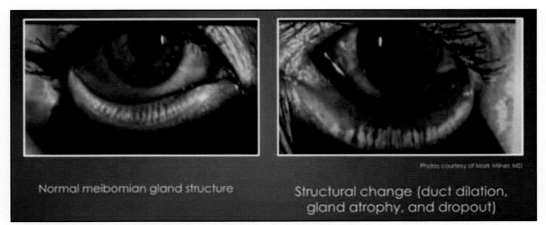

Normal meibomian gland structure

Structural change (duct dilation, gland atrophy, and dropout)

Figure 13-4. Meibography imaging of the lower lids—LipiView (TearScience).

Many point-of-care testing options are now available for diagnosing dry eye. These include tear osmolarity testing, used to quantify tear film hyperosmolarity, which is an indicator of dry eye. Matrix metalloproteinase 9 is a nonspecific marker of inflammation that increases in dry eye. A tear assay is available to determine whether matrix metalloproteinase 9 levels are greater than 41 ng/mL. Meibography is an image of the meibomian glands used to assess the lipid layer and levels of meibomian gland dropout and truncation (Figure 13-4).

These tests are helpful but may not be available in every office. Ultimately, any clinician in any office can diagnose dry eye with a good patient history, a thorough slit-lamp examination, and staining with fluorescein and the vital dyes (rose bengal and lissamine green). Fluorescein stains areas where cells are dead or absent. The vital dyes stain areas where cells are "sick" and there is disruption in the mucin coating. The staining pattern can help with diagnosing dry eye or the diseases that masquerade as dry eye (Figures 13-5 and 13-6). DEWS II discusses aqueous deficient, evaporative, and mixed dry eye.[1] The CEDARS DTS algorithm separates dry eye into 4 diagnostic subcategories.[4] These include aqueous deficiency; evaporative, based on goblet cell or mucin deficiency; blepharitis; both evaporative and nonevaporative; and exposure-related dry eye (Table 13-1).[4] A fifth category of "co-conspirators" is discussed, which includes diseases that masquerade as or contribute to dry eye and should be considered when the clinician is "spinning their wheels" with treatments and not getting results. If clinicians can separate the patient into the 4 categories, keeping in mind that a given patient may have 1, 2, 3, or all 4 of these categories at once, then a more directed treatment approach may provide for a better outcome.

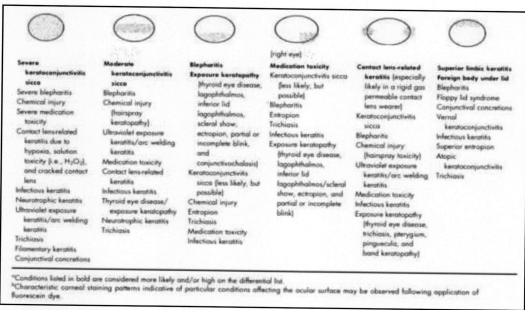

Figure 13-5. Fluorescein staining patterns and the diagnoses associated with each pattern. The most common diagnoses are in boldface. H_2O_2 = hydrogen peroxide. (Reproduced with permission from Milner MS, Beckman KA, Luchs JI, et al. Dysfunctional tear syndrome: dry eye disease and associated tear film disorders–new strategies for diagnosis and treatment. *Curr Opin Ophthalmol.* 2017;28[Suppl 1]:3-47.)

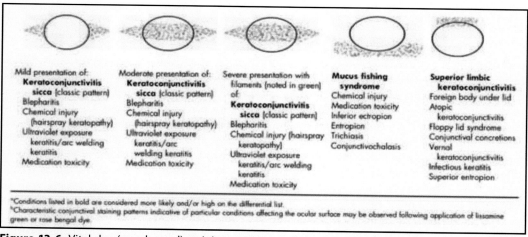

Figure 13-6. Vital dye (rose bengal) staining patterns and the diagnoses associated with each pattern. The most common diagnoses are in boldface. (Reproduced with permission from Milner MS, Beckman KA, Luchs JI, et al. Dysfunctional tear syndrome: dry eye disease and associated tear film disorders–new strategies for diagnosis and treatment. *Curr Opin Ophthalmol.* 2017;28[Suppl 1]:3-47.)

Table 13-1

CEDARS Dysfunction Tear Syndrome Algorithm: Diagnostic-Based Approach by Clinical Findings

Tear Deficiency	Goblet Cell/ Mucin Deficiency	Blepharitis/ MGD	Exposure Keratopathy
Clinical Finding by Dysfunction Tear Syndrome			
1. Decreased Schirmer test	1. Rapid tear breakup time	1. Anterior blepharitis	1. Lagophthalmos
2. Decreased tear lake	2. Conjunctival scarring	2. Posterior blepharitis	2. Poor or partial blink
3. Kerato-conjunctivitis sicca, rose bengal staining	3. Goblet cell deficiency	3. Lid erythema/ debris	3. Lid function

Reproduced with permission from Milner MS, Beckman KA, Luchs JI, et al. Dysfunctional tear syndrome: dry eye disease and associated tear film disorders–new strategies for diagnosis and treatment. *Curr Opin Ophthalmol.* 2017;28(Suppl 1):3-47.

Treatment

Treatment of dry eye disease is not straightforward for the reasons detailed previously, which include difficulty with diagnosis, disparity between signs and symptoms, and the limited number of approved medications for dry eye. Further, clinicians are often frustrated because they have a misconception that the currently available treatments are a panacea for dry eye. Cyclosporine and lifitegrast are both excellent treatments to address the underlying inflammation. They are T-cell immunosuppressive agents that have different mechanisms of action. Many clinicians view a 30% improvement in signs and/or symptoms on either treatment as a failure when, in reality, this is still a success. The common mistake in treating dry eye disease is that clinicians fail to recognize that dry eye, like glaucoma, is often a multitreatment disease. If a glaucoma patient with an intraocular pressure of 27 mm Hg and a target pressure of 17 mm Hg is started on a glaucoma eye drop and the result is a decrease in pressure to 22 mm Hg, the appropriate next step is to add another treatment. A patient with a 30% improvement while on cyclosporine or lifitegrast is often mistakenly instructed to discontinue the drop and is then substituted with another medication. In reality, this is a success, and an additional treatment should be added to the original therapy. In fact, anecdotally, there are many cornea specialists who have successful outcomes with patients on both cyclosporine and lifitegrast simultaneously, as they may have synergistic effects, given that they have different mechanisms of action.

The TFOS DEWS II provides the eye care professional with a stepwise treatment algorithm that is severity based (Table 13-2).[1] The CEDARS algorithm directs treatments based on the 4 diagnostic categories.[4] Each category has first- and second-line treatment options as well as procedural options for each category (Table 13-3). A clinician usually starts with one of the commercially available drugs, as cyclosporine and lifitegrast treat the first 3 categories.

Table 13-2

TFOS DEWS II Dry Eye Treatment Algorithm

Treatment Steps
Step 1: • Education regarding the condition, its management, treatment, and prognosis • Modification of local environment • Education regarding potential dietary modifications (including oral essential fatty acid supplementation) • Identification and potential modification/elimination of offending systemic and topical medications • Ocular lubricants of various types (if MGD is present, then consider lipid-containing supplements) • Lid hygiene and warm compresses of various types

Step 2: If the above options are inadequate, consider:
• Nonpreserved ocular lubricants to minimize preservative-induced toxicity
• Tea tree oil treatment for Demodex (if present)
• Tear conservation
  ○ Punctal occlusion
  ○ Moisture chamber spectacles/goggles
• Overnight treatments (such as ointment or moisture chamber devices)
• In-office, physical heating and expression of the meibomian glands (including device-assisted therapies, such as LipiFlow)
• In-office intense pulsed light therapy for MGD
• Prescription drugs to manage DED [Note: The use of prescription drugs needs to be considered in the context of the individual patient presentation and the relative level of evidence supporting their use for that specific indication, as this group of agents differs widely in mechanism of action.]
  ○ Topical antibiotic or antibiotic/steroid combination applied to the lid margins for anterior blepharitis (if present)
  ○ Topical corticosteroid (limited duration)
  ○ Topical secretagogues
  ○ Topical nonglucocorticoid immunomodulatory drugs (such as cyclosporine)
  ○ Topical LFA-1 antagonist drugs (such as lifitegrast)
  ○ Oral macrolide or tetracycline antibiotics

(continued)

Table 13-2 (continued)

TFOS DEWS II Dry Eye Treatment Algorithm

Treatment Steps

Step 3: If the above options are inadequate, consider:
• Oral secretagogues
• Autologous/allogeneic serum eye drops
• Therapeutic contact lens options
  ○ Soft bandage lenses
  ○ Rigid scleral lenses

Step 4: If the above options are inadequate, consider: • Topical corticosteroid for a longer duration • Amniotic membrane grafts • Surgical punctal occlusion • Other surgical approaches (eg, tarsorrhaphy, salivary gland transplantation)

Reprinted from *Ocul Surf*, 15, Jones L, Downie LE, Korb D, et al, TFOS DEWS II management and therapy report, 575-628, Copyright 2017, with permission from Elsevier.

The patient is then seen at 4 to 6 weeks. If the patient is nearly 100% improved in signs and symptoms, the treatment is continued and the patient is seen at 6 to 12 months. If there is partial improvement, a second treatment is initiated, based on the 4 categories. For example, if a patient is 40% better while on the initial treatment and the Schirmer test is still low, punctal plugs may be an appropriate second option. If the patient achieves 40% success and the Schirmer test is now normal, but there is still significant meibomian gland dysfunction (MGD), the next best treatment may be oral doxycycline, topical azithromycin (off-label), or topical metronidazole ointment (compounded). The severity of disease determines how aggressive a physician should be at each visit. For example, if a patient with severe dry eye presents with graft vs host disease and has 20/200 vision, 3+ punctate staining with filaments, conjunctival scarring with a rapid tear breakup time, and significant MGD with toothpaste-like secretions, this patient may need cyclosporine or lifitegrast, punctal plugs, topical steroids, and topical antibiotics all in the initial visit. Although cyclosporine and lifitegrast are excellent treatments, more options are on the horizon.

The CEDARS algorithm provides additional innovative options.[4] These include topical hormones, such as medroxyprogesterone or dehydroepiandrosterone drops (compounded), or topical albumin drops (compounded) for aqueous deficiency; topical vitamin A ointment (off-label) for goblet cell deficiency; and topical metronidazole ointment (compounded), topical doxycycline drops (compounded), or topical azithromycin drops (off-label) for blepharitis. Procedural treatments provide additional options for each category (see Table 13-3). This is especially true for blepharitis and MGD where there are limited approved treatments.

Table 13-3

CEDARS Dysfunction Tear Syndrome Algorithm: Diagnostic-Based Approach—First Line, Second Line, and Procedure Options

Aqueous Tear Deficiency	*Blepharitis/MGD (Evaporative or Nonevaporative)*	*Goblet Cell/ Mucin Deficiency*	*Exposure- Related DTS*
First Line[a]			
• Tear supplements and lubricants (ie, drops, gels, ointments, sprays, and lubricating inserts) • Nutritional supplements • Topical cyclosporine • Topical lifitegrast • Topical steroids • Topical secretagogues • Moisture chamber eyewear	• Tear supplements and lubricants (ie, drops, gels, ointments, sprays, and lubricating inserts) • Lid hygiene and lid scrubs (ie, cleansers, warm compresses, and massages) • Nutritional supplements • Topical cyclosporine • Topical lifitegrast • Topical erythromycin/ bacitracin • Topical azithromycin • Topical steroids or antibiotics/steroids	• Tear supplements and lubricants (ie, drops, gels, ointments, sprays, and lubricating inserts) • Topical cyclosporine • Topical lifitegrast • Vitamin A ointment – retinoic acid (compounded) • Moisture chamber eyewear • Topical secretagogues	• Tear supplements and lubricants (ie, drops, gels, ointments, sprays, and lubricating inserts) • Taping of the eyelid • Moisture chamber eyewear

(continued)

Table 13-3

CEDARS Dysfunction Tear Syndrome Algorithm: Diagnostic-Based Approach—First Line, Second Line, and Procedure Options

Aqueous Tear Deficiency	Blepharitis/MGD (Evaporative or Nonevaporative)	Goblet Cell/ Mucin Deficiency	Exposure- Related DTS
Second Line[a]			
• Oral secretagogues • Topical hormones (compounded) • Autologous serum (compounded) • Albumin (compounded) • Bandage contact lenses/scleral lenses • Topical dapsone (compounded) • Topical tacrolimus (compounded) • Topical N-acetylcysteine	• Oral doxycycline/ tetracycline • Tea tree oil • Topical metro-nidazole oint-ment of drops (compounded) • Topical doxycycline (compounded) • Topical clindamycin (compounded) • Topical dehydro-epiandrosterone (compounded) • Topical dapsone (compounded) • Topical N-acetylcysteine	• Scleral lenses	• Scleral lenses
Procedures[a]			
• Punctal plugs • Cautery occlusion • Amniotic membrane transplantation	• In-off thermal pul-sation and/or lid massage • Debridement of the lid margin • Intense pulsed light • Meibomian gland probing	—	• Eyelid sur-gery (ie, correction of lid mal-position and tarsor-rhaphy)

[a]The order of treatment in each category is left to the clinical judgment of the clinician and to the preference of the patient.

DTS = dysfunctional tear syndrome.

Reproduced with permission from Milner MS, Beckman KA, Luchs JI, et al. Dysfunctional tear syndrome: dry eye disease and associated tear film disorders – new strategies for diagnosis and treatment. *Curr Opin Ophthalmol.* 2017;28(Suppl 1):3-47.

In addition to LipiFlow, there are several thermal pulsation devices that can heat the lids to above body temperature to change the meibum from solid to liquid as well as massage the glands to express the oils. This results in a "rebooting of the computer" in an attempt to allow the glands to make more "healthy" oils. Intense pulsed light therapy, initially used in dermatology to treat rosacea dermatitis, is another option for posterior blepharitis. An ocular intense pulsed light works by heating the lids and liquefying the lipids like in LipiFlow. The procedure is followed by manual expression of the glands. In addition, the heat closes the vessels, decreasing inflammatory mediators, and may kill the meibomian gland bacteria.

Conclusion

Dry eye disease is a cycle of inflammation with multiple triggers, all leading to signs and symptoms of ocular surface disease. Each risk factor can "jump onto the carousel" from any point, ultimately resulting in inflammation, adding to the complexity of diagnosis and treatment. The CEDARS algorithm provides a simple approach to diagnosis and innovative options to therapy. In the end, there are 3 simple principles for treating the complex dry eye patient in the office. First, treat the trigger if possible. For example, if the dry eye is exacerbated by contact lens overwear, limit the contact lens wear. If the dry eye is a result of rheumatoid arthritis, treat with immunosuppression as needed. The second principle is to treat the inflammation, regardless of the trigger. The cycle of inflammation needs to be broken to improve the signs and symptoms of dry eye. Finally, treat chronically. Dry eye is chronic and progressive in nature, with frequent recurrence off treatment.

References

1. Craig JP, Nichols KK, Akpek EK, et al. TFOS DEWS II definition and classification report. *Ocul Surf.* 2017;15(3):276-283.
2. Behrens A, Doyle JJ, Stern L, et al. Dysfunctional tear syndrome: a Delphi approach to treatment recommendations. *Cornea.* 2006;25(8):900-907.
3. Starr CE, Gupta PK, Farid M, et al. An algorithm for the preoperative diagnosis and treatment of ocular surface disorders. *J Cataract Refract Surg.* 2019;45(5): 669-684.
4. Milner MS, Beckman KA, Luchs JI, et al. Dysfunctional tear syndrome: dry eye disease and associated tear film disorders—new strategies for diagnosis and treatment. *Curr Opin Ophthalmol.* 2017;28(Suppl 1):3-47.

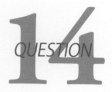
A 51-Year-Old Man Presented With Severe Pain in Both Eyes Upon Awakening in the Morning. He Has Seen Several Other Ophthalmologists With No Resolution. What Could Be Going On, and How Do I Help This Patient?

Steven E. Wilson, MD

A patient with these symptoms is likely having recurrent corneal erosions. The most common cause, especially in bilateral cases, is epithelial basement membrane dystrophy (EBMD),[1] which is also referred to as *map–dot–fingerprint dystrophy*, or *Cogan's microcystic dystrophy*. Some of these cases are genetic, with autosomal dominant inheritance, but many patients have no apparent genetic basis. These recurrent corneal erosions can also occur weeks to years after a traumatic corneal abrasion—and are typically unilateral in this situation.

Diagnosis

The site of recurrent corneal erosions can be detected at the slit lamp with fluorescein if the patient is seen prior to the erosions healing. Even after healing, there is often epithelial surface irregularity and/or punctate epithelial erosions at the site of the newly healed epithelium (Figure 14-1). White epithelial opacities can often be detected at the slit lamp (Figure 14-2) at the base of the epithelium in patients with EBMD and a history of corneal abrasion. These are referred to as *maps*, *dots*, and *fingerprints*, based on their appearance, and represent areas where multiple layers of EBMD (redundant) produce a functional decrease in adhesion of the epithelium to the underlying stroma (more layers of EBMD are not better). Most patients with EBMD detected at the slit lamp via maps, dots, and fingerprints are asymptomatic, but these opacities can be detected in most patients with recurrent corneal erosions. However, it is important to remember that 5% or more of eyes with EBMD do not have maps, dots, or fingerprints detected at the slit lamp. These latter cases may be detected through poor bilateral epithelial adhesion when the

Hardten DR, Hansen MS.
Curbside Consultation in Cornea and External Disease:
49 Clinical Questions, Second Edition (pp 87-89).
© 2022 Taylor & Francis Group.

Figure 14-1. A patient with known recurrent erosions complained of pain in the eye upon awakening the prior morning. Fluorescein staining showed punctate epithelial erosions and spotty negative-stained areas, often noted in an area where the epithelium had recently healed after an abrasion (arrows).

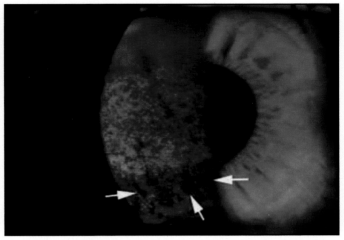

Figure 14-2. Map-dot-fingerprints (arrows) noted at the slit lamp in an eye with epithelial basement membrane dystrophy.

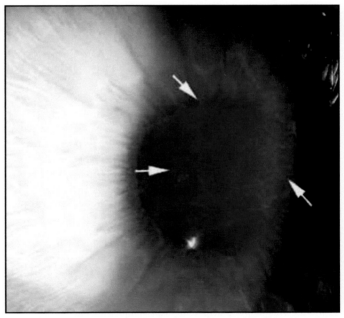

epithelium is scraped for photorefractive keratectomy or epithelial slough when a microkeratome is used in LASIK. Thus, some patients with recurrent erosions without a history of corneal abrasion may have occult EBMD.

Treatment

Initial treatment for recurrent corneal erosion is lubrication of the eye with nonpreserved artificial tears and ointments. In a low-humidity environment, increasing the humidity where the patient sleeps to at least 40% is often helpful (patients produce the least tears during sleep). Treatment of underlying dry eye that promotes adhesion between the tarsal conjunctiva and the corneal epithelium with topical cyclosporine A or lifitegrast is a critical adjuvant consideration. If ocular rosacea is present, it should be treated with mechanical expression of the meibomian glands and oral doxycycline. If recurrent erosions persist despite these measures, or in severe cases, continuous use of a bandage contact lens for 2 to 4 weeks often allows time for the regeneration of mature basement membrane[2] and anchoring fibrils that can bring the episodes to an end. If the recurrent erosions resume after the bandage contact lens treatment, followed by lubrication, then the best option is therapeutic debridement of the epithelium, followed by a continuous bandage contact lens for 3 weeks to allow full recovery of the mature epithelial basement membrane and anchoring fibrils. I recommend removal of all epithelium on the corneal surface to within 1 mm of the limbus for 360 degrees in these cases—taking special care to remove all redundant basement membrane on the stromal surface.

If the recurrent erosions return, despite therapeutic debridement, then phototherapeutic keratectomy (PTK) is the treatment of choice.[3] When PTK is performed, the epithelium to within 1 mm of the limbus is removed with a scalpel (my preference is a #64 Beaver blade), again taking care to remove all normal and redundant basement membrane. The excimer laser PTK facilitates complete removal of all basement membrane that may be missed by the epithelial scrape procedure. In my experience, only 10 to 15 pulses of excimer laser are needed to accomplish this removal without producing a significant hyperopic shift in the refraction, but it is important that these pulses be delivered over the entire cornea, sparing the limbus. Thus, I first use a 6.5-mm beam centered on the pupil for 10 to 15 pulses, and then decrease the beam to 2 mm and treat the periphery for 360 degrees so that each area around the peripheral cornea receives approximately 10 pulses of the excimer laser by using the joystick while also moving the patient's head.

Again, after PTK, a bandage contact lens should be used for 3 weeks to allow full regeneration of the epithelial basement membrane and anchoring fibrils before the tarsal conjunctiva is exposed to the corneal epithelium. After removal of the bandage contact lens, lubrication with nonpreserved artificial tears during the day and ointment at bedtime should be continued for at least several months. Also, make sure the humidity where the patient sleeps is at least 40% by having the patient obtain a hygrometer for the bedside and using a humidifier, if necessary. Phototherapeutic keratectomy can be repeated if necessary. In patients with EBMD, recurrent erosions may return after a few years, and therapeutic debridement and/or PTK may again be needed.

If the erosions occur outside the visual axis, some surgeons recommend anterior stromal micropuncture. In my experience, I prefer PTK because it causes less scarring and is able to treat the whole cornea, which is often abnormal in patients with erosions.

References

1. Laibson PR. Recurrent corneal erosions and epithelial basement membrane dystrophy. *Eye Contact Lens.* 2010;36(5):315-317.
2. Marino GK, Santhiago MR, Santhanam A, Torricelli AAM, Wilson SE. Regeneration of defective epithelial basement membrane and restoration of corneal transparency after photorefractive keratectomy. *J Ref Surg.* 2017;33(5):337-346.
3. Wilson SE, Marino GK, Medeiros CS, Santhiago MR. Phototherapeutic keratectomy: science and art. *J Ref Surg.* 2017;33(3):203-210.

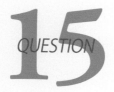

15

A 52-YEAR-OLD MAN WITH OBESITY COMES TO THE OFFICE COMPLAINING OF PAIN AND IRRITATION IN THE RIGHT EYE. THE EXAM SHOWS FLOPPY EYELIDS, 3+ PAPILLAE IN THE UPPER TARSAL CONJUNCTIVA, AND LASH PTOSIS. DOES HE NEED EYELID SURGERY?

Reza Dana, MD, MSc, MPH

Floppy eyelid syndrome (FES) was first described in 1981,[1] exclusively in overweight men presenting with papillary conjunctivitis and floppy eyelids. It is now known that men, women, and even children without obesity can develop FES, but the correlation remains highest with middle-aged obese men.

Symptoms

Symptoms of FES are generally nonspecific. Patients often complain of chronic irritation in one or both eyes, with occasional or constant redness and/or mucus discharge.[2] Itching and chronic eye rubbing are also occasionally noted. Patients often present with a long history of using numerous topical medications/eye drops with little to no relief.

Signs

The cardinal clinical finding in FES is the easily everted upper eyelid. Even gentle lifting of the upper eyelid can lead to lid eversion (Figure 15-1). The lid often has a "rubbery" feel to it, with abnormal thickness, and the tarsus, rather than being rigid, is pliable and soft. Patients almost always have varying degrees of chronic papillary conjunctivitis that is unilateral or bilateral. Sometimes, lash ptosis, ectropion, or blepharoptosis are also seen. The most significant involvement in FES is corneal. This can range from focal punctate epitheliopathy (seen in nearly half of

Hardten DR, Hansen MS.
Curbside Consultation in Cornea and External Disease:
49 Clinical Questions, Second Edition (pp 91-93).
© 2022 Taylor & Francis Group.

Figure 15-1. Clinical photograph demonstrating easy eversion of the upper eyelid in a patient with floppy eyelid syndrome. (Reproduced with permission from Dr. Aaron Fay, Massachusetts Eye and Ear Infirmary, Boston, Massachusetts.)

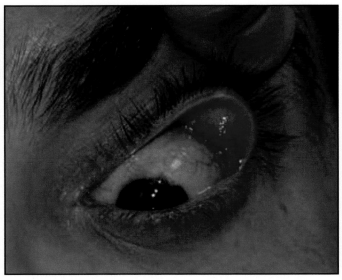

patients) to superficial neovascularization and scarring. Significant thinning, ulceration, and even perforation have also been reported, but these are rare. Up to 10% of patients with FES may also have keratoconus. Eye rubbing, which is commonly seen in many patients with keratoconus, is also seen in many patients with FES, but it is not known whether this is a cause or a consequence of the eyelid pathology.

Histological and cytological studies, although rarely used or needed, can occasionally be helpful in confirming the diagnosis. Pathological examination of resection specimens from the tarsus shows rupture and loss of elastin fibers in the tarsus. Cytological evaluation of the ocular surface shows a nonspecific chronic inflammatory infiltrate in the conjunctival epithelium.[3]

Systemic Associations With FES

It is helpful to consider the various associations with FES, not only in consideration of the differential diagnosis (see the following paragraphs) but also in the overall management of the patients. Most patients with FES are obese, with a significantly elevated body mass index. There is a strong association with obstructive sleep apnea, which itself is also associated with obesity. Only a minority of patients (~2% to 30%) with obstructive sleep apnea have FES, but nearly half of patients with FES have sleep apnea—an important consideration in the management of these patients. Other comorbidities seen in these patients are those commonly seen in obese patients, including systemic hypertension and hyperglycemia.

Pathogenesis

The exact pathogenesis of FES is unknown, but several theories have been proposed.[2] The most common theory relates FES to the mechanical rubbing of the floppy eyelid on the pillow or sheets during sleep, causing eyelid eversion and keratoconjunctivitis. This is supported by the association of FES with the side the patient sleeps on. Another theory proposes that pressure-induced ischemia and reperfusion leads to oxidative injury. Local "ischemia" or hypoperfusion may lead to elevated expression of matrix metalloproteinase enzymes that degrade elastin and cause eyelid floppiness.

Differential Diagnosis

Except for the floppy eyelids, none of the other findings are particularly specific. Chronic ocular irritation, redness, and mucus discharge are also frequently seen in dry eye syndromes, blepharitis, and allergy. For this reason, taking a good history and evaluation of nonophthalmic findings, such as obesity and sleep apnea, can provide important clues to making the correct diagnosis.

Treatment Approaches

Like most other disorders, the most important parameter I consider for guiding me in therapy is the severity of the disease. The guidelines I use are as follows[4]:

- In mild to moderate FES, without corneal thinning or extensive confluent epitheliopathy, conservative approaches often suffice. This involves (1) protecting the eyelid from spontaneous eversion and (2) protecting the cornea. Eyelid taping and/or application of a shield at bedtime can protect the eyelid from eversion in patients who can tolerate these approaches. Application of lubricating gels or ointments is protective of the cornea.

- Similarly, discontinuing chronic use of unneeded and potentially toxic medications, such as antibiotics and anti-inflammatory treatments, including corticosteroids and nonsteroidal anti-inflammatory drugs, is critical in protecting the cornea.

- However, in patients with severe FES or in those who are intolerant of shield application during sleep, surgical treatment is necessary. Surgical treatment typically consists of horizontal tightening procedures—many have been described to treat FES, with a common recommended approach being a pentagonal eyelid wedge resection. Surgical treatment usually is not directed at primarily correcting the ptosis, as this can be improved with decreasing inflammation and lid-tightening procedures alone. Some oculoplastics specialists recommend that patients continue wearing a shield at night to prevent recurrence.

- It is critical to recall that obstructive sleep apnea is a serious and potentially fatal condition associated with cardiac disease and hypoxic organ damage; hence, it should be evaluated in patients with FES, especially those who are obese. Good communication with the primary care physician is critical to ensure appropriate referral, sleep studies, and treatment of sleep apnea if present. Interestingly, it has been reported that treatment of sleep apnea may be associated with reversal of FES without any additional surgical intervention.

References

1. Culbertson WW, Ostler HB. The floppy eyelid syndrome. *Am J Ophthalmol.* 1981;92(4):568-575.
2. Phamm TT, Perry JD. Floppy eyelid syndrome. *Curr Opin Ophthalmol.* 2007;18(5):430-433.
3. Medel R, Alonso T, Vela JI, Calatayud M, Bisbe L, Garcia-Arumi J. Conjunctival cytology in floppy eyelid syndrome: objective assessment of the outcome of surgery. *Br J Ophthalmol.* 2009;93(4):513-517.
4. McNab AA. Reversal of floppy eyelid syndrome with treatment of obstructive sleep apnoea. *Clin Exp Ophthal.* 2000;28(2):125-126.

A Patient Diagnosed With Bell's Palsy 2 Days Ago Presents With Lagophthalmos and Moderate Superficial Punctate Keratopathy Inferiorly on the Cornea. How Should I Treat Them?

Brad H. Feldman, MD and Natalie A. Afshari, MD

Bell's palsy is a peripheral facial nerve paralysis that evolves over hours to days and occurs in the absence of central nervous system disease. It is almost universally unilateral (99.7%), rarely recurrent (< 10%), and typically transient, with nearly all patients improving over time.[1] Remission usually occurs within 4 weeks of the onset of paralysis. However, delayed improvement can be seen for up to 6 months, and up to 17% of patients have some degree of permanent paralysis.[1] It is more common in pregnant women, in patients with diabetes mellitus, and in those with a positive family history.[1] Although considered a diagnosis of exclusion, it accounts for approximately two-thirds of acute facial palsies and is often characterized by a constellation of recognizable symptoms beyond the seventh nerve involvement (Table 16-1).[2]

Reactivation of the herpes simplex virus is now generally thought to be responsible for Bell's palsy. The facial nerve may be particularly susceptible to injury from inflammation because of mechanical compression within the narrow meatal foramen in the temporal bone. Oral prednisone and acyclovir are often given to patients with Bell's palsy early in the disease (ideally, within 72 hours) in attempt to mitigate the disease course.[3] There is no consensus on the effects of these treatments, but the potential benefits and minimal risks support a 10-day course of oral prednisone (60-mg taper) and acyclovir (400 mg 5 times/day) or valacyclovir (1 g 3 times/day).

Evaluation

Care must be taken to examine the external ear, auditory canal, and tympanic membrane for the vesicles that are typical of Ramsay Hunt syndrome from herpes zoster—an entity with

Hardten DR, Hansen MS.
Curbside Consultation in Cornea and External Disease:
49 Clinical Questions, Second Edition (pp 95-99).
© 2022 Taylor & Francis Group.

	Table 16-1

Constellation of Symptoms of Bell's Palsy

Incidence	Symptom
100%	Facial nerve paralysis
80%	Hypersensitivity of face to temperature, wind, and touch
60%	Ear pain
57%	Alterations in taste (dysgeusia)
30%	Decreased tolerance to everyday sounds (hyperacusis)
17%	Decreased tearing

Adapted from Adour KK. Current concepts in neurology diagnosis and management of facial paralysis. *N Engl J Med.* 1982;307:348-351.

a poorer prognosis of facial nerve recovery. Obtaining an audiogram is also important to rule out asymmetric hearing loss from vestibulocochlear involvement. Whenever there is evidence of multiple cranial nerve, bilateral, atypical, or central nervous system involvement, a workup must begin to rule out neoplastic, inflammatory, or autoimmune etiologies. In these cases, magnetic resonance imaging with gadolinium is recommended, as is consultation with an ear, nose, and throat or neurology specialist.

Beyond the disfigurement of the Bell's facial droop, the primary concern for these patients is ocular, secondary to dysfunctional blinking; a widened palpebral fissure; and poor eyelid closure due to a denervated orbicularis oculi and the unopposed eyelid retractors (Figure 16-1). The severity of facial nerve paralysis and lid closure is graded with the House-Brackmann criteria (Table 16-2).[4] Exposure keratopathy from poor lid closure is further exacerbated by a degraded tear film due to increased evaporation; inadequate tear replenishment; disrupted mixing of the mucin, lipid, and aqueous components; and, occasionally, decreased tear production.

Management

The management of exposure keratopathy begins with frequent preservative-free artificial tears throughout the day and more viscous gels or ointments at bedtime. Nocturnal lagophthalmos is addressed most effectively with eyelid taping or placement of a cellophane dressing over the eye to retain moisture. Some patients may benefit from moisture chamber glasses or goggles, and others will require frequent applications of daytime gels or ointments. Slit-lamp examination of these patients typically reveals inferior punctate keratopathy, but this location may vary depending on the degree of nocturnal globe elevation (Bell's phenomenon). Note that in-office testing of Bell's phenomenon does not correlate well with nocturnal globe positioning and is of limited prognostic value.

All patients, including those with only mild exposure keratopathy on initial consultation, are generally seen within 1 week to assess progression. For patients demonstrating persistent moderate to severe exposure keratopathy, aggressive measures, including tarsorrhaphy or gold weight placement, are warranted to avoid corneal scarring, ulceration, or infection. Gold weights provide for

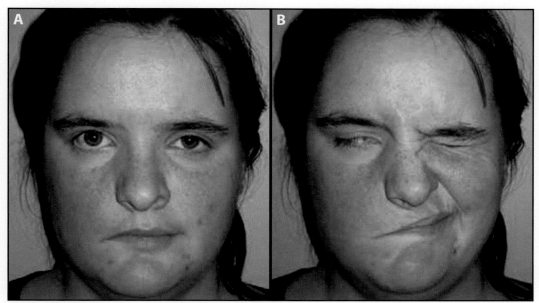

Figure 16-1. (A) Patient with a right facial droop, nasolabial flattening, and widened palpebral fissure. (B) Patient with residual lagophthalmos, despite forceful eyelid closure. (Reproduced with permission from Kumar A, Ryzenman J, Barr A. Revision facial nerve surgery. *Otolaryngol Clin North Am.* 2006;39[4]:815-832.)

Table 16-2
House-Brackmann Grading System for Facial Paralysis

Grade	Definition
I	Normal symmetrical function in all areas
II	Slight weakness, noticeable only on close inspection
	Complete eye closure with minimal effort
	Slight asymmetry of smile with maximal effort
	Synkinesis barely noticeable; contracture or spasm absent
III	Obvious weakness but not disfiguring
	May not be able to lift eyebrow
	Complete eye closure and strong but asymmetrical mouth movement with maximal effort
	Obvious but not disfiguring synkinesis, mass movement, or spasm
IV	Obvious disfiguring weakness
	Inability to lift brow
	Incomplete eye closure and asymmetry of mouth with maximal effort
	Severe synkinesis, mass movement, spasm

(continued)

Table 16-2 (continued)
House-Brackmann Grading System for Facial Paralysis

Grade	Definition
V	Motion barely perceptible
	Incomplete eye closure, slight movement corner mouth
	Synkinesis, contracture, and spasm usually absent
VI	No movement
	Loss of tone
	No synkinesis, contracture, or spasm

Adapted from House JW, Brackmann DE. Facial nerve grading system. *Otolaryngol Head Neck Surg.* 1985;93(2):146-147.

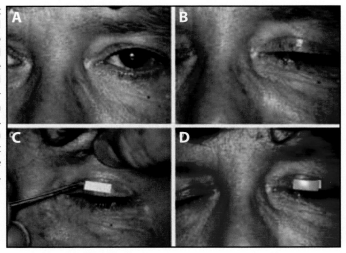

Figure 16-2. Application of lid weight for lagophthalmos. (A) Uncorrected lagophthalmos in the left eye due to Bell's palsy with inferior and lateral injection due to exposure. (B) Three mm of lagophthalmos on forced closure. (C) Application of temporary upper lid weight. (D) Resolution of lagophthalmos with lid weight. (Reproduced with permission from Rahman I, Sadiq SA. Ophthalmic management of facial nerve palsy: a review. *Surv Ophthalmol.* 2007;52[2]:121-144.)

gravitational closure of the upper eyelid, hold a considerable cosmetic advantage over tarsorrhaphy, and do not delay recovery of orbicularis function, even when employed early in the course of disease. To optimize lid positioning, gold weights of 0.6 to 1.8 g can be trialed externally with tape before pretarsal implantation (Figure 16-2). Ninety percent of patients improve with gold weights, even though many have some residual lagophthalmos.[3] Patients must be instructed to elevate their heads at night, and possible complications include migration or extrusion of the implant, as well as associated inflammation.[3]

In severe cases that progress to corneal ulceration, suture tarsorrhaphy is required to ensure adequate corneal coverage and avoid further melting or secondary infection.

After resolution of the ulceration, the tarsorrhaphy can be cautiously opened and reevaluated. At this point, the lagophthalmos may be treated with a combination of lid tightening, loading, and reanimation procedures tailored to the individual. In selected cases of moderate to severe exposure keratopathy, botulinum toxin injection into Müller's muscle and levator can be attempted to achieve an upper lid ptosis lasting for several weeks, but this effect typically takes 4 to 5 days, leads to variable degrees of coverage, and produces a poor cosmetic result. The main advantage is that when the induced ptosis resolves, most patients will have adequate spontaneous recovery of orbicularis function to necessitate no further intervention. For persistent corneal epithelial defects, a human amniotic membrane transplantation can be performed.[5] In cases of coexisting neurotrophic keratitis, new approaches, such as corneal neurotization[6] and nerve growth factor,[7] can be effective therapeutic options.

Infrequently, there is a role for high water–content hydrogel contact lenses or rigid gas permeable scleral lenses, in combination with the frequent use of preservative-free artificial tears to both supplement the tear reservoir and enhance visual acuity through the artificial smooth refractive surface.

References

1. Mattox DE. Clinical disorders of the facial nerve. In: Cummings CW, Flint PW, Harker LA, et al. *Cummings Otolaryngology: Head and Neck Surgery.* 4th ed. Mosby; 2005:3333-3340.
2. Adour KK. Current concepts in neurology diagnosis and management of facial paralysis. *N Engl J Med.* 1982;307(6):348-351.
3. Rahman I, Sadiq SA. Ophthalmic management of facial nerve palsy: a review. *Surv Ophthalmol.* 2007;52(2):121-144.
4. House JW, Brackmann DE. Facial nerve grading system. *Otolaryngol Head Neck Surg.* 1985;93(2):146-147.
5. Soni NG, Pillar A, Margo J, Jeng BH. Management of the persistent corneal epithelial defect. In: Djalilian AR, ed. *Ocular Surface Disease: A Case-Based Guide.* Springer; 2018:221-231.
6. Gennaro P, Gabriele G, Aboh IV, et al. The second division of trigeminal nerve for corneal neurotization: a novel one-stage technique in combination with facial reanimation. *J Craniofac Surg.* 2019;30(4):1252-1254.
7. Pflugfelder SC, Massaro-Giordano M, Perez VL, et al. Topical recombinant human nerve growth factor (cenegermin) for neurotrophic keratopathy: a multicenter randomized vehicle-controlled pivotal trial. *Ophthalmology.* 2020;127(1):14-26.

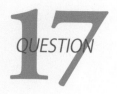
A 68-YEAR-OLD WOMAN WITH RHEUMATOID ARTHRITIS PRESENTS WITH A RED, PAINFUL EYE AND STROMAL MELT AT THE LIMBUS. HOW SHOULD I TREAT HER?

Jesse M. Vislisel, MD

Peripheral ulcerative keratitis (PUK) is a destructive, inflammatory condition of the perilimbal cornea. The typical appearance is a crescent-shaped corneal ulcer with an overlying epithelial defect and an inflammatory infiltrate at its leading edge (Figure 17-1A).[1,2] The peripheral location is likely due to the close proximity to conjunctival vessels that supply disease-causing inflammatory mediators. Most cases of PUK have associated inflammation of the adjacent conjunctiva, episclera, and sclera. These features help differentiate PUK from noninflammatory conditions, such as Terrien's marginal degeneration, which tend to have intact epithelium and minimal active inflammation.

At least half of PUK cases are associated with collagen vascular disease. The most commonly associated disease is rheumatoid arthritis (RA), followed by granulomatosis with polyangiitis (previously known as *Wegener's granulomatosis*). Mooren's ulcer (Figure 17-1B) is a form of PUK, with absence of scleritis and no causative systemic disease. Peripheral microbial keratitis (Figure 17-1C) can cause rapidly progressive PUK, which usually responds to anti-infective medications. PUK or peripheral keratopathy can occur in patients with scleritis (Figure 17-1D). This is a poor prognostic sign because scleritis patients with peripheral keratopathy more often have necrotizing scleritis (NS), decreased vision, anterior uveitis, and impending corneal perforation. The presence of peripheral keratopathy and scleritis also indicates higher likelihood of associated systemic disease.

Hardten DR, Hansen MS.
Curbside Consultation in Cornea and External Disease:
49 Clinical Questions, Second Edition (pp 101-104).
© 2022 Taylor & Francis Group.

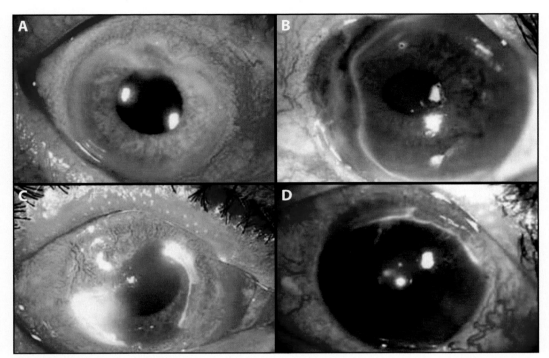

Figure 17-1. (A) PUK associated with granulomatosis with polyangiitis. (Reproduced with permission from EyeRounds.org, University of Iowa.) (B) Mooren's ulcer. Note the overhanging advancing edge and absence of associated scleritis. (C) PUK secondary to *Pseudomonas aeruginosa* infection. Note the extensive infiltrate as opposed to the "clean" ulceration in patients with immune-mediated PUK. (D) Peripheral keratopathy in setting of scleritis.

Significance of Peripheral Ulcerative Keratitis in a Patient With Rheumatoid Arthritis

The development of NS or PUK in patients with RA carries a grim prognosis, not only for the eye, but also for life. It signifies that the destructive vasculitic process is present in the sclera and potentially other extra-articular sites. These patients are at increased risk of death related to visceral vasculitic complications unless treated aggressively with systemic immunosuppressive agents.[3,4]

What Do You Watch for on Eye Examination?

RA patients with scleritis should be closely monitored for the development of signs of NS and PUK. Any peripheral keratopathy in these patients should be followed closely and treated aggressively with appropriate topical and systemic therapy.

Patients with active PUK should be monitored frequently for progressive corneal thinning and perforation due to the potential for rapid progression. Impending or frank corneal perforation often requires surgical intervention to restore tectonic stability to the globe. The clinician should also evaluate for associated uveitis and posterior segment disease at every follow-up visit.

One should also be aware that surgical trauma may trigger inflammatory microangiopathy, resulting in PUK in patients with systemic vasculitis. It is crucial to identify susceptible patients prior to eye surgery to prevent postoperative ocular complications.

Systemic Workup

A thorough medical history and examination are mandatory in the evaluation of PUK. A comprehensive laboratory investigation is also indicated to assess for the presence of occult systemic disease (unless already known), to assess the extent of systemic visceral involvement, and to establish baseline clinical and laboratory data so that treatment-induced side effects can be monitored. The investigation should include corneal cultures and consideration of viral polymerase chain reaction testing, complete blood cell counts with differential, comprehensive metabolic panel, rheumatoid factor, anticyclic citrullinated peptide antibody, antinuclear antibody, antineutrophil cytoplasmic antibody, circulating immune complexes, venereal disease research laboratory test, fluorescent treponemal antibody absorption test, urinalysis, and a chest X-ray or computed tomography. Additional testing might be indicated by review of systems and physical examination. This may include Lyme disease antibody, tuberculin skin testing, hepatitis C antibody, sacroiliac joint x-rays, and sinus imaging.

Treatment

A patient presenting with PUK and RA represents an ophthalmic emergency due to the sight-threatening nature of the condition and potential for rapid progression. Therefore, communication and prompt referral to a rheumatologist who is comfortable with cytotoxic immunosuppressive agents is important. The initial treatment typically involves a combination of systemic corticosteroids and a systemic immunosuppressive agent. Higher doses of corticosteroids are initially needed to achieve rapid control of inflammation, followed by a gradual taper. The long-term goal is to control the inflammation with a steroid-sparing immunosuppressive agent. In addition to controlling the PUK, these medications also reduce the activity of the underlying systemic disease in nonocular locations and improve the survival of corneal grafts, if present.

Topical therapy should include frequent preservative-free lubricants. A prophylactic topical antibiotic should be initiated until the epithelium closes, and a topical cycloplegic agent may be helpful if there is a significant intraocular inflammatory reaction. Topical steroids should be avoided, when possible, due to their potential to contribute to collagenolysis. Oral tetracycline derivatives have beneficial lubricating and anticollagenolytic properties. Topical cyclosporine may also have a role in the treatment of nonhealing ulcers.

Bandage contact lenses may be utilized to reduce discomfort and encourage re-epithelialization. Amniotic membrane grafts may also be helpful. Tissue adhesives may be utilized in the setting of corneal perforation to provide tectonic support and create a barrier between leukocytes and cornea, further preventing stromal melt.

Surgical management may be indicated for severe or refractory PUK. Cases unresponsive to medical therapy may benefit from conjunctival recession to reduce access of leukocytes and other immune mediators to the peripheral cornea. Tarsorrhaphy may be beneficial when there is an exposure component. PUK patients with corneal perforation or thinning that threatens structural integrity of the eye may require corneal transplantation. Surgical options include penetrating keratoplasty, lamellar keratoplasty, or patch graft, depending on the location and extent of involvement. Concomitant systemic immunosuppressive therapy is critical for controlling immune-mediated inflammation and preventing graft melt. Even so, graft survival and visual outcomes after penetrating keratoplasty or patch graft in this patient population remains poor.

References

1. Messemer EM, Foster CS. Vasculitic peripheral ulcerative keratitis. *Surv Ophthalmol.* 1999;43(5):379-396.
2. Ladas JG, Mondino BJ. Systemic disorders associated with peripheral corneal ulceration. *Curr Opin Ophthalmol.* 2000;11(6):468-471.
3. Sangwan VS, Panayotis Z, Foster CS. Mooren's ulcer: current concepts in diagnosis and management. *Indian J Ophthalmol.* 1997;45(1):7-17.
4. Foster CS, Forstot SL, Wilson LA. Mortality rate in rheumatoid arthritis patients developing necrotizing scleritis or peripheral ulcerative keratitis. Effects of immunosuppression. *Ophthalmology.* 1984;91(10):1253-1263.

18

A PATIENT WITH A FILTERING BLEB COMPLAINS OF DISCOMFORT IN THE EYE. THE BLEB IS PROLAPSING ONTO THE CORNEA AND AN AREA OF STROMAL THINNING AND EPITHELIAL STAINING WITH FLUORESCEIN IS ADJACENT TO THE BLEB. WHAT IS THE OPTIMAL MANAGEMENT?

Sonia H. Yoo, MD and Mohamed Abou Shousha, MD, PhD

A successful filtering surgery should not only achieve long-term reduction of intraocular pressure, but should also have a minimal impact on the ocular surface and patient comfort. The morphology of the filtration bleb is an important factor to achieve those aims. Ideally, the bleb should be diffuse, with minimal impact on the ocular surface. However, a large filtering bleb could encroach on the cornea and cause corneal dellen. In most instances, a dellen is a benign lesion. However, in severe cases, a corneal dellen, if untreated, can lead to a descemetocele and corneal perforation.[1]

The term *dellen* is derived from the German word for "dents" and refers to saucer-shaped depressions of the cornea, most commonly at the periphery. The lesion occurs at or near the limbus, adjacent to raised abnormal tissue on the bulbar conjunctiva that prevents the eyelid from adequately resurfacing the cornea with tears during blinking. Localized interruption of the tear film occurs, leading to desiccation of the epithelium and subepithelial tissue. This can also cause the underlying sclera to become markedly thinned and translucent, forming a scleral dellen.

Clinically, a dellen is seen as a saucer-like corneal thinning just anterior to the limbus. Typically, the corneal epithelium remains intact (Figure 18-1), but in severe cases, there may be de-epithelialization. The epithelium exhibits punctate irregularities overlying a thinned area of dehydrated corneal stroma. Fluorescein pools in these depressions but does not stain the stroma. They cause mild discomfort and should be treated with lubrication and close observation.

Dellen have been observed in association with filtering blebs (see Figure 18-1) as well as pingueculae, pterygia, rectus muscle surgery, bullous subconjunctival hemorrhage and injections, limbal tumors, and cataract surgery.

Hardten DR, Hansen MS.
Curbside Consultation in Cornea and External Disease:
49 Clinical Questions, Second Edition (pp 105-108).
© 2022 Taylor & Francis Group.

Figure 18-1. Painful dellen (arrow) in front of an exposed elevated bleb. (Reproduced with permission from Paul Palmberg, MD, Bascom Palmer Eye Institute.)

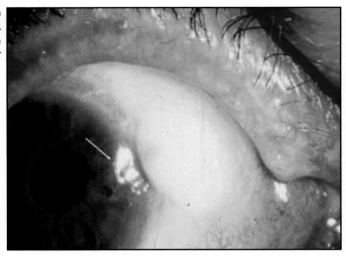

The incidence of dellen after filtering glaucoma surgery was reported in several studies to be between 2% and 30% and, in most instances, are adjacent to large cystic blebs. The wide variation in incidence is probably due to differences in the surgical techniques and thus different sizes of the resulting bleb. The rate of dellen also was reported to be higher in superonasal blebs than superotemporal and least in superior blebs. This could be explained by the observation that filtering bleb dysesthesia occurs more commonly in superonasal blebs.[2]

Dellen with a bleb should not be confused with other causes of peripheral corneal thinning or ulcerative keratitis. Dellen are localized and are always adjacent to the causative conjunctival or limbal elevated lesion. Obviously, infectious infiltrates and ulcers have to be ruled out. Slit-lamp examination of dellen should not reveal any infiltrates. Typically, the eye is very quiet, and the patient complains only of mild discomfort.

In the setting of a filtering glaucoma surgery with adjunctive use of antimetabolites such as mitomycin C, corneal and conjunctival toxicity should be considered. However, such cases will manifest with punctate epithelial erosions and primary conjunctival wound leaks, in addition to the corneal epithelial defects. Worth mentioning are eyes with limbal stem cell deficiency that could also present with persistent epithelial defects. This condition should be differentiated from dellen by the presence of conjunctivalization, surface irregularities, and vascularization of the cornea. Terrien's marginal degeneration could also be confused with dellen, as it produces a quiet peripheral corneal thinning, leaving the epithelium intact. However, that condition is often bilateral and first presents as a peripheral corneal haze that over time exhibits as a slowly progressive peripheral corneal thinning, with a sloping central edge that spares the limbus. Severe dellen that is de-epithelialized with severe stromal thinning and melting could be confused with other causes of peripheral ulcerative keratitis, such as connective tissue diseases, Mooren's ulcer, rosacea keratitis, or severe dry eye. Those causes have to be ruled out from the differential diagnosis.

Management

Treatment of dellen associated with filtering blebs may be complicated by the need to preserve the functioning bleb as opposed to the need to heal the cornea. Medical treatment includes aggressive lubrication with artificial tears and aqueous suppressants. Lubrication in most instances cures the dellen by hydrating the tissue and re-expanding the locally compacted stromal lamellae.

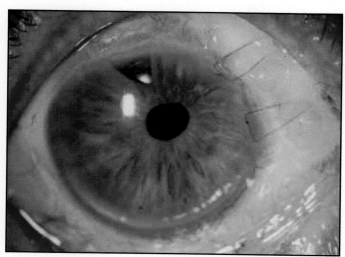

Figure 18-2. Two 9-0 mattress compression sutures were anchored in clear cornea in front of the bleb, anchored in deep Tenon's capsule behind the bleb, and the knot was rotated into the cornea. (Reproduced with permission from Paul Palmberg, MD, Bascom Palmer Eye Institute.)

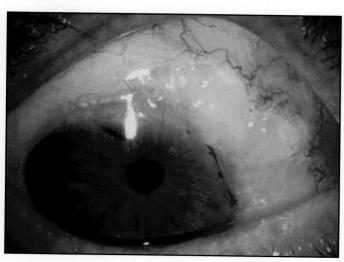

Figure 18-3. Sutures were removed 14 days postoperatively. Intraocular pressure was 8 mm Hg. The bleb contour was changed. Dellen were gone and did not return. (Reproduced with permission from Paul Palmberg, MD, Bascom Palmer Eye Institute.)

Aqueous suppressants could help to decrease the size of the bleb, eliminating the causative factor. In cases of persistent dellen or if there is any sign of de-epithelialization, topical steroids, which are usually prescribed to guard against scarring and failure of the bleb, have to be tapered or discontinued according to the severity of the dellen. In general, blebs become flatter over time, and many dellen with blebs, unlike dellen associated with other limbal elevations, do well without intervention and with conservative treatment only. However, in cases with intractable pain caused by dellen, fluctuation in vision caused by tearing and corneal drying, or persistent dellen with stromal melting, intervention to eliminate the causative factor is warranted. Many techniques have been described for bleb reduction and bleb repair, such as trichloroacetic acid, compression suture (Figures 18-2 and 18-3), and autologous blood injection. Surgical intervention carries a risk of inducing scarring and failure of the bleb and thus should be reserved only for severe cases that are unresponsive to medical therapy.[3,4]

References

1. Baum JL, Mishima S, Boruchoff SA. On the nature of dellen. *Arch Ophthalmol*. 1968;79(6):657-662.
2. Budenz DL, Hoffman K, Zacchei A. Glaucoma filtering bleb dysesthesia. *Am J Ophthalmol*. 2001;131(5):626-630.
3. La Borwit SE, Quigley HA, Jampel HD. Bleb reduction and bleb repair after trabeculectomy. *Ophthalmology*. 2000;107(4):712-718.
4. Haynes WL, Alward WL. Combination of autologous blood injection and bleb compression sutures to treat hypotony maculopathy. *J Glaucoma*. 1999;8(6):384-387.

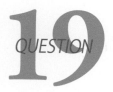

A 53-Year-Old Woman Came to My Office With Sectoral Redness and Pain in One Eye. How Should I Manage Her Eye?

C. Stephen Foster, MD

Episcleritis and scleritis are common conditions that may range from a benign, self-limited, superficial inflammation to a deeper, destructive involvement of the episclera and sclera. It is imperative to differentiate between scleritis and episcleritis because the former is not only associated with underlying systemic disorders, ocular morbidity, and mortality; the treatment modalities differ vastly.

The signs and symptoms of scleritis include pain, globe tenderness to palpation, and ocular redness. The pain is often so intense, it awakens the patient from sleep and tends to radiate to the forehead, jaw, temple, and sinuses.

The redness associated with scleritis usually has a bluish-violaceous tinge, with injection of the deep episcleral blood vessels. It may be localized or diffuse and may occur simultaneously in both eyes.

Peripheral keratopathy in a patient with scleritis is an ominous ocular sign because such patients more often evolve to have necrotizing scleritis and impending corneal perforation.[1]

The classification scheme of Foster and Sainz de la Maza[1] and Watson and Hayreh[2] has divided scleral disorders into scleritis and episcleritis (Figure 19-1).

Posterior scleritis is characterized by flattening of the posterior globe and thickening of the retinochoroidal layer. Posterior scleritis is suspected when patients present with pain (worsened with eye movement) and visualization of serous retinal detachment, swollen optic nerve head, or circumscribed fundus mass. The diagnosis of posterior scleritis can be confirmed with ultrasonographic demonstration of the signs described.

Episcleritis is an acute, localized, self-limited inflammation of the episclera, presenting with a mild pink to red eye. Pain is typically absent, although mild discomfort may be experienced. Slit-lamp examination reveals injection of superficial blood vessels confined to the episcleral

Hardten DR, Hansen MS.
Curbside Consultation in Cornea and External Disease:
49 Clinical Questions, Second Edition (pp 109-115).
© 2022 Taylor & Francis Group.

Figure 19-1. Schematic subcategorization of episcleritis and scleritis types. SINS = surgically induced necrotising sclerokeratitis.

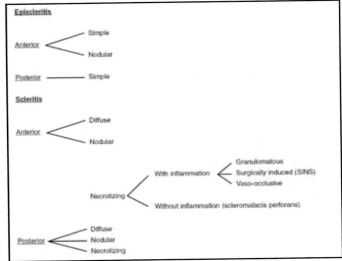

Figure 19-2. Episcleritis. Note the pinkish hue with injection and dilation of the superficial episcleral blood vessels.

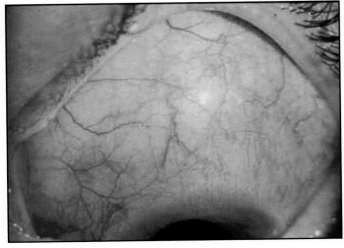

tissue (Figure 19-2). The inflammation vanishes with 10% phenylephrine drops. Recurrences are common, but they decrease in frequency after 4 years. Up to 32% of patients have an underlying systemic disorder (Table 19-1).

What Are the Likely Etiologies of Episcleritis/Scleritis?

An underlying systemic disorder is present in approximately 60% of patients with scleritis (see Table 19-1). Connective tissue or vasculitic diseases are present in nearly 48% of patients; 10% have an infectious etiology; and 2% have atopy, rosacea, or gout.[1,2]

Rheumatoid arthritis (RA) and Wegener's granulomatosis (WG) are the most common systemic associations, followed by relapsing polychondritis, systemic lupus erythematosus (SLE), and arthritis with inflammatory bowel disease.[1] The incidence of scleritis in patients with RA

Table 19-1

Associated Conditions in Episcleritis and Scleritis

Noninfectious	*Infectious*
Connective Tissue Diseases • Rheumatoid arthritis • Systemic lupus erythematosus • Seronegative spondyloarthropathies • Ankylosing spondylitis • Reiter's syndrome • Psoriatic arthritis • Arthritis and inflammatory bowel disease • Relapsing polychondritis **Vasculitides** • Wegener's granulomatosis • Polyarteritis nodosa • Churg-Strauss syndrome • Behcet's disease • Giant cell arteritis • Cogan's syndrome **Miscellaneous** • Atopy • Rosacea • Gout • Foreign body granuloma • Trauma—chemical and/or physical injury • Postsurgical • Drugs	**Bacteria** • Gram positive and gram negative • Mycobacteria • Spirochetes • Chlamydia • Actinomyces • Nocardia **Viruses** • Herpes zoster • Herpes simplex • Mumps **Fungi** • Filamentous fungi • Dimorphic fungi **Parasites** • Acanthamoeba **Toxoplasmosis** • Toxocariasis

is almost 7%,[1] and up to 4% of patients have WG, a potentially fatal multisystem disorder. Necrotizing scleritis, which is associated with an increased risk of mortality, is a common subtype observed in both diseases.[3]

The presence of scleritis is a reasonably accurate guide to systemic activity in a patient with SLE. Sclerotic attacks become aggressive and recurrent as the disease deteriorates and resolve with adequate control of SLE.

Ankylosing spondylitis (AS) has a strong association with human leukocyte antigen B27 (HLA-B27) and a tendency for ocular inflammation. AS scleritis generally takes the form of diffuse scleritis, which, despite recurrences, rarely progresses to necrotizing scleritis.[2]

Psoriatic arthritis (PA) is a triad of psoriasis, inflammatory arthritis, and a negative test for rheumatoid factor (RF). Nail pitting is nearly pathognomonic for the disease. Incidence of scleritis in patients with PA is 1.8%, occurring after years of active arthritis. Although diffuse scleritis is often seen, it may take almost any form.[1,2]

Gastrointestinal and articular manifestations are the hallmarks of inflammatory bowel disease (IBD). Scleritis occurs in 10% of patients with IBD, occurs some years after the onset of intestinal symptoms, and is more common in patients with extraintestinal manifestations.

Although immune-mediated diseases are the main disorders associated with scleritis, less common etiologies, such as infections, should also be considered. Infectious agents cause scleritis through direct invasion or an immune response and should be suspected in patients with indolent progressive scleral necrosis, especially if the past history reveals trauma, chronic topical steroid use, surgical procedures, or systemic disease.

Infections with organisms such as pseudomonas, herpes, or tuberculosis cause severe scleritis that is difficult to treat. Although rare, herpes simplex virus infections and malignancies occasionally masquerade as scleritis and thus are essential to rule out in patients presenting with scleritis of unknown etiology that is unresponsive to conventional therapy.

Episcleritis is often correctly labeled as idiopathic; however, one-third of cases have an underlying systemic association. These diseases are similar to those that cause scleritis and include atopy, gout, and vasculitic autoimmune diseases such as RA, SLE, relapsing polychondritis, and WG. Other common conditions include seronegative arthritic conditions, including IBD and psoriasis. Infectious etiologies, including syphilis and herpes simplex virus, should also be considered.[4]

How Should This Patient Be Worked Up?

Scleritis may be the initial or only presenting clinical manifestation of several potentially fatal disorders. The correct and rapid diagnosis and appropriate therapy are essential to halt the relentless progression of both ocular and systemic processes, preventing globe destruction and possibly saving the patient's life. A detailed history, review of systems, and physical examination, along with appropriate diagnostic tests (Table 19-2), are imperative to confirm or reject any suspected systemic disorder.

In RA, testing for RF, including immunoglobulin (Ig) G and IgA RF (see Table 19-2), in addition to IgM RF, is appropriate in any patient with scleritis who has arthralgias. In WG, detection of antineutrophil cytoplasmic antibodies (ANCA) is the initial and most crucial serologic test, along with urine analysis with microscopy and chest and sinus imaging (computed tomography).[3] Patients with scleritis who are ANCA-positive have aggressive disease and must be treated accordingly. Ocular tissue biopsy may be indicated in some cases of scleritis associated with an underlying systemic condition to establish a diagnosis or in cases of recurrent or refractory scleritis.

For episcleritis, the number of occurrences is an important consideration for treatment. Patients who present with their first episode typically are treated with artificial tears, as idiopathic etiology is the most common and has a self-limited course. All patients presenting with episcleritis should have an extensive review of systems. Patients with a positive review of systems may warrant laboratory investigation while starting treatment with topical lubrication. The initial set of tests are similar to those for scleritis. These tests can be undertaken with the help of the patient's primary care physician.

How Should This Patient Be Treated?

Treatment of scleritis is streamlined to target any underlying systemic disorder, achieve the desired response, and minimize the side effects of therapy. Patients generally do not respond well to topical medications and require systemic therapy with nonsteroidal anti-inflammatory drugs

Table 19-2

Management of Scleritis

	RF	ANCA	ANA	CIC	C	Cryo	X-ray	HLA	Ig	U/A	HBsAg	WBC	BUN and CrCl	ESR/CRP	Urate	Ser
Ankylosing spondylitis	—	—	—	+	—	—	sacro-iliac	+	—	—	—	—	—	—	—	—
Atopy	—	—	—	—	—	—	chest		E	—	—	Eo	—	—	—	—
Behcet's	—	—	—	+	+	—	—	+	—	—	—	—	—	—	—	—
Churg-Strauss	—	—	—	+	—	—	chest	—	E	—	—	Eo	—	—	—	—
Cogan's syndrome	—	—	—	+	+	—	—	—	—	—	—	—	—	—	—	—
Giant cell arteritis	—	—	—	+	—	—	—	—	G	—	—	—	—	+	—	—
Gout	—	—	—	—	—	—	limb	—	—	—	—	—	—	—	+	—
IBD arthritis	—	—	—	—	—	—	limb, sacro-iliac, and abdominal	—	—	—	—	—	—	—	—	—
Infectious	—	—	—	—	—	—	—	—	—	—	—	—	—	—	—	+
PAN	—	—	—	+	+	+	—	—	—	+	+	—	—	—	—	—
Psoriatic arthritis	—	—	—	—	—	—	limb and sacro-iliac	—	—	—	—	—	—	—	—	—

Figure 19-3. Diffuse scleritis. Note the redness with violaceous hue and dilation and injection of the deep episcleral blood vessels.

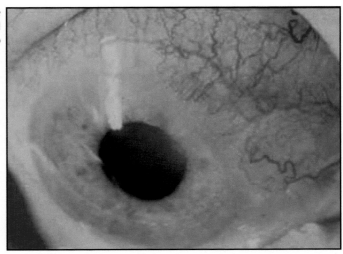

Figure 19-4. Necrotizing scleritis. Note not only the loss of sclera and pronounced avascularity of the necrotized area, but also the surrounding inflammatory signs.

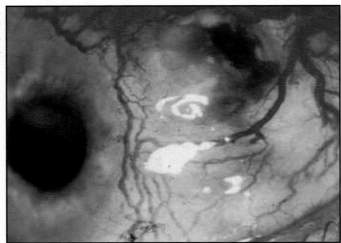

(NSAIDs), steroids, or other immunosuppressive drugs. Oral NSAIDs are the first line of treatment for non-necrotizing anterior scleritis. Up to one-third of patients with diffuse (Figure 19-3) and two-thirds of patients with nodular scleritis respond well to oral NSAIDs within 3 weeks.

Patients with necrotizing (Figure 19-4) and non-necrotizing scleritis with an associated systemic disorder are not likely to respond to oral NSAIDs alone. They require steroids at a dose of 1 mg/kg/day, tapered slowly on clinical remission at the rate of 10 mg/week until 5 mg/day is reached. This is essential to prevent bone loss and other inevitable complications associated with long-term steroid use.

Immunosuppressants are used in case of failure to respond to high-dose steroids or if unacceptably high doses of steroids are needed to maintain remission. This allows a lower dose of steroids to achieve quiescence; hence decreasing the risk of side effects. Up to 25% of patients require treatment with steroid-sparing drugs for long-term control of disease, especially patients with necrotizing scleritis or underlying systemic disorder.

One of the best initial choices of immunosuppressant therapy is methotrexate at a dose of 15 to 30 mg/week, which is efficacious, has a more favorable side effects profile, and has lower oncogenic potential compared with alkylating agents. Azathioprine 2 mg/kg/day or mycophenolate mofetil 1 g twice daily is also effective. Alkylating agents, such as cyclophosphamide 2 mg/kg/day, along with steroids, are used as a last-line effort or as a first-line therapy in patients with WG or polyarteritis nodosa.

Alternately, intravenous high-dose methylprednisolone 1 g/day 3 times within the first week, with dose reduction weekly thereafter, can be used with or without immunosuppressive agents. The use of periocular injection of steroids for non-necrotizing scleritis has been limited by side effects, including increased intraocular pressure, cataract formation, exacerbation of scleral melting, and globe perforation.[5]

Current research is focused on the use of biologics. These are monoclonal antibodies, such as infliximab (tumor necrosis factor alpha inhibitor), daclizumab (an IgG monoclonal antibody that binds to CD25 of the interleukin-2 receptor), and rituximab (anti-CD20 B-cell monoclonal antibody) used in the treatment of scleritis.

Episcleritis, a self-limiting disease, requires no treatment. Some patients may benefit from the use of artificial tears and oral NSAIDs. Topical NSAIDs may help in some instances, and while topical steroids may seem like magic, their use is an unwise approach because this strategy can prolong the total duration of the patient's problem.

References

1. Foster CS, Sainz de la Maza M. *The Sclera*. Springer-Verlag; 1994.
2. Watson PG, Hayreh SS. Scleritis and episcleritis. *Br J Ophthalmol*. 1976;60(3):163-191.
3. Joshi L, Hamour S, Salama AD, Pusey CD, Lightman S, Taylor SRJ. Renal and ocular targets for therapy in Wegener's granulomatosis. *Inflamm Allergy Drug Targets*. 2009;8(1):70-79.
4. Akpek EK, Uy HS, Christen W, Gurdal C, Foster CS. Severity of episcleritis and systemic disease association. *Ophthalmology*. 1999;106(4):729-731.
5. Jabs D, Mudun A, Dunn J, Marsh MJ. Episcleritis and scleritis: clinical features and treatment results. *Am J Ophthalmol*. 2000;130(4):469-476.

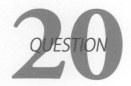

A 72-Year-Old Woman Has Conjunctival Injection in Both Eyes and Symblepharon and Trichiasis in the Right Eye. The Right Cornea Has Moderate Punctate Staining. Should I Just Pull Out the Lashes or Do a Wedge Resection of the Lower Lid to Tighten It Up?

David D. Verdier, MD

The answer is neither. The trichiasis needs proper treatment, but it is not this patient's major concern. The red flag in her examination, in flashing neon lights, is the finding of symblepharon. The most common and feared diagnosis associated with symblepharon is mucous membrane pemphigoid (MMP), also known as *ocular cicatricial pemphigoid*, when there is predominant involvement of the conjunctiva. Untreated, MMP often leads to blindness and can even lead to death from pharyngeal or esophageal stricture. Even with proper treatment, up to 50% of patients with MMP have progressive conjunctival cicatrization and vision loss.

Etiology, Course, and Treatment of Mucous Membrane Pemphigoid

MMP is an immune-related progressive systemic disease that affects the mucous membranes of the eye, nose, mouth, trachea, esophagus, genitalia, and skin. It is characterized by linear deposition of immunoglobulins and/or complement in the basement membrane, causing subepithelial blistering and cicatrization. Ocular involvement is present in 70% of patient with MMP.[1] Up to 80% of patients with MMP with ocular involvement develop nonocular systemic findings, most commonly gingivitis or mouth and nasopharyngeal ulcers or blisters, as well as esophageal strictures, cutaneous blisters, and erythematous plaques.[2,3]

Ocular MMP is usually bilateral. It most often occurs between ages 30 and 90 years, with peak involvement in the seventh decade of life. There is a slight female preponderance.

Hardten DR, Hansen MS.
Curbside Consultation in Cornea and External Disease:
49 Clinical Questions, Second Edition (pp 117-120).
© 2022 Taylor & Francis Group.

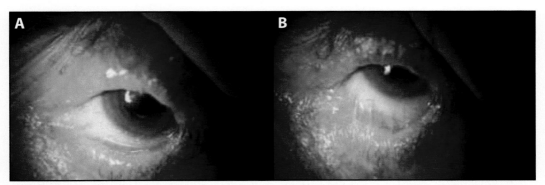

Figure 20-1. (A) Difficult-to-appreciate cicatrization in primary gaze. (B) Cicatrization is easily demonstrated with retracting the lower lid inferiorly with same eye in upgaze.

Signs of ocular MMP include chronic, often episodic conjunctivitis, which is a sign of active disease. Subepithelial fibrosis causes conjunctival foreshortening, which can progress to symblepharon and often entropion and trichiasis. Caruncle and plica semilunaris scarring are often early findings. Meibomian gland and lacrimal duct obstruction cause dry eye problems, often contributing to corneal ulceration, scarring, and neovascularization. In end-stage disease, the cornea can become opacified and keratinized and the lids fused.

Patients with active autoimmune-driven conjunctival inflammation require systemic immunosuppression to limit disease progression. Topical steroids are of little value. Because of the considerable morbidity, mortality, and long-term expense of systemic immunosuppression, strong consideration should be given for the patient to have mucous membrane or skin biopsy with immunohistochemistry studies demonstrating immunoglobulin G, immunoglobulin A, or complement components along the basement membrane zone. However, negative or inconclusive biopsy results do not exclude the diagnosis of MMP in the presence of characteristic clinical features. The diagnostic sensitivity of immunofluorescence alone is 50%, and immunoperoxidase techniques may improve sensitivity to 83%.[3]

Differential Diagnosis for Cicatrizing Conjunctivitis

MMP is often a diagnosis of exclusion. Our patient requires a thorough history and physical examination, including review of systems. The differential diagnosis of cicatrizing conjunctivitis includes past lid surgery or trauma, radiation, chemical or thermal burns, Stevens-Johnson syndrome, Sjögren's syndrome, trachoma, atopic keratoconjunctivitis, post-infectious conjunctivitis, rosacea, graft vs host disease, lichen planus, conjunctival squamous or sebaceous cell carcinoma, and paraneoplastic pseudopemphigoid. An association between chronic use of glaucoma medications and cicatrizing conjunctivitis has also been referred to as *pseudopemphigoid*.

The first order of business in our patient is to establish her diagnosis. A careful history and physical examination should rule in or out most non-MMP causes of cicatrizing conjunctivitis. Does the patient have a positive history of esophageal stricture or problems swallowing? Does she have any skin or oral mucosa findings? What are the frequency, duration, and clinical findings of her conjunctivitis? Look for subtle evidence of cicatrization in either eye, assisted by successively pulling each lid away from the field of gaze (Figure 20-1). Some corneal consultants believe that any patient with a history suggestive of MMP should be biopsied. However, biopsy is not without risk, as disrupting the conjunctiva in a patient with cicatrizing conjunctivitis may cause flare-up of the disease. Oral mucosa lesions may offer a less risky biopsy site. I may hold off on

Table 20-1 Mucous Membrane Pemphigoid Treatment Options	
Mild to Moderate Disease	Dapsone or mycophenolate mofetil; alternatives: sulfapyridine, methotrexate
Moderate Disease	Mycophenalate mofetil or azathioprine
Severe Disease	Cyclophosphamide plus short-course oral steroids
Refractory Disease	Consider intravenous immunoglobulin or combination intravenous immunoglobulin/rituximab
All Patients	• Consider combination therapy • Co-manage with oncologist, rheumatologist, or dermatologist

biopsy, especially if the disease appears quiet, in which case I may also hold off on treatment. Furthermore, if the disease presentation is strongly consistent with the diagnosis of MMP, I might skip the biopsy, as I will likely initiate treatment even if the biopsy is negative, given the 20% to 50% chance of a false-negative result.

Management

Our 72-year-old patient has active bilateral conjunctival involvement that has progressed to the point of symblepharon formation. In the absence of likely explanation for a non-MMP etiology, consider biopsy and begin systemic immunosuppressive therapy. A team approach is optimal, including an ophthalmologist to follow ocular disease activity and progression and a specialist (usually an oncologist, rheumatologist, or dermatologist) with experience in systemic immunosuppressive therapy. Treatment should be tailored to each patient with a stepwise approach (Table 20-1).[1,2,4-6] At each visit, I like to grade and record conjunctival injection in each quadrant to document the degree of active ocular disease. Disease progression can be measured by staging, based on the extent of conjunctival foreshortening and symblepharon (Table 20-2).[7]

The treatment plan must also include supportive care for the ocular surface, including aggressive dry eye and blepharitis treatment and correction of lid anomalies, including trichiasis. Trichiasis in patients with MMP is often associated with entropion formation. Adhering to the team approach for this very serious disease, I would refer our patient to an oculoplastics consultant. They might advocate a lid-splitting technique, with or without mucous membrane grafting, to treat both entropion and misdirected lashes, with care to minimize conjunctival disruption.[8] Frequent epilation may be considered to manage our patient until systemic immunosuppression therapy has controlled the inflammation. Surgical treatment is then more likely to succeed without activating the cicatricial process. Sparing the conjunctiva is preferable.

Wedge resection is less desirable for our patient because it adds to conjunctival shortening and may involve more direct conjunctival contact. Manual epilation offers no long-term solution. Treatment of trichiasis should include a more permanent approach, such as electrocautery or radiofrequency ablation.

Table 20-2 **Staging of Mucous Membrane Pemphigoid**	
Stage I	Conjunctival inflammation and subepithelial fibrosis
Stage II	Shrinkage of conjunctiva with foreshortening of fornices
Stage III	Symblepharon formation
Stage IV	Ankyloblepharon formation

Corneal transplantation should be avoided in most patients with MMP because of the very high risk of failure from both ocular surface compromise and rejection. I would consider corneal transplantation or keratoprosthesis as a last resort and only if vision loss is bilateral and severe.

Should our patient develop significant cataract, she will likely do well with cataract surgery, as long as the eye is quiet and a clear corneal incision approach is used. Control of MMP by immunosuppressive therapy should be optimized prior to cataract surgery, and it can be augmented by a perioperative course of oral or intravenous steroids (eg, a 10-day course of oral prednisone 60 mg daily starting 3 days prior to surgery).

References

1. Georgoudis P, Sabatino F, Szentmary N, et al. Ocular mucous membrane pemphigoid: current state of pathophysiology, diagnostics and treatment. *Ophthalmol Ther*. 2019;8(1):5-17.
2. Saw VPJ, Dart JKG, Rauz S, et al. Immunosuppressive therapy for ocular mucous membrane pemphigoid. *Ophthalmology*. 2008;115(2):253-261.
3. Foster CS. Ocular cicatricial pemphigoid. *Medscape*. Updated July 16, 2019. Accessed October 10, 2021. https://emedicine.medscape.com/article/1191261
4. Thorne JE, Woreta FA, Jabs DA, Anhalt GJ. Treatment of ocular mucous membrane pemphigoid with immunosuppressive drug therapy. *Ophthalmology*. 2008;115(12):2146-2152.
5. Wang K, Seitzman G, Gonzales JA. Ocular cicatricial pemphigoid. *Curr Opin Ophthalmol*. 2018;29(6):543-551.
6. Foster CS, Chang PY, Ahmed AR. Combination of rituximab and intravenous immunoglobulin for recalcitrant ocular cicatricial pemphigoid: a preliminary report. *Ophthalmology*. 2010;117(5):861-869.
7. Foster CS. Cicatricial pemphigoid. *Trans Am Ophthalmol Soc*. 1986;84:527-663.
8. Koreen IV, Taich A, Elner VM. Anterior lamellar recession with buccal mucous membrane grafting for cicatricial entropion. *Ophthalmic Plast Reconstr Surg*. 2009;25(3):180-184.

A Patient Who Suffered a Chemical Burn in the Left Eye 2 Years Ago Complains of Persistent Blurry Vision and Photophobia. There Is Corneal Neovascularization and Conjunctivalization Extending 5 mm From the Limbus. Do They Need Limbal Stem Cell Transplantation?

Manachai Nonpassopon, MD;
Muanploy Niparugs, MD; and Ali R. Djalilian, MD

Diagnosis

Limbal stem cell deficiency (LSCD) is a condition where the cornea is unable to maintain (regenerate) the corneal epithelium due to an inadequate number/function of the limbal epithelial stem cells. Patients may complain of redness, irritation, photophobia, and decreased vision. Early slit-lamp findings include loss of the palisades of Vogt, late staining of the epithelium with fluorescein, corneal neovascularization, and the development of peripheral pannus. Over time, corneal findings may progress to involve the central cornea. The epithelium becomes irregular and hazy, and persistent epithelial defects may lead to stromal scarring. Conjunctivalization results from invasion of the corneal surface by conjunctival tissue due to the absence of the limbal barrier.

The hallmark sign for diagnosis of LSCD is the presence of conjunctival epithelium on the corneal surface. This is evident by an opaque epithelium that stains with fluorescein in a whorl pattern. Over time, there is superficial neovascularization and stromal scarring (early disease may not have neovascularization). In cases where the clinical diagnosis is in question, additional testing can be used to document the presence of conjunctival epithelium. These tests include tissue biopsy, impression cytology, and in vivo confocal microscopy.

A practical approach for staging ocular surface disease in such cases must consider several factors, including the laterality (unilateral vs bilateral), the extent of the LSCD (partial vs total), and the involvement of the conjunctiva.[1]

Hardten DR, Hansen MS.
Curbside Consultation in Cornea and External Disease:
49 Clinical Questions, Second Edition (pp 121-126).
© 2022 Taylor & Francis Group.

Treatment

The patient presented in this question is in the chronic phase of a chemical burn and clearly has LSCD. Generally, chemical injuries not only cause LSCD, but they also damage the other parts of the ocular surface, including conjunctiva, meibomian glands, and eyelids/eyelashes. Moreover, glaucoma should always be considered in these patients, especially alkali-associated injuries. A multidisciplinary approach, involving cornea, oculoplastics, and glaucoma specialists, may be required in some cases.

OPTIMIZING THE HEALTH OF THE OCULAR SURFACE

In many cases of chemical injury, it is most important to optimize the health of the surface to prevent further damage to the remaining limbal stem cells and/or to improve the success of any future surgical intervention. In general, there are 2 main causes for persistent damage to limbal stem cells: (1) persistent dryness and inflammation and (2) concomitant conjunctival and lid disease. Nonpreservative artificial tears (or autologous serum when available) and other immune-modulatory drugs, such as a topical steroid or cyclosporine, should be considered for all patients. Topical vitamin A ointment 0.01% used once at night is also another useful adjunct in patients with partial limbal stem cell deficiency. It is useful to consider high-Dk (oxygen permeability) bandage contact lens or scleral lens in severe dry eye patients presenting with chronic severe punctate erosion (alternatively, lateral tarsorrhaphy can be used). Conjunctival scarring, presenting with forniceal shortening or symblepharon, may lead to inadequate tear film and eyelid/eyelash abnormalities. Entropion, ectropion, trichiasis, or other abnormalities of lid contour can cause mechanical trauma, poor blink, and exposure. Fornix and eyelid reconstruction, with or without amniotic membrane or mucous membrane graft, along with tarsorrhaphy, will restore a more normal ocular surface environment and help to preserve the remaining limbal stem cells or prepare the surface for future limbal procedures. Likewise, toxicity from drops should be minimized by the use of benzalkonium chloride or preservative-free antiglaucoma drugs. Patients requiring multiple eye drops may be considered for surgical management of glaucoma to decrease the burden of the drops prior to any other surface intervention.

Patients with partial limbal stem cell deficiency, without involvement of the central cornea, can often be monitored and will not require surgical intervention. In patients where the conjunctival epithelium extends into the visual axis, causing reduced acuity, a sectoral procedure may be considered.

SECTORAL INTERVENTIONS FOR PARTIAL LIMBAL STEM CELL DEFICIENCY

In cases of partial LSCD with annoying symptoms, such as photophobia, irritation, or decreasing vision due to conjunctival growth into the central cornea, it may be possible to restore a corneal epithelial phenotype by scraping the conjunctiva and allowing the corneal epithelium to grow in from the adjacent healthier areas. Two different procedures have been described for such cases. Sequential sector conjunctival epitheliectomy (SSCE) is a procedure for removal of conjunctival epithelium, wherein covering a sector of cornea and limbus is repeated sequentially until the desired endpoint is obtained.[2,3] This is done by brushing off conjunctiva-derived epithelium with a dry Weck-Cel sponge. Conjunctival epithelium is characteristically very loose, and gentle brushing can remove the epithelium (more adherent epithelium that does not come off by brushing is typically corneal and should not be removed). After the initial scraping, the patient should be seen in follow-up every 1 to 2 days to monitor the epithelial regeneration, and any conjunctival epithelial regrowth (coming from the limbus) is removed again, allowing corneal epithelium from

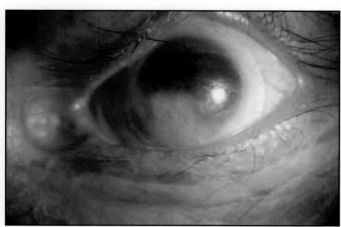

Figure 21-1. Patient with partial limbal stem cell deficiency and central corneal scar from acid chemical burn after fitting a scleral contact lens. Visual acuity improved to 20/50. (Reproduced with permission from Ellen Shorter, OD, University of Illinois Eye and Ear Infirmary, Chicago, Illinois.)

the adjacent areas to heal the defect. SSCE is most successful in patients with focal LSCD that is generally less than 4 to 6 clock hours; otherwise, cases with more extensive limbal stem cell disease are not likely to be successful. In addition, SSCE is not appropriate for corneas with a dense fibrovascular pannus, and/or unhealthy corneal stromal bed may result in persistent epithelial defect, risking corneal melting and perforation. For such cases, an amniotic membrane transplantation may be considered. Amniotic membrane has some important properties, such as promoting epithelialization, and reducing inflammatory, cicatricial, and angiogenic processes. Several reports have demonstrated that amniotic membrane can help preserve and expand the remaining limbal epithelial stem cell population in case of partial LSCD.[4,5] The surgical procedure involves conjunctival peritomy, removing subconjunctival fibrotic tissue in area of LSCD followed by debridement of superficial fibrovascular tissue, abnormal corneal epithelium, and pannus. After suitable hemostasis, the amniotic membrane graft is oriented basement membrane–up and secured on denuded sclera and corneal surface by suture or fibrin glue. By this method, if patients still have adequate residual limbal stem cells, new ocular surface should be clearer with less fibrovascular tissue. Moreover, scleral lens or Prosthetic Replacement of the Ocular Surface Ecosystem (PROSE; Boston Sight) may have a role for better visualization if irregularity of cornea is still present (Figure 21-1).

LIMBAL STEM CELL TRANSPLANTATION

In patients with extensive LSCD (ie, more than 270 degrees), with involvement of the central cornea, limbal transplantation must be considered. First, the most important issue is that limbal stem cell transplantation (LSCT) should not be performed during active inflammation and must be postponed until the ocular surface inflammation has subsided or is well controlled by steroid or immunosuppressive drugs. Moreover, as mentioned earlier, conjunctival or eyelid abnormalities should be addressed before considering LSCT. In patients with unilateral LSCD, the harvested limbal stem cell can be taken from autologous or nonautologous sources. However, the autologous graft is preferred because of the low risk of immunologic rejection and no complication from immunosuppressive drugs. Conjunctival limbal autograft (CLAU), taken from 2 pieces—2 clock hours each—from the completely healthy fellow eye is considered the most effective surgical procedure in patients with total unilateral LSCD. Large CLAU case series have shown that this procedure produces excellent results, often with complete regression of corneal neovascularization such that successful re-epithelialization and functional vision was achieved in about 80% of patients.[6,7] The risk of inducing LSCD in a completely healthy donor eye is extremely low.[8] The

Figure 21-2. The patient with partial limbal stem cell deficiency after simple limbal epithelial transplantation. (Reproduced with permission from Drs. Geetha Iyer and Sankara Nethralaya, Tamil Nadu, India.)

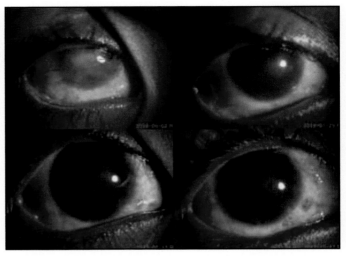

other 2 options to reduce the risk of LSCD in a donor eye are simple limbal epithelial transplantation (SLET) and cultivated limbal epithelial transplantation (CLET; Figure 21-2).

Both SLET and CLET are procedures that harvest only a small piece of limbus (not more than 4 mm). SLET involves taking a small piece of healthy limbus and splitting it into 8 to 10 pieces. Six to 8 pieces of limbus are glued peripherally and 2 to 3 are glued paracentrally on amniotic membrane that is glued over recipient cornea. After that, a large bandage contact lens (or a second amniotic membrane) is used to cover the donor tissue, again to prevent the grafts from falling off. In contrast to SLET, CLET involves expanding a small piece of limbal graft in the laboratory for a few weeks, after which the cultured epithelial sheet is transplanted to the patient again. The donor tissue has to be harvested from the contralateral eye but also from ipsilateral eye if there is enough healthy tissue remaining.[9] A large cohort study from Basu et al[10] of unilateral LSCD described the success rate, in terms of complete epithelization and a stable corneal surface without progressive conjunctivalization encroaching on the central cornea, as 76% after a mean follow-up period of 35.5 months. These outstanding results seem to be comparable with the outcomes of CLET in other large series.[11-13] The major advantages of SLET over CLET are the single-step procedure and that it does not require an expensive laboratory setup for ex vivo cell cultivation.

Although SLET has many impressive advantages, CLAU may be preferred in the patients who have severe conjunctival deficiency because a large piece of the donor's conjunctiva can be harvested and used to reconstruct the conjunctiva. Moreover, if the patients have a likelihood of needing a keratoplasty in the future due to extensive corneal scarring or thinning, SLET may not be a good choice because many pieces of limbal tissue will be lost during the corneal host trephination (CLAU is the preferred procedure).

Conclusion

In the presented case, if the central cornea is spared and the vision is good, the best option is to optimize the surface and observe. If there is central corneal involvement in the setting of partial LSCD, with at least 180 degrees of healthy limbus, then either SSCE or sectoral pannus removal with amniotic membrane is considered—an ipsilateral CLAU or SLET can be performed if the sectoral procedure fails. If there is extensive (near total) LSCD, then a contralateral CLAU (or SLET) may be considered (Figure 21-3).

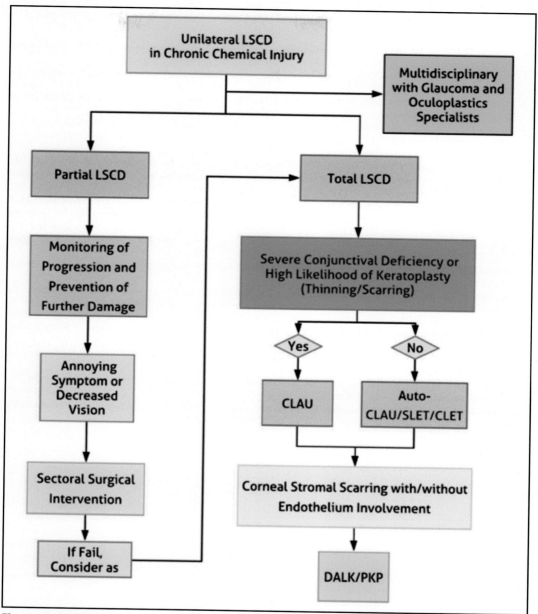

Figure 21-3. Algorithm for the management of unilateral limbal stem cell deficiency.

References

1. Holland EJ, Mannis MJ, Lee WB, eds. *Ocular Surface Disease: Cornea, Conjunctiva and Tear Film*. Saunders Elsevier; 2013.
2. Dua HS, Miri A, Said DG. Contemporary limbal stem cell transplantation—a review. *Clin Exp Ophthalmol*. 2010;38(2):104-117.
3. Dua HS. Sequential sectoral conjunctival epitheliectomy (SSCE). In: Mannis MJ, Holland EJ, eds. *Ocular Surface Disease: Medical and Surgical Management*. Springer; 2002:168-174.
4. Gomes JAP, dos Santos MS, Cunha MC, Mascaro VLD, de Nadai Barros J, de Sousa LB. Amniotic membrane transplantation for partial and total limbal stem cell deficiency secondary to chemical burn. *Ophthalmology*. 2003;110(3):466-473.
5. Tseng SC, Prabhasawat P, Barton K, Gray T, Meller D. Amniotic membrane transplantation with or without limbal allografts for corneal surface reconstruction in patients with limbal stem cell deficiency. *Arch Ophthalmol*. 1998;116(4):431-441.
6. Barreiro TP, Santos MS, Vieira AC, de Nadai Barros J, Hazarbassanov RM, Gomes JAP. Comparative study of conjunctival limbal transplantation not associated with the use of amniotic membrane transplantation for treatment of total limbal deficiency secondary to chemical injury. *Cornea*. 2014;33(7):716-720.
7. Kenyon KR, Tseng SC. Limbal autograft transplantation for ocular surface disorders. *Ophthalmology*. 1989;96(5):709-722.
8. Holland EJ. Management of limbal stem cell deficiency: a historical perspective, past, present, and future. *Cornea*. 2015;34 Suppl 10:S9-S15.
9. Vazirani J, Basu S, Kenia H, et al. Unilateral partial limbal stem cell deficiency: contralateral versus ipsilateral autologous cultivated limbal epithelial transplantation. *Am J Ophthalmol*. 2014;157(3):584-590.e1-2.
10. Basu S, Sureka SP, Shanbhag SS, Kethiri AR, Singh V, Sangwan VS. Simple limbal epithelial transplantation: long-term clinical outcomes in 125 cases of unilateral chronic ocular surface burns. *Ophthalmology*. 2016;123(5):1000-1010.
11. Vazirani J, Ali MH, Sharma N, et al. Autologous simple limbal epithelial transplantation for unilateral limbal stem cell deficiency: multicentre results. *Br J Ophthalmol*. 2016;100(10):1416-1420.
12. Rama P, Matuska S, Paganoni G, Spinelli A, De Luca M, Pellegrini G. Limbal stem-cell therapy and long-term corneal regeneration. *N Engl J Med*. 2010;363(2):147-155.
13. Sangwan VS, Basu S, Vemuganti GK, et al. Clinical outcomes of xeno-free autologous cultivated limbal epithelial transplantation: a 10-year study. *Br J Ophthalmol*. 2011;95(11):1525-1529.

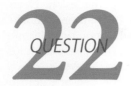

A 47-Year-Old Man Has a Growth in the Nasal Corner of His Right Eye. Should His Pterygium Be Removed Surgically?

Kyle Jones, MD and Jessica Chow, MD

Pterygia are wing-shaped folds of conjunctiva and fibrovascular tissue that grow from the bulbar conjunctiva onto the cornea, most commonly in the interpalpebral area. They are most frequently seen in individuals from equatorial regions with higher levels of sunlight exposure. They are usually asymptomatic. However, they may cause irritation in some individuals and, as they grow, can induce corneal astigmatism and directly obstruct the visual axis.

If a patient presents with a pterygium, obtaining a detailed history is important. How long has the lesion been present? Pterygia are often noted to be present for months to years. However, rapid growth, atypical pigmentation, the presence of prominent feeder vessels, or a gelatinous or leukoplakic appearance should raise concern for ocular surface squamous neoplasia. Is the pterygium symptomatic? The earliest symptoms may be those of dry eye, such as ocular burning, itching, tearing, and redness, related to irregular distribution of the tear film on the ocular surface. For this, lubricating drops and gels, topical cyclosporine, and a short course of topical corticosteroids can be effective at reducing these symptoms. Surgery is rarely needed except in cases of persistent discomfort, despite these measures.

Pterygium Treatment

Surgical intervention may be required if the pterygium grows and causes loss of best-corrected visual acuity through corneal astigmatism and/or direct extension into the visual axis. In rare cases, the pterygium may become so large it restricts extraocular movements. A pterygium larger than 3 mm may induce astigmatism, and one more than halfway to the center of the pupil of a typical cornea (> 3.5 mm) is likely to be associated with at least 1 diopter of astigmatism.[1] Corneal

Hardten DR, Hansen MS.
Curbside Consultation in Cornea and External Disease:
49 Clinical Questions, Second Edition (pp 127-130).
© 2022 Taylor & Francis Group.

topography can be obtained to identify irregular astigmatism induced by the lesion. Detailed discussion of the risks and benefits of surgical excision is critical. Risk of recurrence should be discussed with the patient and has been significantly reduced with various modifications of the bare sclera excision technique. Adherence to a regimen of postoperative corticosteroid drops to prevent recurrence and reduce inflammation should also be stressed prior to surgery.

Compared to pterygium excision, leaving bare sclera exposed, the application of a graft over the sclera has been shown to significantly reduce recurrence. Conjunctival autograft and amniotic membrane graft are the 2 main options available. If the bare sclera defect is small, a sliding flap of contiguous conjunctiva can be rotated to cover the defect, or a free graft can be excised from the superior bulbar conjunctiva and secured to the bordering conjunctiva with 10-0 nylon (non-absorbable) or 8-0 polyglactin (absorbable) sutures.

Four randomized clinical trials comparing recurrence rates of conjunctival autografts with amniotic membrane grafts have shown lower recurrence rates with the conjunctival autograft.[2] In a systematic review of 20 randomized, controlled trials comparing recurrence rates in the presence of conjunctival autografts and amniotic membrane grafts 6 months after surgery, the rate in the conjunctival autograft group varied from 3.3% to 16.7%, and the amniotic membrane graft group varied from 6.4% to 42.3%.[3]

A conjunctival autograft of sufficient quality requires that Tenon's layer be adequately dissected away, which can be time consuming. The main advantage of an amniotic membrane graft is that it avoids needing to harvest conjunctiva, and the procedure is therefore shorter and technically easier. Amniotic membrane grafts would be preferred over conjunctival autograft in patients where both temporal and nasal pterygia need to be removed in the same eye because the conjunctival graft required would likely be very large.

Mitomycin C serves as a potent inhibitor of fibroblast proliferation. Its use intraoperatively or postoperatively as an adjuvant during pterygium excision has also been demonstrated to reduce recurrence rate compared with the bare sclera technique. In a study of 45 patients at almost 3 years of follow-up, patients treated with pterygium excision with intraoperative 0.02% mitomycin C demonstrated a significantly lower rate of recurrence compared with those with excision and bare sclera alone (12.5% vs 35.6%).[4] However, larger concentration or duration of exposure of mitomycin C has been associated with a higher rate of vision-threatening complications, such as scleral ulceration and delayed conjunctival epithelialization. After the application of mitomycin C is complete, thoroughly irrigating the area with balanced salt solution can help ameliorate those complications. There are numerous methods for using mitomycin C. A Merocel sponge soaked in mitomycin C 0.02% applied to bare sclera for 2 to 5 minutes has been reported.[5] Other methods have been described, including injection of 0.02% mitomycin C directly into the subconjunctival space. Mitomycin C eye drops taken postoperatively has been previously described but has fallen out of favor due to higher rates of complications. One trial of 41 eyes that underwent pterygium excision demonstrated that the rate of recurrence with intraoperative mitomycin C was not sig-nificantly different compared with conjunctival autograft alone.[5] Further studies are needed to determine the optimal duration of treatment and route of administration.

Sutures and fibrin glue are the main methods of securing a graft in position after pterygium excision. Nylon sutures have been used to secure both conjunctival and amniotic membrane grafts, but they do not absorb and have to be removed postoperatively. Polyglactin suture is absorbable but tends to cause more inflammation, which can increase the rate of recurrence. Suturing also prolongs operation time and may increase postoperative discomfort as well as suture-related com-plications. Meta-analyses have shown that fibrin glue may result in less recurrence, shorten surgery duration, and cause less postoperative pain than sutures alone.[6] The main disadvantages of using fibrin glue include increased cost as well as risk of dislodging of the graft during the postoperative period. Placing cardinal sutures, along with the fibrin glue, may help prevent this complication.

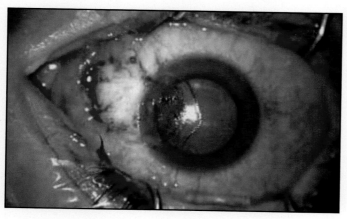

Figure 22-1. Bare sclera after pterygium excision.

Recently, a novel technique has been described, involving graft with amniotic membrane and limbal epithelial stem cells termed *minor ipsilateral simple limbal stem cell* transplantation.[7] The procedure involves an amniotic membrane graft over bare sclera fixed with fibrin glue, as well as placement of small pieces of limbal epithelial tissue on the conjunctival side of the limbus over the fixed amniotic membrane. These pieces are then secured in place with fibrin glue and covered by a second smaller amniotic membrane. In a study where this technique was performed on 10 eyes, there were no signs of early recurrence in an 8-month follow-up period, and no major vision threatening complications were reported. This technique may offer an advantage in that less conjunctival tissue is needed, which may be helpful if another surgery is required in the future, and the presence of the limbal stem cells may help to reduce recurrence rates.

Surgical Technique

Our preferred surgical technique in pterygium excision is to use a crescent blade to dissect a smooth plane between the pterygium and cornea starting at its most anterior edge on the cornea and dissecting toward the limbus. Ideally, Bowman's layer should be left intact. We polish the corneal defect with a corneal burr. We dissect down to bare sclera near the limbus but use caution when dissecting Tenon's tissue farther posteriorly, near the medial rectus insertion (Figure 22-1). Due to its lower recurrence rate compared with an amniotic membrane graft, we prefer to use conjunctival autograft transplantation during pterygium excision, and we prefer to use tissue from the superotemporal bulbar conjunctiva. The area of conjunctiva to be harvested should be marked 0.5 mm to 1.0 mm larger than the bare sclera defect to ensure full coverage of the defect (Figure 22-2). During the transplant, it is important to maintain the orientation of the conjunctiva so that the limbal aspect of the graft is adjacent to the cornea when fixed over the excision site. We secure the conjunctival graft with 3 cardinal 10-0 nylon sutures at the limbal border of the graft (Figure 22-3). We prefer nonabsorbable sutures due to less invoked postoperative inflammation compared with absorbable polyglactin suture. In most cases, we also prefer to place fibrin glue under the graft. In cases of recurrent pterygium, we treat with 0.02% mitomycin C–soaked sponges under the edges of the dissected conjunctiva for 45 seconds, followed by thorough irrigation with balanced salt solution. We also secure an amniotic membrane graft over the conjunctival graft with fibrin glue.

In the postoperative period, control of inflammation with topical steroids is critical to prevent recurrence, and we taper topical steroids slowly over the course of 10 to 12 weeks after surgery. If there is significant pain due to the corneal epithelial defect, we may place a soft bandage contact lens and continue topical antibiotics.

Figure 22-2. Harvesting of a superior bulbar conjunctival autograft. Care is taken to dissect conjunctiva away from Tenon's layer.

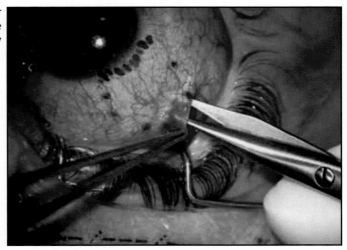

Figure 22-3. Conjunctival autograft in place with fibrin glue and 3 cardinal sutures located at the limbus.

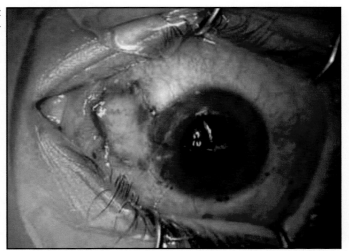

References

1. Khan FA, Niazi SPK, Khan DA. The impact of pterygium excision on corneal astigmatism. *J Coll Physicians Surg Pak*. 2014;24(6):404-407.

2. Kaufman SC, Jacobs DS, Lee WB, Deng SX, Rosenblatt MI, Shtein RM. Options and adjuvants in surgery for pterygium: a report by the American Academy of Ophthalmology. *Ophthalmology*. 2013;120(1):201-208.

3. Clearfield E, Hawkins BS, Kuo IC. Conjunctival autograft versus amniotic membrane transplantation for treatment of pterygium: findings from a Cochrane Systematic Review. *Am J Ophthalmol*. 2017;182:8-17. doi:10.1016/j.ajo.2017.07.004

4. Mastropasqua L, Carpineto P, Ciancaglini M, Gallenga PE. Long term results of intraoperative mitomycin C in the treatment of recurrent pterygium. *Br J Ophthalmol*. 1996;80(4):288-291.

5. Sheppard JD, Mansur A, Comstock TL, Hovanesian JA. An update on the surgical management of pterygium and the role of loteprednol etabonate ointment. *Clin Ophthalmol*. 2014;8:1105-1118. doi:10.2147/OPTH.S55259

6. Romano V, Cruciani M, Conti L, Fontana L. Fibrin glue versus sutures for conjunctival autografting in primary pterygium surgery. *Cochrane Database Syst Rev*. 2016;12(12):CD011308. doi:10.1002/14651858.CD011308.pub2

7. Hernandez-Bogantes E, Amescua G, Navas A, et al. Minor ipsilateral simple limbal epithelial transplantation (mini-SLET) for pterygium treatment. *Br J Ophthalmol*. 2015;99(12):1598-1600.

A 67-Year-Old Woman Complains of Constant Eye Irritation. The Exam Shows Conjunctivochalasis of the Lower Bulbar Conjunctiva. Should I Excise the Redundant Conjunctiva?

Benjamin B. Bert, MD

As we age, the tissues in our bodies lose their elasticity. The ocular surface is not exempt from this phenomenon, and one of the most common signs of this degradation is conjunctivochalasis. In 1942, Wendell Hughes, MD, coined the term *conjunctivochalasis*, meaning relaxation of the conjunctiva.[1] However, the entity itself was described previously in 1908 by Anton Elschnig, MD, as loose, nonedematous conjunctiva.[2] We currently define conjunctivochalasis as loose, redundant conjunctiva, most often located on the inferior globe.

Clinical Diagnosis

While conjunctivochalasis increases in incidence and magnitude with age,[3] its appearance and location can vary. However, conjunctivochalasis is most often seen in the inferotemporal bulbar conjunctiva (Figure 23-1).[4] The symptoms of conjunctivochalasis present similarly to the complaints of dry eye disease, including eye pain, blurred vision, epiphora, dryness, and the presence of subconjunctival hemorrhages. If symptoms worsen in downgaze, the culprit is likely the redundant conjunctiva of conjunctivochalasis.[4] Symptoms of blurred vision and eye pain also worsen with frequent blinking if conjunctivochalasis is to blame. One explanation for this phenomenon is that the upper eyelids are not dipping into the inferior tear meniscus but only touching the redundant conjunctiva (Figure 23-2) and then returning to their open position, without spreading a new tear film over the ocular surface. Combining a faster tear break-up time[4] with compromised tear replenishing puts symptomatic conjunctivochalasis patients at a distinct disadvantage.

Hardten DR, Hansen MS.
*Curbside Consultation in Cornea and External Disease:
49 Clinical Questions, Second Edition* (pp 131-135).
© 2022 Taylor & Francis Group.

Figure 23-1. Note the ridge of conjunctiva on top of the lid margin. The tear lake is visible, resting on top of the unstable conjunctivochalasis, when it should normally be along the lid margin. The conjunctiva is also blocking the normal view of the inferior limbus.

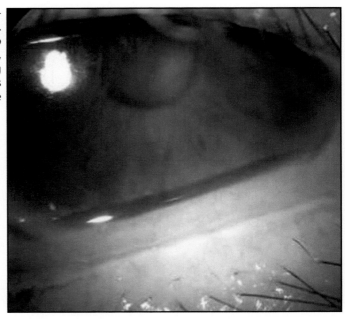

Figure 23-2. Slit-beam view of the excess conjunctiva that has filled the space where the tear lake should normally rest. The conjunctivochalasis in this area also blocks any transfer of tears from the fornix.

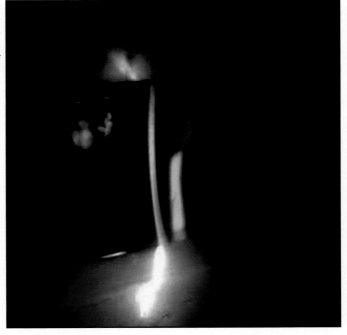

Conjunctivochalasis is hypothesized to contribute to epiphora in 2 ways. First, the reduplicated folds of conjunctiva disrupt the inferior tear lake, and, second, the conjunctiva itself can cause a mechanical blockage of the inferior punctum.[5,6] Blockage of the tear drainage keeps inflammatory cytokines on the ocular surface longer, particularly interleukin-1b and tumor necrosis factor alpha. These cytokines can then cause activation of matrix metalloproteinases 1 and 3 in conjunctival fibroblasts, causing additional breakdown of the conjunctival elasticity and furthering the progression of conjunctivochalasis.[7] This hypothesis is in direct contradiction to one of the standard treatments of dry eye disease, which would be to place punctal plugs and purposefully obstruct tear outflow. Histologically, loss of elastic fibers in the conjunctiva was demonstrated, regardless of the location of the conjunctivochalasis.[8]

Treatment

Not all patients with conjunctivochalasis will be symptomatic; however, a patient who is complaining of burning, irritated, or dry eyes should be examined closely for the presence of conjunctivochalasis. Treatments should be tailored to the patient and their specific pathology, giving a better chance for success.

MEDICAL TREATMENT

The medical treatment of conjunctivochalasis can be separated into the following categories:

- Mild: The finding of conjunctivochalasis alone does not warrant treatment. If the patient is asymptomatic, observation is the appropriate treatment.

- Moderate: The goal is to correct the disruption of the tear film. Lubricants tend to be the first-line medications. The different viscosities and their effects in conjunctivochalasis have not been studied, but one hypothesis would be that a thicker gel/ointment would be more beneficial due to it being able to stay suspended on the redundant folds and create a pseudo tear lake for blinking.

- Severe: With extreme conjunctivochalasis, the excess conjunctiva can be exposed, even when the eyelids are closed. To prevent desiccation, it is imperative to use artificial tear ointment or patch the eyes at night.[9] These patients may also require ointment during the day.

Underlying conjunctival inflammatory diseases should also be addressed to prevent progression of the conjunctivochalasis. For example, allergic conjunctivitis should be treated with topical antihistamines/mast cell stabilizers, and general elevated inflammation should be treated with topical steroids.[9] If patients remain symptomatic despite medical treatment, then surgery becomes a reasonable option.

SURGICAL TREATMENT

Numerous different techniques have been published to correct conjunctivochalasis. Some are minimally invasive and can be done in the office, whereas others require a controlled environment like a procedure room or operating room.

CAUTERY

Most in-office procedures involve thermal-induced shrinkage or thermal-assisted excision to get rid of the redundant folds of conjunctiva. One study described using thermocautery as a way to excise the excess conjunctiva at the slit lamp, with results showing greater than 90% improvement in both subjective and objective findings.[9] The technique used in the study involved grasping the redundant conjunctiva with nontoothed forceps and then excising the grasped portion with a handheld, low-temperature cautery. Scarring was noted postoperatively in 15% of their patients, which did not have any sequelae.

Another study described using a bipolar electrocautery forceps to apply the treatment directly to the symptomatic fold itself, which the authors identified by positive lissamine green staining.[10] The procedure utilized a traction suture through the inferior limbus to rotate the eye superiorly, so this would require a controlled environment. After anesthetizing the area, the stained portion of conjunctiva is elevated, and its base is grasped using the bipolar forceps. Energy is applied to the area directly at a rate of 30 mA until "complete shrinkage" is achieved. The benefit of this technique is that you target the exact area where the symptoms are coming from for that individual patient, whether it is nasal, inferior, or temporal. All the patients in that study had complete resolution of their symptoms, without scar development.[11]

ARGON LASER

Argon laser has also been used to "shrink" the redundant conjunctiva. For the treatments, the 532-nm argon green laser was set at 500 μm and ranged in power from 600 to 1200 mW for a duration of 0.5 seconds to apply treatment to the inferior conjunctiva. Approximately 100 pulses of the laser were delivered during the treatment, using "proper shrinkage" as their endpoint. The results showed a statistically significant improvement in the Ocular Surface Disease Index and in tear break-up time, improving from 9.2 seconds to 10.2 seconds. The treatments were more successful in mild and moderate cases.[12]

INCISIONAL/GLUE APPROACHES

In the operating room, the redundant conjunctiva can be removed in numerous ways, previously described in the literature, including simple excision with direct closure[6]; injection of fibrin glue subconjunctivally, then pinching and excising[13]; and a technique where a limbal peritomy is made with radial relaxing incisions, allowing the loose conjunctiva to be pulled anteriorly and excised with subsequent approximation of the cut edge of conjunctiva to the limbus.[14]

However, the goal with any surgical procedure is to restore the normal anatomy. Thus, it is best to not only excise or tighten the redundant folds of conjunctiva, but also to reestablish the fornix. Restoring the depth of the fornix to its physiologic baseline allows improved tear film function. Many believe fixing the fornix is as important as removing the redundant conjunctiva itself. The importance of the fornix was emphasized in a study that showed the tear reservoir in the inferior fornix will rapidly replenish the tear meniscus in normal patients but it cannot in patients where it is blocked by redundant conjunctiva.[15] The researchers then showed that surgical repair and deepening of the inferior fornix reestablished the normal function of the reservoir and thus provides better resolution of dry eye and ocular surface discomfort symptoms than excision alone.

To normalize the fornix during excision of the conjunctiva, the researchers made a crescentic excision of the loose inferior bulbar conjunctiva starting with a peritomy approximately 2 mm posterior to the limbus. All the loose and thin conjunctival tissue was excised, allowing the remaining conjunctiva to recess into the fornix. The bare scleral defect was covered with cryopreserved amniotic membrane and anchored using either sutures[16] or fibrin glue.[17] Glue has become more preferred due to less inflammation and better patient comfort. In a retrospective review by the same researchers, there was significant improvement in dry eye symptoms and clinical findings. An added benefit was that 56% of the patients who had a prior diagnosis of aqueous deficient dry eye had normalized on their fluorescein clearance testing.[18] The hypothesis was that the conjunctivochalasis caused so much disruption and blockage in the fornix that it had created an aqueous-deficient state.

Conclusion

Ocular surface discomfort is a common and often frustrating condition for both patients and physicians. It is important to look at the entire ocular surface to diagnose and appropriately treat a patient's symptoms. With targeted treatment, there is a much better chance for success. To that effect, do not overlook the role that conjunctivochalasis contributes to these symptoms. After trying conservative management with topical medications, if a patient is still symptomatic, then it is beneficial to take them to the operating room. By surgically returning the ocular surface to a more normal state, the body can then successfully maintain homeostasis.

References

1. Hughes WL. Conjunctivochalasis. *Am J Ophthalmol.* 1942;25:48-51.
2. Elschnig A. Beitrag zur aetiologie und therapie der chronischen konjunktivitis. *Dtsch Med Wochenschr.* 1908;34:1133-1155.
3. Gumus K, Pflugfelder SC. Increasing prevalence and severity of conjunctivochalasis with aging detected by anterior segment optical coherence tomography. *Am J Ophthalmol.* 2013;155(2):238-242.
4. Balci O. Clinical characteristics of patients with conjunctivochalasis. *Clin Ophthalmol.* 2014;28;8:1655-1660.
5. Liu D. Conjunctivochalasis. A cause of tearing and its management. *Ophthalmic Plast Reconstr Surg.* 1986;2(1):1:25-28.
6. Erdogan-Poyraz C, Mocan MC, Irkec M, Orhan M. Delayed tear clearance in patients with conjunctivochalasis is associated with punctal occlusion. *Cornea.* 2007;26(3):3:290-293.
7. Wang Y, Dogru M, Matsumoto Y, et al. The impact of nasal conjunctivochalasis on tear functions and ocular surface findings. *Am J Ophthalmol.* 2007;144(6):930-937.
8. Harbiyeli II, Erdem E, Erdogan S, Kuyucu Y, Polat S, Yagmur M. Investigation of conjunctivochalasis histopathology with light and electron microscopy in patients with conjunctivochalasis in different locations. *Int Ophthalmol.* 2019;39(7):1491-1499.
9. Meller D, Tseng SC. Conjunctivochalasis: literature review and possible pathophysiology. *Surv Ophthalmol.* 1998;43(3):225-232.
10. Nakasato S, Uemoto R, Mizuki N. Thermocautery for inferior conjunctivochalasis. *Cornea.* 2012;31(5):514-519.
11. Arenas E, Muñoz D. A new surgical approach for the treatment of conjunctivochalasis: reduction of the conjunctival fold with bipolar electrocautery forceps. *ScientificWorldJournal.* 2016;2016:6589751.
12. Yang HS, Choi S. New approach for conjunctivochalasis using an argon green laser. *Cornea.* 2013;32(5):574-578.
13. Doss LR, Doss EL, Doss RP. Paste-pinch-cut conjunctivoplasty: subconjunctival fibrin sealant injection in the repair of conjunctivochalasis. *Cornea.* 2012;31(8):959-962.
14. Serrano F, Mora LM. Conjunctivochalasis: a surgical technique. *Ophthalmic Surg.* 1989;20(12):883-884.
15. Huang Y, Sheha H, Tseng SC. Conjunctivochalasis interferes with tear flow from fornix to tear meniscus. *Ophthalmology.* 2013;120(8):1681-1687.
16. Otaka I, Kyu N. A new surgical technique for management of conjunctivochalasis. *Am J Ophthalmol.* 2000;129(3):385-387.
17. Kheirkhah A, Casas V, Blanco G, et al. Amniotic membrane transplantation with fibrin glue for conjunctivochalasis. *Am J Ophthalmol.* 2007;144(2):311-313.
18. Cheng AMS, Yin HY, Chen R, et al. Restoration of fornix tear reservoir in conjunctivochalasis with fornix reconstruction. *Cornea.* 2016;35(6):736-740.

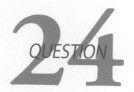
I HAVE A PATIENT WITH A PAPILLOMATOUS, WAXY, CONJUNCTIVAL AND CORNEAL LESION. SHOULD I BE CONCERNED ABOUT CONJUNCTIVAL INTRAEPITHELIAL NEOPLASIA?

Brian D. Alder, MD

Conjunctival and corneal lesions are commonly encountered in the clinic. In some cases, these lesions represent ocular surface squamous neoplasms (OSSN). OSSN is a general term that encompasses a variety of abnormal growth patterns of squamous epithelial cells on the surface of the eye, ranging from benign conjunctival papilloma to mild conjunctival intraepithelial neoplasia (CIN) to squamous cell carcinoma.[1]

Diagnosis

Patients with OSSN typically present with the complaint of a growth in the eye, with symptoms ranging from no pain to mild foreign body sensation to severe pain. Clinically, OSSN can have a variety of appearances, including lesions that are waxy, gelatinous, leukoplakic, and papillomatous (Figures 24-1 through 24-5). Lesions tend to be located on the interpalpebral bulbar conjunctiva or cornea. They often have feeder vessels and can be flat or raised. During slit-lamp examination, staining of the lesion with rose bengal can help to differentiate OSSN lesions from other entities, as rose bengal stains the devitalized epithelium of OSSN lesions. As imaging modalities continue to improve, high- or ultra-high–resolution optical coherence tomography may begin to play an important role in the clinical assessment of conjunctival lesions, as it has been shown to be helpful in the differentiation of OSSN from other lesions.[2]

The incidence of OSSN varies widely, depending on geographic location, and has been reported to be between < 0.2 cases/million/year in the United Kingdom and 35 cases/million/year in Uganda.[3] In the Western world, OSSN is most commonly found in older, White men,[4] whereas

Hardten DR, Hansen MS.
Curbside Consultation in Cornea and External Disease:
49 Clinical Questions, Second Edition (pp 137-141).
© 2022 Taylor & Francis Group.

Figure 24-1. Flat, gelatinous, highly vascularized OSSN with feeder vessel.

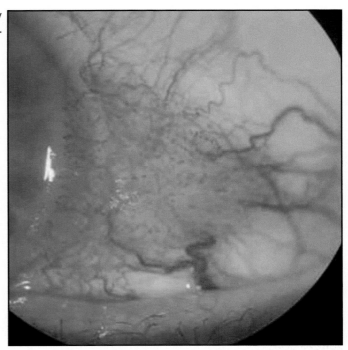

Figure 24-2. Raised conjunctival papilloma.

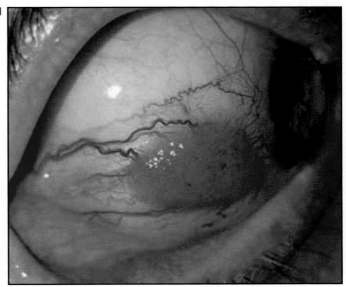

in Africa, patients are often diagnosed at a younger age.[3] Other risk factors for the development of OSSN include exposure to ultraviolet light, HIV positivity, exposure to petroleum chemicals, and heavy smoking.[5,6] While there is a clear causal relationship between human papillomavirus (HPV) and the development of cervical cancer, the association of HPV with the development of OSSN is unclear, although it is thought to play a role in certain patients.[7]

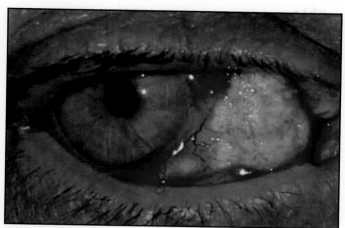

Figure 24-3. Large, raised, leuko-plakic, conjunctival lesion. Further examination showed extension into the inferior fornix, and imaging showed deep extension into the orbit.

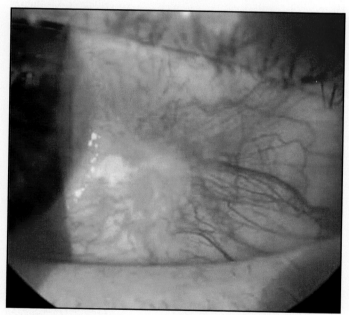

Figure 24-4. Flat conjunctival lesion with focal yellow-appearance centrally and highly vascularized adjacent conjunctiva.

Although clinical evaluation is crucial in the diagnosis and management of OSSN, definitive diagnosis of OSSN is made on histopathology following an incisional or excisional biopsy. In some settings, where cytopathologists with expertise in ocular pathology are available, impression cytology may play an important role in confirming histologic diagnosis, without the need for incisional biopsy.[8] When the diagnosis is in doubt, incisional biopsy can easily be performed in the clinic at the slit lamp or minor procedure room.

The histopathology of OSSN lesions is important for prognosis and can range from preinvasive lesions (termed *conjunctival* or *corneal intraepithelial neoplasia*) to invasive OSSN. The key pathologic finding differentiating CIN lesions from invasive OSSN is the breaching of the basement membrane and the spread of dysplastic epithelium into the substantia propria found in invasive OSSN. CIN lesions can be graded as mild, moderate, or severe, depending on the depth of dysplasia found on histology. CIN lesions with full-thickness involvement, or severe dysplasia, are often termed *carcinoma in situ*.[9]

Figure 24-5. Leukoplakic conjunctival OSSN at the corneal limbus.

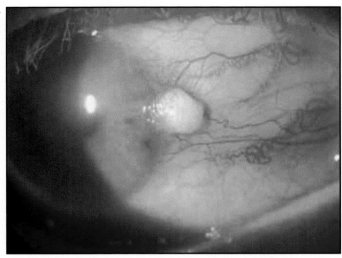

Treatment

Treatment for OSSN has evolved over the past 2 decades and can involve medical treatment with topical agents, surgical excision, or a combination of the two. A survey in 2013 of ophthalmologists who frequently treat OSSN showed that topical agents were being used more frequently as either monotherapy or in combination with surgical excision compared with 2003. Despite this trend to more frequent usage of topical agents, respondents still reported that surgical excision would be used as either monotherapy or in combination with topical agents in most of the cases.[10]

The currently available topical agents include interferon alpha 2b, mitomycin C, and 5-fluorouracil.[11-13] In the same 2013 survey, interferon alpha 2b had replaced mitomycin C as the topical agent of choice in 2013 compared with 2003.[10] Interferon alpha 2b, used 4 times daily, has been shown to be effective in achieving clinical resolution of CIN lesions in more than 95% of cases, with minimal, self-limited side effects[12] The most frequent side effect reported with the usage of interferon alpha 2b is transient flu-like symptoms. Interferon alpha 2b is available only from compounding pharmacies, and its considerable expense may be an obstacle for some patients.

The surgical technique should include excision of the lesion, with wide margins of up to 4 mm of tumor-free conjunctiva to maximize total lesion removal. Cryotherapy should be applied to the limbus and to the conjunctival edges, preferably in a double freeze-thaw method. In cases of deep extension, sclerotomy should be performed. When the lesion extends onto the cornea, treatment with absolute alcohol is recommended. The conjunctival defect is typically closed with either amniotic membrane or conjunctival autograft.[14]

Careful monitoring of patients after treatment is important for early detection of possible recurrence. With surgical excision monotherapy and negative margins, the recurrence rates vary between 5% and 33%. If margins are not clear, the recurrence rate is as high as 53%.[15] For patients treated with topical monotherapy, recurrence rates ranged between 3% and 14%.[12,16]

The recurrence rates of surgical monotherapy vs medical treatment of OSSN were compared in a retrospective, matched, case-controlled study. There were no statistically significant differences in the recurrence rate between the medically and surgically treated groups, with a median follow up of 21 to 24 months, with a 1-year recurrence rate of 3% to 5%.[14] Side effects in the 2 groups were also compared, with no significant differences found.[14]

OSSN lesions are commonly encountered in the clinic and deserve careful evaluation. Overall prognosis for OSSN is good with appropriate treatment and follow-up.

References

1. Sayed-Ahmed IO, Palioura S, Galor A, Karp CL. Diagnosis and medical management of ocular surface squamous neoplasia. *Expert Review of Ophthalmology.* 2016;12(1):11-19. doi:10.1080/17469899.2017.1263567
2. Thomas BJ, Galor A, Nanji AA, et al. Ultra high-resolution anterior segment optical coherence tomography in the diagnosis and management of ocular surface squamous neoplasia. *Ocul Surf.* 2014;12(1):46-58. doi:10.1016/j.jtos.2013.11.001
3. Kiire CA, Srinivasan S, Karp CL. Ocular surface squamous neoplasia. *Int Ophthalmol Clin.* 2010;50(3):35-46. doi:10.1097/iio.0b013e3181e246e5
4. Basti S, Macsai MS. Ocular surface squamous neoplasia: a review. *Cornea.* 2003;22(7):687-704. doi:10.1097/00003226-200310000-00015
5. Napora C, Cohen EJ, Genvert GI, et al. Factors associated with conjunctival intraepithelial neoplasia: a case control study. *Ophthalmic Surg.* 1990;21(1):27-30.
6. Lee GA, Williams G, Hirst LW, Green AC. Risk factors in the development of ocular surface epithelial dysplasia. *Ophthalmology.* 1994;101(2):360-364. doi:10.1016/s0161-6420(94)31328-5
7. Di Girolamo N. Association of human papilloma virus with pterygia and ocular-surface squamous neoplasia. *Eye.* 2012;26(2):202-211. doi:10.1038/eye.2011.312
8. Nolan GR, Hirst LW, Bancroft BJ. The cytomorphology of ocular surface squamous neoplasia by using impression cytology. *Cancer.* 2001;93(1):60-67.
9. Lee GA, Hirst LW. Ocular surface squamous neoplasia. *Surv Ophthalmol.* 1995;39(6):429-450. doi:10.1016/s0039-6257(05)80054-2
10. Adler E, Turner JR, Stone DU. Ocular surface squamous neoplasia: a survey of changes in the standard of care from 2003 to 2012. *Cornea.* 2013;32(12):1558-1561. doi:10.1097/ico.0b013e3182a6ea6c
11. Hirst LW. Randomized controlled trial of topical mitomycin C for ocular surface squamous neoplasia. *Ophthalmology.* 2007;114(5):976-982. doi:10.1016/j.ophtha.2006.09.026
12. Schechter BA, Koreishi AF, Karp CL, Feuer W. Long-term follow-up of conjunctival and corneal intraepithelial neoplasia treated with topical interferon alfa-2b. *Ophthalmology.* 2008;115(8):1291-1296.e1. doi:10.1016/j.ophtha.2007.10.039
13. Joag MG, Sise A, Murillo JC, et al. Topical 5-fluorouracil 1% as primary treatment for ocular surface squamous neoplasia. *Ophthalmology.* 2016;123(7):1442-1448. doi:10.1016/j.ophtha.2016.02.034
14. Nanji AA, Moon CS, Galor A, Sein J, Oellers P, Karp CL. Surgical versus medical treatment of ocular surface squamous neoplasia. *Ophthalmology.* 2014;121(5):994-1000. doi:10.1016/j.ophtha.2013.11.017
15. Erie JC, Campbell RJ, Liesegang TJ. Conjunctival and corneal intraepithelial and invasive neoplasia. *Ophthalmology.* 1986;93(2):176-183. doi:10.1016/s0161-6420(86)33764-3
16. Besley J, Pappalardo J, Lee GA, Hirst LW, Vincent SJ. Risk factors for ocular surface squamous neoplasia recurrence after treatment with topical mitomycin C and interferon alpha-2b. *Am J Ophthalmol.* 2014;157(2):287-293.e2. doi:10.1016/j.ajo.2013.10.012

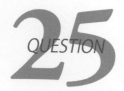

A 13-Year-Old Adolescent Girl Is Complaining of an Enlarging Brown Spot on Her Eye. The Exam Shows a Flat Conjunctival Pigmented Nevus That Is 3 mm in Diameter, Surrounded by Mild Conjunctival Injection. Should I Be Worried About Malignancy?

Frederick (Rick) W. Fraunfelder, MD

The differential diagnosis of pigmented conjunctival lesions includes congenital conjunctival freckles, melanocytosis, conjunctival nevi, racial melanosis, primary acquired melanosis (PAM), and malignant melanoma.[1] There are also many secondary causes of pigmented conjunctival lesions, such as drug-related pigment deposits and metabolic diseases leading to pigmented conjunctiva. Pigmented lesions of the ocular surface are relatively common and are typically benign. Because they can arise from a number of cell types and can be influenced by a variety of environmental factors, lesion characteristics and patient history are helpful in making the correct diagnosis.

Benign Conjunctival Nevus

The case presented here most likely represents a benign conjunctival nevus. The history and examination findings for our 13-year-old patient are most consistent with this diagnosis, as conjunctival nevi typically appear in childhood as small, flat, circumscribed lesions near the limbus in the interpalpebral region (Figure 25-1). They are found less often at the caruncle or semilunar fold and rarely involve the palpebral conjunctiva or lid margin. They may or may not be pigmented, and they can vary in color from pink to yellow-tan to dark brown.

Incidence is 1.2:10 million people/year in all races. Conjunctival nevi are hamartomas and are described by their histological configuration as junctional, compound, or subepithelial.

Hardten DR, Hansen MS.
*Curbside Consultation in Cornea and External Disease:
49 Clinical Questions, Second Edition* (pp 143-146).
© 2022 Taylor & Francis Group.

Figure 25-1. Conjunctival nevus with cysts.

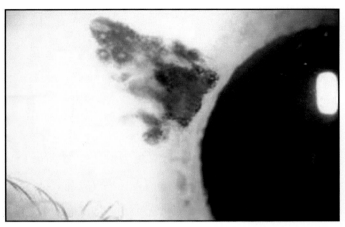

Junctional nevi are located only within the epithelium and are rarely found except in children. They are difficult to distinguish histopathologically from PAM. Compound nevi are more common and involve both epithelium and subconjunctival connective tissue. Approximately 50% of these contain small epithelial inclusion cysts, which are lined by cuboidal cells and goblet cells. Subepithelial nevi are typically nonpigmented and often have a cobblestone appearance.

Before discussing management, it may be worthwhile to describe the other possibilities in the differential diagnosis.

Conjunctival Freckles

Ephelis, or conjunctival freckles, are flat brown patches typically found on the bulbar conjunctiva near the limbus. They are typically small and do not carry malignancy potential. Ephelis are more common in darkly pigmented individuals and may arise in early childhood rather than at birth. Their pigmentation remains stable over time, and the surrounding conjunctiva is normal. Histologically, the conjunctival epithelium appears normal, aside from a well-circumscribed area of hyperpigmented basal cells.

Ocular Melanocytosis

Ocular melanocytosis is another common congenital condition, occurring in 1/2500 individuals and found most typically in Black, Hispanic, and Asian populations. Typically unilateral and affecting the episclera, this condition presents with nonmobile, slate-grey patches that are visible through normal conjunctiva. The iris and choroid may be involved, and many patients have ipsilateral dermal involvement in the cranial nerve V distribution (oculodermal melanocytosis, or Nevus of Ota). There is some risk of malignant transformation, with a lifetime risk of uveal melanoma of about 1 in 400. Secondary glaucoma occurs in 10% of affected eyes.

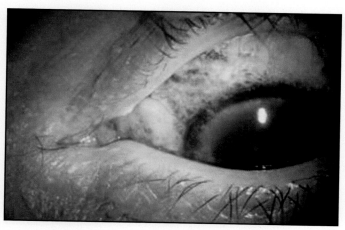

Figure 25-2. Diffuse primary acquired melanosis.

Benign Racial Melanosis

Benign melanosis, also known as *racial melanosis*, is a bilateral, diffuse, patchy increase in pigmentation of the bulbar conjunctiva. Typically found in middle-aged patients with dark skin, the incidence varies: 92.5% in Black, 36% in Asian, 28% in Hispanic, and 4.9% in White populations. These lesions represent melanocytic hyperplasia, which may be triggered by sunlight exposure or other stimuli. Typically flat and affecting the perilimbal and interpalpebral bulbar conjunctiva, these lesions do not carry malignancy potential.

Primary Acquired Melanosis

PAM typically affects White middle-aged patients and initially appears as flat, brown lesions of the conjunctival epithelium (Figure 25-2). These lesions are unilateral and may affect any part of the bulbar or palpebral conjunctiva. They may be analogous to lentigo maligna of the skin (also known as *Hutchinson's melanotic freckle*) and are therefore considered to be a premalignant condition. PAM is relatively common, affecting approximately 36% of White patients. Histology demonstrates a spectrum of epithelial involvement by abnormal melanocytes, ranging from mild increased pigmentation of the basal epithelium to formation of melanocytic nests to microinvasion of the substantia propria (signifying melanoma). PAM with atypia—a histologic description based on biopsy—is a strong predictor for malignant transformation. Studies indicate that 33% to 46% of these lesions will progress to melanoma within an average time of 2.5 years.

There are many other secondary causes of benign acquired melanosis. Melanin-like pigmentation of the conjunctiva may appear in patients taking certain topical and systemic medications, such as epinephrine ("adrenochrome deposits"), tetracycline, or silver-containing compounds. Trauma or chronic inflammation may induce migration of melanocytes or melanin-containing macrophages into the superficial conjunctiva, causing patchy pigmentation. Metabolic diseases, such as ochronosis or hemochromatosis, are potential causes, as are copper or iron-containing metallic foreign bodies.

Figure 25-3. Conjunctival malignant melanoma.

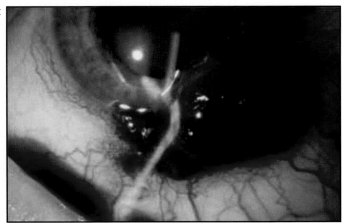

Malignant Melanoma

Malignant melanoma of the conjunctiva may arise from PAM, from acquired nevi, or de novo from normal conjunctiva. It is the second most common malignant neoplasm of the conjunctiva after squamous cell carcinoma. With a prevalence of 1:2 million among the White population, it is a relatively rare condition and is exceedingly rare in children or adolescents.[2] These lesions tend to grow in a nodular fashion and are highly vascularized, so they may bleed (Figure 25-3). They may invade the globe or orbit, although rates of metastasis are lower than that for cutaneous melanoma. Melanomas of the bulbar conjunctiva carry a better prognosis than those on the palpebral conjunctiva or caruncle. Occasionally, melanomas of the uvea may erode through the sclera and mimic a conjunctival lesion.

Management

Increased mucin production by the goblet cells contained in nevus cysts may cause abrupt but benign enlargement of the lesion. Inflammation can also induce an increase in nevus size, and a nevus may grow in a benign fashion during puberty (as in our case) or pregnancy. Rapid growth of a pigmented lesion outside of these circumstances, increase in nodularity, bleeding, or involvement of the cornea or palpebral tissues are more concerning for risk of malignancy. A new lesion arising from an area of PAM is similarly concerning. In these cases, excisional biopsy and/or cryotherapy is recommended.[3] If no concerning features are present and the lesion presents no cosmetic problem to the patient, then observation is warranted.

References

1. Shields CL, Dermirci H, Karatza E, Shields JA. Clinical survey of 1643 melanocytic and nonmelanocytic conjunctival tumors. *Ophthalmology.* 2004;111(9):1747-1754.
2. Jakobiec FA, Rini FJ, Fraunfelder FT, Brownstein S. Cryotherapy for conjunctival primary acquired melanosis and malignant melanoma. Experience with 62 cases. *Ophthalmology.* 1988;95(8):1058-1070.
3. Fraunfelder FW. Liquid nitrogen cryotherapy for surface eye disease (an AOS thesis). *Trans Am Ophthalmol Soc.* 2008;106:301-324.

A PATIENT HAS IRRITATION IN THEIR NONSEEING, BLIND EYE. THE EXAM SHOWS MILDLY INFLAMED CONJUNCTIVA AND DIFFUSE CORNEAL EPITHELIAL AND STROMAL EDEMA WITH LARGE BULLAE. WHAT SHOULD I RECOMMEND?

Jill S. Melicher, MD

Pain in a blind eye can present a difficult situation for both the patient and the clinician. Patients hold on to hope that the vision will return or the eye will become comfortable once again. They often want to undergo any surgical procedure necessary to retain or restore the eye, even if they understand a poor visual outcome will remain. Physicians are left with the difficult discussion around the impact that a surgery on a nonseeing eye can present for the patient. We may not understand to the fullest extent the psychological impact, and sometimes the cultural impact, that losing an eye presents for our patients and their families. There are 2 main considerations in caring for a patient with a nonseeing eye. The first consideration is optimizing pain control. Pain may result from surface irritation from ruptured bullae or elevated intraocular pressure. Patients with diffuse corneal edema and bullous keratopathy have often been living with discomfort and constant eye drops for long periods of time. Treating both etiologies is often necessary. The second consideration is your patient's desire for an aesthetic outcome. Patients with a blind, nonseeing eye often have a disorganized or discolored cornea, drawing more attention to the eye than they like.

Patients faced with a blind eye are often interested in maximizing comfort, minimizing the need for eye drops, and decreasing the number of appointments they need to attend. The medical and surgical management of a blind, nonseeing eye will be discussed herein.

Hardten DR, Hansen MS.
*Curbside Consultation in Cornea and External Disease:
49 Clinical Questions, Second Edition* (pp 147-149).
© 2022 Taylor & Francis Group.

Medical Management

The goal of medical therapy is to minimize the bullae and maximize surface and ocular comfort. Topical medication, including hyperosmotic ointments and drops (0.5% sodium chloride) and lubrication may be sufficient for mild bullous disease. Patients with large bullae find comfort in corneal coverage. A bandage contact lens may provide temporary relief. Coupled with low-dose steroids and pulse doses of broad-spectrum antibiotics, bandage contact lenses may be sufficient for coverage until the bullae scar and the corneal heals.

Endothelial cell function may be compromised by increased intraocular pressure. Maximal medical control of intraocular pressure is important in the management of bullous keratopathy, although some topical medications (prostaglandin analogs, carbonic anhydrase inhibitors, and Rho kinase inhibitors) can be irritants to the ocular surface or effect corneal isoenzymes, exacerbating corneal edema and keratopathy.

Intractable pain can also be managed by retrobulbar injection of Thorazine (chlorpromazine) or ethyl alcohol.[1] A retrobulbar injection of lidocaine with 1:100,000 epinephrine is administered, using a stopcock to allow injection into the same retrobulbar space, after which 1 mL of 100% ethyl alcohol or 1 mL of Thorazine (25 mg/mL) is administered. Retrobulbar injections are effective in reducing pain in two-thirds of patients with ocular discomfort; they can be effective for 3 to 12 months and may be repeated as necessary.[1,2]

Surgical Management

Several options exist for the surgical management of pseudophakic bullous keratopathy in the blind, painful eye. Minimizing the use of penetrating intraocular surgery in this patient population is optimal to decrease, albeit small, the risk of sympathetic ophthalmia.

Conjunctival/Gunderson Flap

Conjunctival flap surgery is useful in eyes with light perception or no-light perception with bullous keratopathy. The corneal epithelium is removed limbus to limbus, and subconjunctival dissection is performed deep into the superior fornix and inferior fornix, as thin as possible, without buttonholing the conjunctiva, for mobilization of the conjunctiva over the cornea. The conjunctival flap is advanced over the cornea and anchored with 8-0 or 10-0 Vicryl sutures (Ethicon US, LLC) at the limbus. Topical broad-spectrum antibiotics and steroids are used for 1 month postoperatively. A bandage contact lens is placed until the sutures are removed or dissolve. These patients are comfortable very quickly after surgery. Consideration for a scleral shell or painted contact lens following conjunctival flap surgery may improve the overall aesthetic outcome for the patient.[3]

Evisceration/Enucleation Surgery

Patients with poor mobility in their conjunctiva due to trauma or previous surgery are better candidates for evisceration or enucleation surgery for treatment of their pain. My preference in technique is evisceration, due to the superiority in ocular prosthetic motility following surgery. Evisceration surgery treats not only the ocular pain but often also aesthetically improves the appearance of the corneal edema, blue hue, in the blind eye. During surgery, I remove all hardware and implants (ie, tube shunts, encircling bands) prior to evisceration and implant placement. Severely phthsical eyes are better treated with enucleation to maximize the implant size, thus minimizing a superior sulcus deformity.

Evisceration surgery may be performed under retrobulbar and facial block, with light intravenous sedation. A conjunctival peritomy is performed with sub-Tenon's dissection in all 4 quadrants. A super sharp blade is introduced into the anterior chamber, and right and left corneal scissors are used to perform a keratectomy. An evisceration spatula is swept 360 degrees, as well as posteriorly, to remove the ocular contents. The scleral shell is cleaned with 100% ethyl alcohol to remove all retinal pigment epithelial cells. Bipolar cautery is used for hemostasis at the nerve and vortex veins. Relaxing incisions are created circumferentially around the optic nerve and in all 4 quadrants in the posterior sclera. Two distinct scleral flaps are created anteriorly with Stevens scissors. Sizers are placed in the scleral shell to identify the appropriate implant size. The evisceration implant is placed, and the anterior flaps are advanced in a layered fashion with buried 5-0 Mersilene suture (Ethicon US, LLC) over the implant. Tenon's capsule is approximated over the scleral flaps with 5-0 Vicryl sutures. The conjunctiva is closed with 7-0 Vicryl sutures in running, locking fashion. A conformer is placed, and a temporary tarsorrhaphy is performed with 7-0 Vicryl suture. The tarsorrhaphy is left in place for 1 month.[4]

Aesthetically, evisceration surgery may be helpful in improving the overall appearance of a nonseeing, blind painful eye.

In summary, medical and surgical management can be used in the treatment of a blind, painful eye with corneal edema and bullous keratopathy. The approach is determined by your patient's pain level, desire to minimize appointments and drops, and comfort level with definitive eye removal surgery.

References

1. Chen TC, Ahn Yuen SJ, Sangalang MA, Fernando RE, Leuenberger EU. Retrobulbar chlorpromazine injections for the management of blind and seeing painful eyes. *J Glaucoma.* 2002;11(3):209-213.
2. Galindo-Ferreiro A, Akaishi P, Cruz A, et al. Retrobulbar injections for blind pain eyes: a comparative study of retrobulbar alcohol versus chlorpromazine. *J Glaucoma.* 2016;25(11):886-890.
3. Gundersen T. Conjunctival flaps in the treatment of corneal disease with reference to a new technique of application. *AMA Arch Ophthalmol.* 1958;60(5):880-888.
4. Migliori M. Enucleation versus evisceration. *Curr Opin Ophthalmol.* 2002;13(5):298-302.

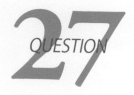

A Patient Had LASIK 2 Months Ago and Has Persistent Pain in the Eyes That Does Not Seem to Be Related to Surface Issues or Other Anatomical Abnormalities. How Do I Diagnose and Manage This?

Wendy Liu, MD and Konstantinos D. Sarantopoulos, MD, PhD

Persistent pain in the eyes after LASIK may be caused by diverse and complex pathophysiological mechanisms that involve interactions between the cornea and somatosensory, optic, and autonomic neural circuits.[1] A sensitized peripheral and central nervous system may be the main contributing factor to pain and sensitivity to light.[2] Not infrequently, various mechanisms coexist, such as in cases of concomitant inflammatory and neuropathic contributors to pain. Yet, in most chronic cases, centralized pain as a result of sensitization and hyperexcitability of central neurons, subsequent to nociceptive input, may further contribute to chronicity and intractability of pain. High prevalence of other chronic painful and/or psychiatric illnesses or cognitive–behavioral abnormalities in patients with pain in the eyes further confound their diagnostic and therapeutic approach. These considerations highlight the need for interdisciplinary diagnostic and therapeutic approaches, involving eye and pain specialists, mental health specialists, physical therapists, and other health professionals.

Diagnosis

Many patients complaining of pain after LASIK (especially those without surface issues or anatomical abnormalities) have a neuropathic component that contributes to their symptoms in variable degrees. Early identification of neuropathy may guide the delivery of proper treatments, may reduce suffering, and may improve long-term outcomes (by attenuating any processes leading to central sensitization and to expansion and chronicity of pain).[1,2]

Hardten DR, Hansen MS.
Curbside Consultation in Cornea and External Disease:
49 Clinical Questions, Second Edition (pp 151-155).
© 2022 Taylor & Francis Group.

Figure 27-1. Testing for tactile (touch) cutaneous allodynia in patients with eye pain. This can be tested by applying a nonpainful stimulus, such as gentle touch or stroking, onto the eyelids or periocular skin compared with a more distal or contralateral site as control. Patients with allodynia report the sensation as painful.

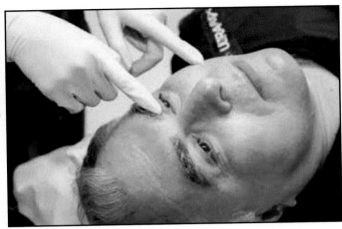

Ideally, patients should first receive a detailed evaluation by an ophthalmologist to rule out any pertinent ocular pathology; yet, in many patients, despite extensive workup, minimal or no objective abnormalities are found. In those patients, the discrepancy between minimal or no signs from the ocular examination and the high intensity of symptoms is indicative of predominantly neuropathic pain.[2] In patients with minimal signs but with intense symptoms ("pain without stain"), the pain is likely driven by neuropathic mechanisms and central sensitization,[2] which leads the management toward antineuropathic therapeutic choices.

Neuropathic ocular pain is further suggested by pertinent descriptors of pain, such as "burning," "stinging," or "shooting"; "electrical shock"; or "foreign body"-like sensations in the eyes or within both the eyes and the periocular tissues. Painful sensations may be spontaneous and/or evoked in response to normally nonpainful stimuli, such as wind (wind allodynia), cold (cold allodynia), light (photophobia), or touch onto the surrounding skin.[2,3] Avoidance behaviors, such as wearing sunglasses, avoidance of sunlight, or preferring dark rooms, are common.

Medical history should look for coexisting painful or mental health illnesses, such as headaches, neck and back pain, musculoskeletal pain, fibromyalgia, posttraumatic stress disorder, and depression. The review of systems may also reveal pertinent symptoms that may suggest neurological dysfunction (numbness, weakness) or a more generalized or systemic disorder, such as an autoimmune disease.

Because pain in the eye may be primary or referred from other sites, subsequent to illness of the brain (tumor, demyelinating or neurovascular disorder) or of the trigeminal system (trigeminal neuralgia or neuropathy), a detailed neurological examination should always be a part of the initial assessment. Motor or sensory deficits should be investigated further by appropriate imaging or referral to a neurologist. Sensory deficits in the trigeminal innervation may be suggestive of a compression neuropathy or a demyelinating condition. Balance impairment, hearing loss, or tinnitus accompanying pain in the eye or around the eye may also raise the suspicion of a cerebellopontine angle tumor.

Allodynia (pain elicited by nonpainful stimuli) can be detected on the eyelids and periocular cutaneous areas simply using gentle palpation with a fingertip, in comparison with the contralateral side or with an adjacent site (Figure 27-1). Hyperalgesia (exaggerated pain response to mildly uncomfortable stimuli) can also be tested in a comparative manner, using a gentle scratchy stimulus with the folded tip of a piece of paper (Figure 27-2). Allodynia and hyperalgesia are usually suggestive of the presence of neuropathy or central sensitization.[2]

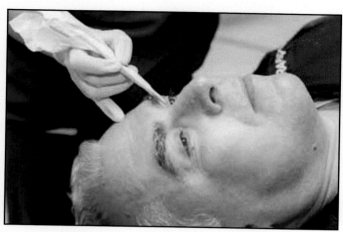

Figure 27-2. Testing for mechanical hyperalgesia in patients with eye pain. This can be tested by applying a slightly painful stimulus, such as scratching with the tip of a folded paper towel, onto the eyelids or onto periocular skin compared with a more distal or contralateral site as control. Patients with hyperalgesia report the sensation as more painful than control.

Overall, the following criteria guide the suspicion of neuropathic eye pain:

- Discrepancy between signs and symptoms
- Allodynia, hyperalgesia, and/or photophobia
- Absence of response to topical anesthetic drops to the cornea[2]
- Minimal or no relief from artificial tears[2]

Additional testing may include:

- Brain imaging by magnetic resonance imaging and/or magnetic resonance angiography to rule out any central nervous system lesions, such demyelinating conditions, or intracranial masses
- Blood tests, such as complete blood count and comprehensive metabolic panel, to determine choices and doses for drugs
- Electrocardiography to determine the QT interval if antidepressants are considered
- Other more specialized tests, such as orbit imaging, thermography, or tests to rule out autoimmune disorders

Treatment

Patients with pain in their eyes usually benefit significantly from comprehensive, multimodal therapeutic approaches.[3]

In addition to other anti-inflammatory therapies (doxycycline, topical steroids, cyclosporine A, and tacrolimus, or autologous serum tears), systemic nonsteroidal anti-inflammatory drugs may help. These include celecoxib, which is safer in patients with gastrointestinal intolerance, or drugs with more potent anti-inflammatory properties, such as indomethacin or diclofenac that possess antineuropathic actions.

Opioids should be avoided. Concerns about their long-term efficacy, poor outcomes, paradoxical worsening of pain (opioid-induced hyperalgesia), and safety issues—including opioid-related deaths and problems of diversion and abuse—limit their use.

Drugs for neuropathic pain may be used alone as monotherapies or in combinations.[3] These include antiepileptics, such as the α2δ ligands (gabapentin, pregabalin),[3,4] other anticonvulsants (topiramate, carbamazepine), or some antidepressants with analgesic properties (amitriptyline, nortriptyline, or duloxetine).[3] Selection may be guided by descriptors of pain (anticonvulsants for

Figure 27-3. Needle placement onto the supraorbital ridge for supraorbital nerve block. Needle is guided by palpation to the supraorbital notch, and, after negative aspiration, 1 mL of a local anesthetic solution, with or without steroid, is injected slowly.

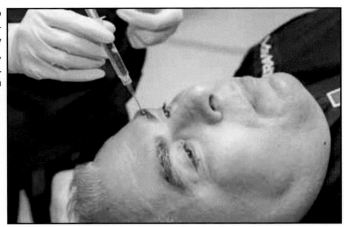

Figure 27-4. Needle placement for supratrochlear nerve block at a site 1 cm medial to the supraorbital notch onto the supraorbital ridge. After negative aspiration, 0.5 to 1 mL of a local anesthetic solution, with or without steroid, is injected slowly.

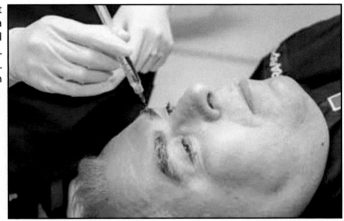

"electrical-like," "shooting," or paroxysmal pain vs antidepressants for constant "burning" pain) by coexisting conditions (depression), as well as by the side effects profile of each individual agent. For example, α2δ ligands are preferred because of a mild side effects profile, but their use requires caution in those with renal insufficiency, while antidepressants are contraindicated in patients with glaucoma, urinary retention, cardiac disease, or seizures.

Unwanted effects from a drug may necessitate switching to another. Doses are gradually titrated up to recommended maximal doses for each drug. In case of satisfactory response, the drug should be continued for a few months; however, in cases of failure, the drug should be discontinued and then a new therapy should ensue with a different agent. In case of incomplete response, another agent of another category may be added. Combination therapy is often required in refractory cases of eye pain, and combined therapy of gabapentin or pregabalin with nortriptyline or duloxetine may be helpful.[3]

Neural blockade can be used for diagnostic and therapeutic purposes. Relief of pain after a nerve block suggests the contribution of the blocked nerve to the maintenance of pain. Uninjured nerves, adjacent to those injured by noxious events (such as those affected by LASIK), may lead to pain also, and blocking these adjacent periorbital nerves can provide relief[4,5] (Figures 27-3 through 27-5).

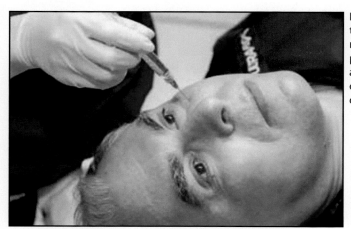

Figure 27-5. Needle placement onto the infraorbital ridge for infraorbital nerve block. Needle is guided by palpation to the infraorbital notch, and, after negative aspiration, 1 mL of a local anesthetic solution, with or without steroid, is injected slowly.

Several nerve blocks have been described, such as supraorbital (see Figure 27-3), supratrochlear (see Figure 27-4), infraorbital (see Figure 27-5),[4,5] lacrimal nerve blocks, or, rarely, blocks at the trigeminal ganglion. Sometimes, long-lasting results can be obtained by repeating these nerve blocks, with the inclusion of corticosteroids as necessary.[4,5] Stellate ganglion blocks or sphenopalatine ganglion blocks may also be very beneficial, whereas botulinum toxin A injections can help selected patients.

A multimodal regimen may also include desensitization therapy, moisture chamber glasses, and nutritional supplements (omega-3 fatty acids, α-lipoid acid). Nonpharmacological techniques include transcutaneous electrical nerve stimulation, which, applied periorbitally, improves pain and dryness and reduces the use of tears.

It should be noted that patients with chronic ocular pain may also suffer from other chronic pain conditions, such as migraines, back or musculoskeletal pain, as well as emotional disorders. Aggressive treatment of these conditions may have a positive impact on the alleviation of eye pain. Therefore, referral to and comanaged with a mental health specialist should be considered as an essential component of a multimodal treatment plan.

We promote the notion that optimal approaches to eye pain after LASIK should be patient-centered and tailored to the individual, multidisciplinary, and multimodal treatments, including proper pharmacotherapy, neural blockade, psychotherapy, and physical therapy. This comprehensive, multispecialty care should be initiated by ophthalmologists and, if necessary, subsequently carried out in specialized, tertiary oculofacial pain clinics for patients with intractable pain.

References

1. Galor A, Levitt RC, Felix ER, Martin ER, Sarantopoulos CD. Neuropathic ocular pain: an important yet underevaluated feature of dry eye. *Eye (Lond)*. 2015;29(3):301-312.
2. Crane AM, Feuer W, Felix ER, et al. Evidence of central sensitisation in those with dry eye symptoms and neuropathic-like ocular pain complaints: incomplete response to topical anaesthesia and generalised heightened sensitivity to evoked pain. *Br J Ophthalmol*. 2017;101(9):1238-1243. doi:10.1136/bjophthalmol-2016-309658
3. Goyal S, Hamrah P. Understanding neuropathic corneal pain—gaps and current therapeutic approaches. *Semin Ophthalmol*. 2016;31(1-2):59-70.
4. Small LR, Galor A, Felix ER, Horn DB, Levitt RC, Sarantopoulos CD. Oral gabapentinoids and nerve blocks for the treatment of chronic ocular pain. *Eye Contact Lens*. 2020;46(3):174-181. doi:10.1097/ICL.0000000000000630
5. Duerr ER, Chang A, Venkateswaran N, et al. Resolution of pain with periocular injections in a patient with a 7-year history of chronic ocular pain. *Am J Ophthalmol Case Rep*. 2019;14:35-38.

SECTION IV

INFECTION

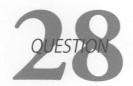
A Patient Presents With Corneal Ulcer. What Workup and Treatment Would You Recommend?

Note: This particular question is unique in this book, as there is 1 question and 2 different responses. We did this because there can be different approaches to an apparent corneal ulcer, based on the location and available antibiotics. This book is intended to be helpful to physicians around the world. We chose authors from India and the United States to provide 2 different perspectives.

Prashant Garg, MD

A corneal ulcer is characterized by an epithelial defect associated with underlying stromal infiltrate (Figure 28-1). Because it can be caused by a variety of infective and noninfective conditions, patients with ulcerative keratitis present both a diagnostic and therapeutic challenge to ophthalmologists. A systematic approach can help ophthalmologists to better manage this condition.

Diagnosis

A detailed history and thorough clinical examination using the slit-lamp biomicroscope are important steps in the diagnosis of corneal ulcer. Pay attention to mode of onset of symptoms, duration, and rate of progression. If the patient has been treated elsewhere, note the details of the treatment and the response. If the patient wears contact lenses, it is important to know the type of lenses (rigid gas permeable lenses or soft lenses), the wearing schedule (especially if the patient sleeps wearing lenses), and cleaning regimens, including information on care of the lens case.

Hardten DR, Hansen MS.
Curbside Consultation in Cornea and External Disease:
49 Clinical Questions, Second Edition (pp 159-168).
© 2022 Taylor & Francis Group.

Figure 28-1. Corneal ulcer.

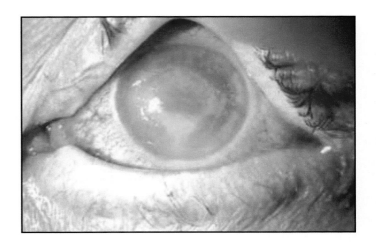

Figure 28-2. Schematic documentation of a case of corneal ulcer.

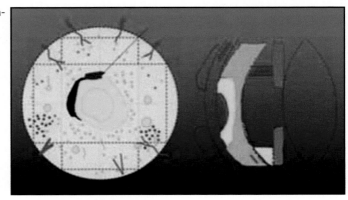

Inquire about any systemic illness, duration of the disease, and the treatment. This is important because systemic diseases, such as rheumatoid arthritis and other collagen vascular diseases, can cause ulcerative keratitis. Similarly, acne rosacea and other dermatological conditions can also produce sterile ulcerative keratitis.[1]

While you elicit the patient history, pay attention to structures around the eyes. This will help you to rule out disorders such as herpes zoster, acne rosacea, proptosis, and exposure keratitis or lagophthalmos.

Perform a thorough systematic slit-lamp examination, with special attention to lids, including eyelashes, intermarginal strip, and posterior lid margin; lacrimal sac; tear film; conjunctiva; sclera; cornea; anterior chamber; pupil; and posterior segment. While examining the cornea, note the location of the ulcer, size of epithelial defect and infiltrate, nature of the infiltrate and the character of the edge, depth of stromal involvement, and associated thinning or perforation. Examine the surrounding cornea for evidence of satellite lesions, immune rings, or radial keratoneuritis. Look for evidence of limbal or scleral involvement.

Try to document all findings in a schematic diagram, as shown in Figure 28-2. This will help you properly analyze all the clinical signs and assess the response to therapy during follow-up visits.

Although clinical signs may be insufficient to confirm infection, to be safe, a break in the continuity of the epithelium associated with underlying stromal suppuration should be considered infectious unless proven otherwise. Although viral infection is the leading cause of corneal ulcer

Table 28-1

Differential Diagnosis of Microbial Keratitis

Slowly Progressive Localized Infiltrate Bacteria	*Rapidly Progressive Diffuse Suppurative Infiltrate Bacteria*

• Gram-positive
 ○ *Staphylococcus epidermidis*
 ○ α-hemolytic streptococci
 ○ *Actinomycetales*
  i. *Actinomyces*
  ii. *Nocardia*
  iii. *Mycobacterium*
• Gram-negative
 ○ *Moraxella*
 ○ *Serratia*
	• Gram-positive
	 ○ *Staphylococcus aureus*
	 ○ *Streptococcus pneumoniae*
	 ○ ß-hemolytic streptococci
	• Gram-negative
	 ○ *Pseudomonas*
	 ○ *Enterobacteriaceae*
	• Mixed infection
	• Drug toxicity

Fungi

• Filamentous fungi (*Fusarium, Aspergillus,* dematiaceous)
• Yeast (*Candida*)

Protozoa

• *Acanthamoeba*
• Microsporidia

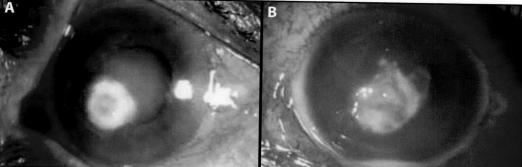

Figure 28-3. Corneal ulcer caused by (A) gram-positive bacteria *Streptococcus pneumoniae* and (B) gram-negative bacteria *Pseudomonas aeruginosa.*

in developed nations, bacteria, fungi, and *Acanthamoeba* all can invade the cornea to cause suppurative keratitis. A good practical approach to arriving at a diagnosis can be looking at the rate of progression and nature of infiltration (Table 28-1).

Some of the characteristic clinical pictures of infection by various organisms are shown in Figures 28-3 through 28-5.

Figure 28-4. Corneal ulcer caused by *Nocardia* asteroids.

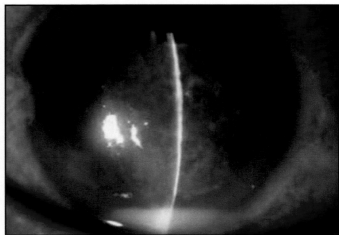

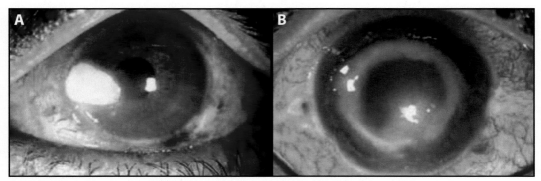

Figure 28-5. Corneal ulcer caused by (A) filamentous fungi and (B) *Acanthamoeba*.

It is important to remember that the clinical appearance of suppurative keratitis depends on many variables, and it is often difficult to arrive at an etiological diagnosis based entirely on slit-lamp examination.[2] Laboratory investigations are therefore required if the causative organism is to be identified. It consists of corneal scraping using a #15 surgical blade or Kimura spatula and inoculating it on various culture media that promote the growth of bacteria, fungi, and parasites, as shown in Figure 28-6. The initial management is based on smear examination.

Management

Facilities for detailed microbiology workup may not be available to many ophthalmologists, and because bacteria cause a significant percentage of suppurative keratitis cases and most antibacterial drugs are bactericidal, a practical approach could be used to perform laboratory workup only in patients with severe keratitis (corneal infiltrates more than 6 mm in size) or cases that show unusual clinical features.[3] In other cases, the following approaches can be adopted:

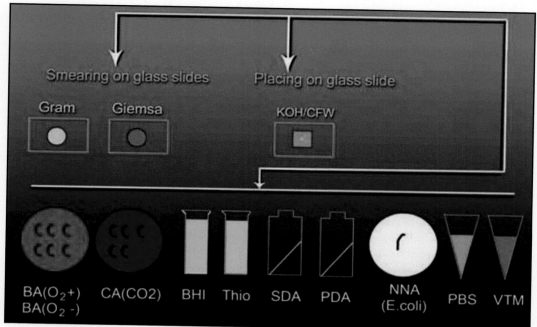

Figure 28-6. Schematic diagram of microbiology workup in corneal ulcer.

- Nonsevere keratitis (infiltrates less than 2 mm in size) and no clinical signs of fungal or *Acanthamoeba* infection: Treat empirically with broad-spectrum antibacterial therapy. Treatment can be started with one of the commercially available fourth-generation fluoroquinolones.

- Keratitis with infiltrates that are between 2 and 5 mm and no clinical signs of fungal or *Acanthamoeba* infection: Treat with either fourth-generation fluoroquinolones or a combination of fortified cefazolin (5%) and ciprofloxacin 0.3%.

- Nonsevere keratitis (infiltrate size less than 5 mm) with clinical evidence of fungal or *Acanthamoeba* infection and in geographical locations where such infections are common: Perform corneal scrapings and examine the material under a light microscope using 10% potassium hydroxide. Treatment with antifungal and anti-*Acanthamoeba* drugs should be started only if the smear is positive for these infections.

All antimicrobial drugs must be instilled frequently in the initial phase. Patients with severe keratitis may warrant inpatient treatment, whereas others can typically undergo outpatient treatment. However, we must review these patients almost every day for the first 3 to 4 days.

In addition to antimicrobial drugs, prescribe one of the cycloplegic agents and a systemic analgesic (if the patient has pain). Antiglaucoma drugs are necessary only if intraocular pressure is high.

In addition to antimicrobial therapy, one must treat associated conditions that result in persistence or progression of ulcerative keratitis, such as conjunctival foreign body, lagophthalmos, meibomitis, dacryocystitis, or drug toxicity.

Treatment Adjustment

The following modifications of treatment are based on the patient's clinical response and culture results:

- If the patient is responding to initial therapy, reduce the frequency of instillation to maintain therapeutic corneal concentrations of the drugs.

- If the patient is not responding to initial therapy and microbiology workup was not done, perform a detailed microbiology workup or refer the patient to a center where such facilities exist.

- If the patient is not responding to initial therapy and microbiology workup was performed, review the results of the culture and antimicrobial susceptibility and modify therapy accordingly. Repeat the microbiology test or perform a corneal biopsy if the tests are negative. In vivo confocal microscopy can be useful in patients with suspected fungal or *Acanthamoeba* keratitis.[4]

All patients with advanced disease or failed medical treatment will require surgical treatment in the form of full-thickness penetrating or lamellar keratoplasty.[5]

The patient presented herein has a large central corneal ulcer associated with inflammation of the lid margin. The infiltrate size is more than 6 mm, so we must perform corneal scrapings in this case. Initial treatment must be based on results of the microscopic examination of smears. In addition to antimicrobial therapy, this patient will require treatment for lid inflammation.

References

1. Sadowsky AE. Dermatological disorders. In: Krachmer JH, Mannis MJ, Holland EJ, eds. *Cornea*. Mosby; 1997:989-1002.
2. Thomas PA, Leck AK, Myatt M. Characteristic clinical features as an aid to the diagnosis of suppurative keratitis caused by filamentous fungi. *Br J Ophthalmol*. 2005;89(12):1554-1558.
3. McLeod SD, DeBacker CM, Viana MA. Differential care of corneal ulcers in the community based on apparent severity. *Ophthalmology*. 1996;103(3):479-484.
4. Kanavi MR, Javadi M, Yazdani S, Mirdehghanm S. Sensitivity and specificity of confocal scan in the diagnosis of infectious keratitis. *Cornea*. 2007;26(7):782-786.
5. Anshu A, Parthasarathy A, Mehta JS, Htoon HM, Tan DTH. Outcomes of therapeutic deep lamellar keratoplasty and penetrating keratoplasty for advanced infectious keratitis: a comparative study. *Ophthalmology*. 2009;116(4):615-623.

Celine E. Satija, MD and David R. Hardten, MD

The patient in Figure 28-1 shows a corneal epithelial defect with an underlying stromal infiltrate and a hypopyon, which is highly suspicious for an infectious corneal ulcer. This corneal ulcer does not have characteristic features that would point us to one organism; therefore, we would treat broadly and narrow our differential.

We start with a detailed history of the onset and duration of the patients' eye irritation and vision changes. We ask about an ocular history, including any recent surgeries; trauma; the use of contact lenses (eg, the type of contact lenses and routine hygiene of these lenses); ocular conditions such as dry eye, recurrent epithelial erosions, or herpetic or neurotrophic keratitis; and recent activities such as freshwater swimming, gardening, or handling of vegetative matter. We ask about systemic disease such as diabetes mellitus, malignancy, immunocompromised state, or use of immunocompromising drugs. We take note of the symptoms including pain, photophobia, redness, and discharge. We then perform a careful slit-lamp examination, and would start by evaluating the eyelids for any signs of inflammation or trauma. We evaluate for conjunctival injection, discharge, size of the infiltrate, size of the overlying epithelial defect, any satellite lesions, the character of the infiltrate (whether it is soupy like necrotic tissue or firm), corneal thinning, vascularization, surrounding corneal edema, amount of intraocular inflammation, keratic precipitates, and hypopyon. We measure corneal sensation using a cotton swab or esthesiometer, as any asymmetry in corneal sensation could suggest a herpetic or neurotrophic component. Finally, we carefully document these findings with colored drawings or, if available, slit-lamp photos, with and without fluorescein.

Workup

To identify the infectious source, we perform corneal scrapings for Gram staining, anaerobic and aerobic cultures, and fungal prep.[1] We typically use a drop of proparacaine to numb the eye, then scrape the ulcer from the base and rim with Kimura spatulas. If you do not have access to Kimura spatulas, you can also use a round knife, surgical blade, or large needle. We use these inoculated spatulas to form C shapes on the culture plates (blood agar, chocolate agar, and Sabouraud agar) and in the liquid broth (thioglycolate broth; Table 28-2). If we have a clinical suspicion for *Acanthamoeba* such as in a contact lens wearer with a ring ulcer or chronic ulcer, we also send an *Acanthamoeba* culture on a non-nutrient agar plate with *Escherichia coli* overlay both from the patient's eye and from the contact lens case. In addition, we perform confocal microscopy on the patient looking for *Acanthamoeba* cysts. If we suspect a viral or neurotrophic component, we send a culturette for polymerase chain reaction for herpes simplex virus. Ideally, these cultures would be completed prior to starting any treatment. Table 28-3 shows some common pitfalls to avoid in corneal culture.

Table 28-2
Methods Used in Laboratory Diagnosis of Infectious Keratitis

Smears	Gram stain	Bacteria
	Blankophor	Fungi
	Fresh mount, trichrome	*Acanthamoeba*
Media	Blood agar	Most bacteria, yeast, fungi
	Chocolate agar	Most bacteria, *Haemophilus*, *Neisseria*, *Moraxella*
	Chopped meat broth	Aerobic and anaerobic bacteria
	Sabouraud agar	Most fungi and yeast
	1.5% non-nutrient agar	*Acanthamoeba*
Polymerase Chain Reaction	—	Herpes simplex virus

Table 28-3
Pitfalls During the Process of Laboratory Diagnosis

Scrapes and Swabs	Only superficial debris on the surface of ulcer are taken Contamination Cotton swabs are inappropriate
Media	Old, inappropriate, or cold plates are used. The plates should stay 30 minutes at room temperature
Transport	Culture media are not kept room temperature during the transport (BenEzra)
Interpretation of the Result	Overestimation of nonpathogenic organisms and nonsignificant number of organisms

Treatment

We start treatment when cultures are obtained. In the case of small peripheral corneal ulcers with minimal anterior chamber reaction, we start moxifloxacin 0.5% (Vigamox; Novartis Pharmaceuticals) every 1 to 2 hours. We would then follow this patient closely, initially daily, until improvement is seen and then we start to taper the antibiotic after 48 hours or when the ulcer started to show improvement. After 48 hours of antibiotic usage, we consider adding a topical steroid.

Table 28-4

Preparation of Different Types of Fortified Antibiotics for the Treatment of Corneal Ulcers

Fortified Antibiotic	Instructions for Preparation
Gentamicin or tobramycin, 14 mg/mL	Add 2 mL of parenteral antibiotic (40 mg/mL) to a 5-mL bottle of gentamicin or tobramycin 3 mg/mL.
Vancomycin, 50 mg/mL	Withdraw 2 mL of balanced salt solution (BSS) or an artificial tear solution from a 10-mL bottle and inject it into the vial of powdered vancomycin 500 mg. When in solution, withdraw the entire volume and inject back into the bottle that contains 8 mL of BSS or artificial tears.
Cefazolin, 50 mg/mL	Add 10 mL of BSS or artificial tears to 500 mg of cefazolin dry powder to form a 10-mL solution of cefazolin 50 mg/mL, which is injected into a sterile eye drop bottle.

Adapted from Chandler JW, Sugar J, Edelhauser HF. External diseases: cornea, conjunctiva, sclera, eyelids, lacrimal system. In: Podos SM, Yanoff M, eds. *Textbook of Ophthalmology.* Vol 8. Mosby; 1994:11.8.

If the ulcer is greater than 1 mm, centrally located, and with significant anterior chamber reaction, we treat with fortified antibiotics every hour for 48 hours (vancomycin 50 mg/mL and tobramycin 14 mg/mL are most readily available in our region; Table 28-4).[2] Some clinicians use subconjunctival gentamicin or tobramycin daily for several days. We instruct patients to use a lot of lubricating drops, as the fortified antibiotics can irritate the conjunctiva significantly. We also prescribe a cycloplegic agent until the anterior chamber reaction resolves to reduce synechiae formation. While many patients can perform this care as an outpatient, some patients require inpatient admission due to frequency of drops or concern for drop compliance. We follow patients daily with slit-lamp examinations. Slit-lamp photos can be helpful for monitoring progress and showing patients their progress as well. Sometimes, it seems that the patients' eye looks worse on day 1 rather than better due to the increased injection from fortified antibiotics. We continue to see them every day until the ulcer starts to improve, taking note of the interval change in the size of the epithelial defect, amount of anterior chamber reaction, and consolidation of the infiltrate. We watch carefully to ensure that the area of ulceration is not becoming so thin that it may perforate. If the patient has a large corneal perforation, we perform an urgent penetrating keratoplasty.

When the ulcer starts to improve and the patient has had 48 hours of antibiotic therapy, we start to reduce the frequency of drops to every 2 hours during the day and every 4 hours at night. As cultures come back, we narrow our antibiotic choice based on sensitivities. As the ulcer improves, we continue to taper antibiotic frequency.

If the ulcer is not improving after 2 to 3 days of intensive antibacterial therapy, we start to think of alternative etiologies such as fungal or *Acanthamoeba*, especially if the patient is a contact lens wearer.[3] We consider reculturing the cornea or performing confocal microscopy to look for fungal or *Acanthamoeba* elements. If fungal keratitis is suspected, we add natamycin or amphotericin B every 1 or 2 hours. Oral ketoconazole, voriconazole, or fluconazole can also be given and are well tolerated. If the fungal keratitis does not improve, we consider intrastromal voriconazole or amphotericin B. If *Acanthamoeba* is suspected, we start the patient on polyhexamethylene biguanide every hour and propamidine (Brolene; Sanofi) every 2 hours. Patients with *Acanthamoeba* require treatment for at least 3 months and often up to 1 year. Polymicrobial infections can and do occur and are thought to create more inflammation with worse prognosis.[4]

When the ulcer starts to improve, we start adjunctive therapy with prednisolone acetate to reduce corneal scarring.[5] We start slowly, initially concurrent with antibiotics, as the local immunosuppression prevents migration of neutrophils and decreases opsonization, thereby potentially promoting infection.[6] If an epithelial defect becomes persistent once the ulcer is considered sterile, we place a bandage contact lens, and, if still not healed, we consider using amniotic membrane or a ring (ProKera; Bio-Tissue Inc) to help heal the epithelial defect.

References

1. Cohen EJ, Rapuano CJ. Bacteria keratitis, fungal keratitis, *Acanthamoeba*, herpes simplex virus, herpes zoster virus. In: Kunimoto DY, Kanitkar KD, Maker MS, Friedberg MA, Rapuano CJ, eds. *The Wills Eye Manual: Office and Emergency Room Diagnosis and Treatment of Eye Disease.* 4th ed. Lippincott Williams & Wilkins; 2004:52-65.
2. Chandler JW, Sugar J, Edelhauser HF. External diseases: cornea, conjunctiva, sclera, eyelids, lacrimal system. In: Podos SM, Yanoff M, eds. *Textbook of Ophthalmology.* Vol 8. Mosby; 1994:11.8.
3. Por YM, Mehta JS, Chua JL, et al. Acanthamoeba keratitis associated with contact lens wear in Singapore. *Am J Ophthalmol.* 2009;148(1):7-12.e2.
4. Tu EY, Joslin CE, Nijm LM, Feder RS, Jain S, Shoff ME. Polymicrobial keratitis: acanthamoeba and infectious crystalline keratopathy. *Am J Ophthalmol.* 2009;148(1):13-19.
5. Srinivasan M, Mascarenhas J, Rajaraman R, et al. The steroids for corneal ulcers trial (SCUT): secondary 12-month clinical outcomes of a randomized controlled trial. *Am J Ophthalmol.* 2014;157(2):327-333.e3. doi:10.1016/j.ajo.2013.09.025
6. O'Brien TP. Bacterial keratitis. In: Foster CS, Azar DT, Dohlman CH, eds. *Smolin and Thoft's The Cornea: Scientific Foundations and Clinical Practice.* 4th ed. Lippincott Williams & Wilkins; 2005:235-288.

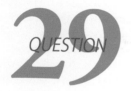

A 22-Year-Old Woman Complaining of Blurry Vision in One Eye Has Deep Sectoral Corneal Stromal Neovascularization With Stromal Infiltrate and Lipid Deposits in the Center of the Cornea. How Should I Manage This Patient?

Cullen D. Ryburn, MD and Derek W. DelMonte, MD

The most important aspect of appropriate management in this case is determining the etiology for the stromal infiltrate and neovascularization (NV). When corneal NV is associated with lipid deposits, it often indicates a chronic process. However, the original inciting event that led to the NV can vary widely, from a primary inflammatory process to an infectious cause. Other forms of keratitis, including neurotrophic or traumatic, as well as medication toxicity or contact lens overwear could also be considered.

A more complete history is required to filter this differential into a useful resource. For example, a rapid onset of pain and redness would suggest an acute inflammatory or infectious cause, whereas a history of poor contact lens hygiene may suggest contact lens overwear, or a lack of pain may indicate a neurotrophic etiology.

The physical examination is also helpful when evaluating the cause of corneal NV. Before looking at the cornea, make sure to take a good look at the eyelids and lashes. Staphylococcal marginal keratitis is a common and underdiagnosed entity originating from hyperreactivity to staphylococcal antigens as a result of overgrowth at the lid margin from poor meibomian gland health. One misconception regarding this disease comes from the belief that staphylococcal marginal disease should only exist perilimbal, where the lid margin and the cornea meet, but in severe and chronic cases, epithelial defects, NV, and lipid exudation can extend over the entirety of the cornea.

The next important aspect is the health of the epithelium overlying the infiltrate. Classically, the absence of epithelium indicates active disease in many disease processes, while some exceptions do exist, including syphilitic interstitial keratitis, herpetic stromal keratitis, and, occasionally, fungal keratitis. Make sure to measure and document the size of the epithelial defect and the stromal infiltrate separately, as this will be used as an objective clinical indicator for improvement.

Hardten DR, Hansen MS.
*Curbside Consultation in Cornea and External Disease:
49 Clinical Questions, Second Edition* (pp 169-171).
© 2022 Taylor & Francis Group.

If an epithelial defect with stromal infiltrate is present, corneal cultures are indicated. However, one must remember that persistent epithelial defects can cause significant NV in the absence of inflammation or infection. This is most commonly seen in neurotrophic disease and medication toxicity. To add another level of complexity, medication toxicity (overuse of fortified antibiotics or prolonged use of topical antivirals) can lead to a secondary neurotrophic keratitis. In patients with prior chemical injury or exposure to mitomycin-C (eg, history of refractive surgery, pterygium removal, glaucoma filtering surgery), limbal stem cell deficiency would also be included in the differential diagnosis for unhealthy epithelium.

If the epithelium is intact and the suspicion remains high for an infectious etiology with a deep stromal infiltrate, the most common etiologies would include fungal, herpetic, syphilitic, infectious crystalline keratitis from group A *Streptococcus* and *Acanthamoeba*. Again, a thorough history (including questions regarding contact lens wear, recent freshwater exposure, or history of oral or genital lesions) would be important when evaluating for these conditions. To aid in diagnosis, use an 8-0 Vicryl (or similarly braided) suture (Ethicon) by passing the needle and suture through the infiltrate. The suture material is then cut into pieces and placed on the appropriate culture media. A corneal biopsy could also be considered in difficult cases.

One should also examine the entire cornea, looking for other areas of stromal haze with or without underlying ghost vessels, which can be suggestive of a recurrent herpetic cause, and is often associated with decreased corneal sensation. Intraocular inflammation, such as anterior chamber cells or endothelial keratic precipitates as well as sectoral iris atrophy, would also be common findings in a herpetic cause.

Treatment Options

Treatment should be guided by the most likely cause of the NV. These can be difficult cases, so do not be afraid to change or adapt therapy if there is no response after a reasonable treatment duration. That being said, we try to avoid continually adding of therapy without tapering or removing failed therapy, as this can contribute to overmedication and toxicity.

Infectious corneal ulcers should have care directed toward their suspected microbial etiology. However, we would advocate that antifungal or antiparasitic agents should not be initiated without a confirmed positive culture. If the suspicion for fungal infection is high and cultures have been negative, then evaluation with a suture biopsy, corneal punch biopsy, or confocal microscopy can aid in diagnosis. If herpetic disease is suspected, the most common treatment pattern is using oral acyclovir or valacyclovir for 10 to 14 days. Patients with stromal scarring from repeated episodes of herpetic disease should have consideration for lifelong therapy at prophylactic dosing. The addition of topical steroids to control the inflammatory component in an active infectious ulcer remains controversial and should be used with caution.

Noninfectious epithelial defects with stromal infiltrate with NV presents unique challenges as well. Neurotrophic keratitis can be a difficult disease to treat. Epithelialization can be slow, even in aggressively treated cases, and chronic exposure generates stromal haze and NV. Until recently, the favored treatment patterns have focused on frequent lubrication with preservative-free artificial tears, serum tears, or placement of amniotic membranes. These conservative measures are excellent when they work, but in severe disease, the epithelium may break down and relapse despite aggressive treatment. More recently, there have been several treatment breakthroughs, including the topical application of recombinant human nerve growth factor. One such medication received US Food and Drug Administration approval in 2018, marking a significant advancement in the treatment of neurotrophic keratitis.[1] The other major change in treatment of neurotrophic keratitis involves a surgical approach. Corneal neurotization involves placing a nerve transplant or graft to provide new nerve fascicles to the corneal limbus.[2]

When discussing treatment for the NV itself, several medical and surgical approaches have been used with varying success. Topical corticosteroids are important in suppression of new NV in an acute inflammatory event; however, they have not been shown to be an effective treatment for mature NV. Use of topical nonsteroidal anti-inflammatory medications is also controversial and without good data to guide treatment patterns.[3] Recent research on the use of anti-vascular endothelial growth factor in corneal NV has shown that both topical and subconjunctival applications of bevacizumab can achieve significant reduction in NV.[4] Another recent study demonstrated reduced corneal NV and statistically significant improvement in vision by placement of 1% bevacizumab into a Prosthetic Replacement of the Ocular Surface Ecosystem (PROSE; Boston Sight) contact lens, with daily wear of 10 to 16 hours.[5] Gene-based therapies have been promising in animals studies, and antisense oligonucleotides targeting corneal NV have entered human clinical trials.[6] Fine-needle diathermy has been described as helpful for treating large feeder vessels. However, care must be taken to avoid too much thermal energy to the corneal-limbal area, which can lead to worsening inflammation and NV.[7]

In regard to NV from limbal stem cell deficiency, surgical interventions, such as limbal stem cell transplantation, have been shown to improve NV and visual acuity.[8] In cases of mild limbal stem cell deficiency, placement of amniotic membrane has also been shown to decrease NV and improve vision, with the benefit of avoiding the need for systemic immunosuppressive medications required for allogenic limbal stem cell transplantation.

Visual rehabilitation can begin when the active process is controlled and the NV has been minimized. Although contact lenses can be the cause of corneal NV if abused, they can also be helpful in the treatment and visual rehabilitation of these patients. Rigid gas permeable lenses or scleral lenses can help minimize higher-order aberrations induced by corneal scarring. Scleral lenses have made significant improvements in fit and comfort, decreasing the need for full-thickness corneal transplantation in scarred or ectatic corneas.

References

1. FDA approves first drug for neurotrophic keratitis, a rare eye disease. *FDA News Release.* August 22, 2018. Accessed October 13, 2021. https://www.fda.gov/news-events/press-announcements/fda-approves-first-drug-neurotrophic-keratitis-rare-eye-disease
2. Elbaz U, Bains R, Zuker RM, Borschel GH, Ali A. Restoration of corneal sensation with regional nerve transfers and nerve grafts: a new approach to a difficult problem. *JAMA Ophthalmol.* 2014;132(11):1289-1295.
3. Gupta D, Illingworth C. Treatments for corneal neovascularization: a review. *Cornea.* 2011;30(8):927-938.
4. Papathanassiou M, Theodoropoulou S, Analitis A, Tzonou A, Theodossiadis PG. Vascular endothelial growth factor inhibitors for treatment of corneal neovascularization: a meta-analysis. *Cornea.* 2013;32(4):435-444.
5. Yin J, Jacobs JD. Long-term outcome of using Prosthetic Replacement of Ocular Surface Ecosystem (PROSE) as a drug delivery system for bevacizumab in the treatment of corneal neovascularization. *Ocul Surf.* 2019;17(1):134-141.
6. Liu S, Romano V, Steger B, Kaye SB, Hamill KJ, Willoughby CE. Gene-based antiangiogenic applications for corneal neovascularization. *Surv Ophthalmol.* 2018;63(2):193-213.
7. Trikha S, Parikh S, Osmond C, Anderson DF, Hossain PN. Long-term outcomes of fine needle diathermy for established corneal neovascularisation. *Br J Ophthalmol.* 2014;98(4):454-458.
8. Tseng SC, Prabhasawat P, Barton K, Gray T, Meller D. Amniotic membrane transplantation with or without limbal allografts for corneal surface reconstruction in patients with limbal stem cell deficiency. *Arch Ophthalmol.* 1998;116(4):431-441.

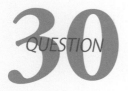

A Corneal Infiltrate Is Unresponsive to Topical Fluoroquinolones. Could This Be Acanthamoeba?

Elmer Y. Tu, MD

Acanthamoeba are free-living amoebae that form a resilient thick-walled cyst in harsh conditions. Keratitis is its most common human disease and should be considered in any patient with a corneal infiltrate that does not respond appropriately to traditional topical antibiotics, especially in contact lens wearers (comprising > 85% to 90% of *Acanthamoeba* keratitis [AK] cases in Western countries).[1] Exposure to nonsterile water as well as outdoor trauma are also common risk factors.[1] However, antibacterial resistance is not restricted to AK, so this differential must include viral, fungal, other parasitic, and increasingly fluoroquinolone-resistant bacterial pathogens, such as *Streptococcus* species and methicillin-resistant *Staphylococcus aureus*.

Evaluation and Diagnosis

The clinical presentation of AK may range from diffuse epitheliitis; mild foreign body sensation, with little or no stromal involvement (Figure 30-1) to the stromal ring-shaped infiltrate; radial keratoneuritis; and severe intractable pain nearly diagnostic of the infection (Figure 30-2). Disease is bilateral in up to 10% of AK cases and may be polymicrobial, previously identified concomitantly with viral, fungal, and bacterial pathogens. Because of the specificity and long duration of therapy, definitive microbiologic diagnosis is preferred, including histologic smears of corneal scrapings (Giemsa stain, Wright stain, Diff-Quik stain, KOH prep, Calcofluor White stain, and others) or culture (non-nutrient agar with *Enterobacter* overlay). Of these methods, sensitivity and specificity is highest for histologic methods, while cultures are positive in only 0% to 50% of clinical cases of AK. Increasing validation of polymerase chain reaction has promise in confirming the diagnosis of AK.[2]

Hardten DR, Hansen MS.
*Curbside Consultation in Cornea and External Disease:
49 Clinical Questions, Second Edition* (pp 173-176).
© 2022 Taylor & Francis Group.

Figure 30-1. Slit-lamp photo of a contact lens wearer with AK that is clinically restricted to the epithelial layer. Smears and confocal microscopy were grossly positive for the organism.

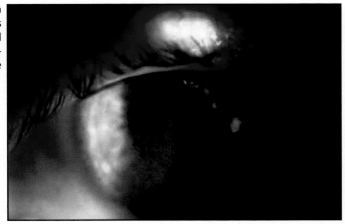

Figure 30-2. Slit-lamp photo of advanced AK showing a classic immune ring infiltrate with central haze and minimal necrosis, nearly pathognomonic for AK.

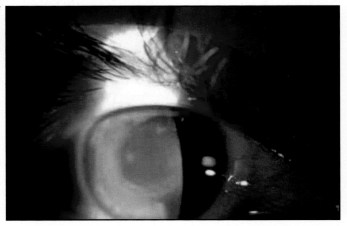

Confocal microscopy has been extensively used in the diagnosis of AK, but commercial availability of the units is becoming limited. These instruments offer en face serial sections of the cornea with high magnification and resolution, allowing in vivo imaging at a cellular level. Cysts are characteristically bright, reflective, circular opacities, often with internal structure visible (Figure 30-3). In centers familiar with its use, both the sensitivity and specificity of confocal microscopy in the diagnosis may exceed 90%.[2] Other imaging modalities have limited utility in AK.

Management

In the United States, no commercially available topical medications are known to be effective for AK. I strongly recommend mechanical debridement of any clinically involved epithelium to debulk the infectious load and obtain tissue samples. Rarely, this alone may be curative in epitheliitis, but I use this only as an adjunct to specific medical therapy. Primary topical therapy for AK has been either compounded chlorhexidine gluconate 0.02% (CHG) or polyhexamethylene biguanide 0.02% (PHMB; Bacquacil).[3] I maintain hourly dosing for the first 3 to 7 days, with a gradual taper over the first month to 4 times/day, continued for several months with a more

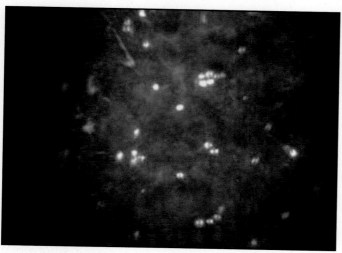

Figure 30-3. Confocal microscopy showing multiple bright, centered cysts in the anterior stroma (upper and right portions). Note that the appearance varies significantly with lighting and position.

gradual taper. However, the management is highly dependent on response to these medications, with some patients being treated for as little as a few weeks and others, usually those with deeper stromal involvement, requiring frequent dosing for an extended period of time. Because these agents have similar mechanisms of action, I do not initially use them together, preferring to vary concentration and/or frequency. I prefer CHG because it is better tolerated and can be increased in concentration to 0.04% or 0.06% if needed, although some patients with AK may be responsive to a change to PHMB.

The diamidines, propamidine isethionate 0.1% (Brolene; Sanofi) and hexamidine isethionate 0.1% (Desmodine; Bausch + Lomb), are mostly effective against the trophozoites, and are prescribed hourly for the first few days, with a rapid taper over the first month before surface toxicity ensues. However, these drugs are not currently available in the United States.

Other previously described topical agents (eg, neomycin, clotrimazole) have a minimal role in the current treatment algorithm for routine AK.

When Should Systemic Therapy, Steroids, or Therapeutic Keratoplasty Be Considered?

Because topical therapy is usually sufficient, routine systemic therapy is unnecessary. In advanced or poorly responding cases of AK, oral itraconazole (suspension preferred for greater absorption) has been described, although my own experience has been disappointing. Intravenous pentamidine and some of the newer systemic antifungal agents may be more effective but have not been extensively studied. Of these, systemic oral voriconazole 200 mg twice daily or higher dose, depending on serum levels, has shown some effect.[4] The approval of miltefosine, an alkyl-phosphocholine, for systemic leishmaniasis in the United States, has brought its designation by the US Food and Drug Administration in December of 2015 as a drug that can be used systemically for AK. I find the drug to more efficacious than previously described agents for severe disease.[5]

Therapeutic keratoplasty is reserved for recalcitrant cases or in impending perforations but with a guarded prognosis for failure, secondary glaucoma, and recurrent infection.[6] Lamellar keratectomy—manual, laser, or combined with keratoplasty—may be successful if infections are restricted to the anterior layers of the cornea. There is no role for collagen cross-linking as a primary treatment for AK and success as an adjunctive therapy when used with anti-*Acanthamoeba* drugs has been decidedly mixed. It may relieve pain by denervating the cornea, but it has been noted to have severely detrimental effects in more advanced cases. The role of corticosteroids and other immunosuppressant agents, both topical and systemic, has been clarified somewhat, with recent studies confirming that their use prior to effective anti-AK therapy is detrimental to prognosis, but concomitant use after 2 or more weeks of anti-AK therapy is helpful and necessary in patients with severe inflammatory sequelae, especially in those with intractable limbitis, scleritis, and/or uveitis.[7] Practically, I attempt to rapidly discontinue or reduce to the lowest effective level of topical and systemic corticosteroids in patients presenting with AK.

How Should the Clinical Response Be Assessed and Duration of Treatment Determined?

The assessment of clinical response can be challenging in AK. The presence of epithelial infestation and radial keratoneuritis is easy to assess and usually resolves rapidly, although radial keratoneuritis may uncommonly scar exuberantly. Stromal disease is more difficult to evaluate because the borders of the keratitis are diffuse and inflammation does not always correlate with infectious activity. While some cases of post-infectious sterile corneal inflammation have been described, persistent keratitis, unlike the extracorneal manifestations, should be considered infectious unless proven otherwise. When corticosteroids are used, a constant level should be maintained to permit interval assessments of inflammatory activity as an indirect indicator of disease activity. It should be noted that viable amoeba have been recovered months to years after initial symptoms, but usually with continuing treatment. By convention, a period of 3 months of quiescence off of all medications should be observed before a cure is assumed, but recurrences may rarely occur after this period.

References

1. Joslin CE, Tu EY, Shoff ME, et al. The association of contact lens solution use and *Acanthamoeba* keratitis. *Am J Ophthalmol.* 2007;144(2):169-180.
2. Tu EY, Joslin CE, Sugar J, Booton GC, Shoff ME, Fuerst PA. The relative value of confocal microscopy and superficial corneal scrapings in the diagnosis of *Acanthamoeba* keratitis. *Cornea.* 2008;27(7):764-772.
3. Papa V, Rama P, Radford C, Minassian DC, Dart JKG. *Acanthamoeba* keratitis therapy: time to cure and visual outcome analysis for different antiamoebic therapies in 227 cases. *Br J Ophthalmol.* 2020;104(4):575-581.
4. Tu EY, Joslin CE, Shoff ME. Successful treatment of chronic stromal *Acanthamoeba* keratitis with oral voriconazole monotherapy. *Cornea.* 2010;29(9):1066-1068.
5. Avdagic E, Chew HF, Veldman P, et al. Resolution of *Acanthamoeba* keratitis with adjunctive use of oral miltefosine. *Ocul Immunol Inflamm.* 201929(2):278-281.
6. Robaei D, Carnt N, Minassian DC, Dart JK. Therapeutic and optical keratoplasty in the management of *Acanthamoeba* keratitis: risk factors, outcomes, and summary of the literature. *Ophthalmology.* 2015;122(1):17-24.
7. Dart JKG, Saw VPJ, Kilvington S. *Acanthamoeba* keratitis: diagnosis and treatment update 2009. *Am J Ophthalmol.* 2009;148(4):487-499.e482.

A Corneal Infiltrate of a Farmer Hit by a Tree Branch Is Not Clearing on Topical Fluoroquinolone Drops. What Should I Do Next?

Erik Letko, MD

This patient is at risk for infectious keratitis—bacterial, fungal, or both. Corneal injury with an organic matter, such as a tree branch in this case, increases the suspicion of fungal infection. One should keep this possibility in mind at the initial visit and during the follow-up period, particularly if the patient does not respond to empiric topical antibiotics.

Epidemiology

The most common risk factors for fungal keratitis comprise corneal trauma with organic matter, eye conditions, including prior penetrating keratoplasty; ocular surface pathology; contact lens wear; use of corticosteroids; and systemic conditions such as diabetes mellitus, compromised immune system, chronic illness, or hospitalization. According to one report, the rate of contact lens–related keratitis doubled in recent years.[1] It is noteworthy that the incidence of fungal keratitis is higher in places with a warm and humid climate. A detailed medical and ocular history and examination play a critical role in assessing the degree of suspicion of fungal keratitis. Fungal keratitis varies, depending on geographic region, between 6% and 20% of all infectious keratitis cases in the United States.[2] *Aspergillus* (Figure 31-1), *Candida*, and *Fusarium* species are the most common pathogens.

Hardten DR, Hansen MS.
*Curbside Consultation in Cornea and External Disease:
49 Clinical Questions, Second Edition* (pp 177-179).
© 2022 Taylor & Francis Group.

Figure 31-1. *Aspergillus* keratitis. Note the irregular surface of the lesion.

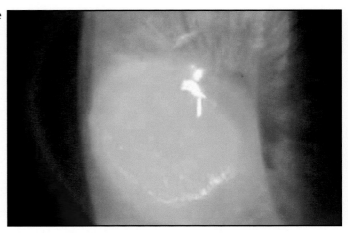

Signs and Symptoms

The symptoms of fungal keratitis typically do not present as acutely as those of bacterial keratitis. Clinical signs can vary widely, but certain slit-lamp findings, such as corneal lesions with feathery margins, satellite or branching lesions, irregular surface, or intact epithelium, are suspicious of fungal keratitis. However, one should keep in mind that all of these findings could be present with bacterial keratitis. Therefore, the presence of any or all of these signs raises the likelihood of fungal keratitis but does not confirm it. For these reasons, the diagnosis of fungal keratitis represents a challenge and is heavily dependent on laboratory methods.

Diagnosis

Harvesting a good specimen for stains and cultures plays a critical role in prompt diagnosis and treatment. The specimen should be obtained using a metal instrument, such as a spatula or surgical blade. The surgical blade might be preferable in cases where deeper scraping is needed. The specimen should contain a good sample of corneal epithelium and stroma from the area of the lesion. Removal of the involved epithelium and stroma plays not only a diagnostic role, but also a therapeutic one. In addition to Gram stain used routinely by most microbiology laboratories, special stains such as Giemsa and/or calcofluor may increase the chance of identifying fungus. The culture media should include sheep blood agar, Sabouraud agar, chocolate agar, and thioglycollate broth. Although not routinely used, brain-heart infusion broth could be requested to increase the diagnostic yield, particularly when routine cultures were negative and the degree of suspicion remains high.

In cases where stains and cultures of specimens scraped from the cornea are negative, corneal biopsy is indicated. If available, confocal microscopy can also be helpful. The biopsy could be performed with a 2- or 3-mm dermatologic trephine, lamellar keratectomy, or by passing a needle or suture through the involved stroma. The biopsy specimen should involve the infiltrated as well as normal tissue. It is important to keep in mind that fungi can penetrate intact Descemet's membrane and, in the presence of hypopyon or posterior corneal plaque, an anterior chamber tap may help address the question of whether the fungus invaded intraocularly. These diagnostic tools are important not only in establishing the diagnosis, but also in guiding the treatment.

Treatment

Difficulties with diagnosis, lack of commercially available topical antifungal agents, and poor penetration of these agents to deeper layers of the cornea, particularly if the epithelium is intact, represent challenges when treating fungal keratitis. The most common antifungal topical agents include polyenes (natamycin and amphotericin B) and azoles (eg, ketoconazole and voriconazole). Additionally, antiseptics such as polyhexamethylene biguanide, povidone-iodine, chlorhexidine, and benzalkonium showed some effect against fungal pathogens, but the literature data are limited.

Pimaricin (natamycin), the only commercially available antifungal eye drops in the United States, is typically used as a first-line agent once diagnosis of fungal keratitis is established. Amphotericin B (for *Candida* keratitis) and an azole (for *Aspergillus* keratitis) can be added as a second agent, particularly in cases where response to natamycin is not satisfactory. Intraocular antifungal agents can be used at the time of anterior chamber or vitreous tap in patients where suspicion of endophthalmitis exists. The use of systemic antifungal agents has to be judicial because their therapeutic effect on fungal keratitis or endophthalmitis is limited due to poor penetration and systemic side effects profile. The systemic use of voriconazole showed some promise in a recent study.[3] The length of treatment for fungal keratitis varies widely, depending on response. The minimum length of treatment is typically 1 month, but it is not unusual to use antifungal agents for several months. Repeat cultures or corneal biopsy might help determine when it is safe to cease the therapy. In patients who do not respond to antifungal agents, therapeutic keratoplasty might be needed.

Fungal keratitis represents diagnostic and therapeutic challenges. A thorough history, examination, and multiple diagnostic tests, often repeated, are required to establish the diagnosis and monitor treatment.

References

1. Jurkunas U, Behlau I, Colby K. Fungal keratitis: changing pathogens and risk factors. *Cornea*. 2009;28(6):638-643.
2. Alfonso EC, Rosa RH, Miller D. Fungal keratitis. In: Krachmer JH, Mannis MJ, Holland EJ, eds. *Cornea*. 2nd ed. Elsevier Mosby; 2005:1101-1114.
3. Bunya VY, Hammersmith KM, Rapuano CJ, Ayres BD, Cohen EJ. Topical and oral voriconazole in the treatment of fungal keratitis. *Am J Ophthalmol*. 2007;143(1):151-153.

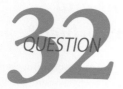

I Have a Patient With Shingles Over the Right Side of Their Face and Around the Eye Treated With Oral Antivirals for 10 Days. Does This Protect Them From Eye Involvement?

Celine E. Satija, MD and David R. Hardten, MD

Varicella zoster virus (VZV) is one of 8 DNA herpes viruses that cause disease in humans. In its most common manifestation as childhood chickenpox, VZV characteristically causes vesicular, pruritic, disseminated lesions at varying stages of maturity. Herpes zoster, or shingles, is a reactivation of the VZV, which typically lays dormant in the dorsal ganglion cells of the central nervous system. When it affects the nasociliary branch of the trigeminal nerve (V1), it is termed *herpes zoster ophthalmicus* (HZO) and can affect the eye. The typical presentation of HZO begins with a prodromal phase, with headache, photophobia, and malaise. Localized skin reactions, such as itching or tingling, can occur up to 1 week before the presentation of a painful rash that typically appears on the forehead, respects the midline, and is characterized by vesicles in different stages.[1] This rash can be accompanied by significant pain and a burning sensation. Vesicles on the tip or side of the nose, or the Hutchinson's sign, are indicative of V1 involvement and can help indicate that the globe may subsequently become involved. In the past, HZO was thought to primarily affect immunocompromised and older patients. Recent studies indicated that immunocompetent and younger patients are presenting with HZO. The mean age of onset is now in the sixth decade.[2]

The mainstay of treatment at this time is oral antiviral agents. Approved treatments for herpes zoster include acyclovir 800 mg 5 times/day for 7 to 10 days, famciclovir 500 mg 3 times/day for 7 days, or valacyclovir 1000 mg 3 times/day for 7 days, although immunocompromised patients may require longer durations of treatment. Acyclovir has been shown to shorten the duration of viral shedding, halt the rate and duration of new lesion formation, and decrease the overall pain level.[1] It is important to start treatment early, as starting treatment before 72 hours of disease onset has been shown to reduce eye disease at 6 months from 50% to 30%.[1]

Hardten DR, Hansen MS.
Curbside Consultation in Cornea and External Disease:
49 Clinical Questions, Second Edition (pp 181-183).
© 2022 Taylor & Francis Group.

How Does Eye Involvement Present and How Often Should the Patient Be Examined?

Ocular involvement in HZO most commonly presents with blepharoconjunctivitis. Blepharoconjunctivitis can be managed supportively with cool compresses and frequent lubrication. Skin lesions around the eye can be treated with antibiotic ointment such as erythromycin ointment or bacitracin ointment. HZO can also commonly affect the cornea and cause epithelial keratitis with branching, infiltrate dendrites with tapered ends. These are differentiable clinically from the herpes simplex dendrites, which are ulcerative and have terminal bulbs. Both herpes viruses can cause corneal denervation. Patients with keratitis can also develop a keratouveitis, with redness, photophobia, and blurred vision. Upon initial suspicion, plan to see the patient back within 1 week to monitor for keratitis or keratouveitis, which can develop as early as 1 to 2 days after the appearance of a rash (punctate epithelial keratitis) and as late as several months following the rash (deep stromal keratitis). Uveitis is managed typically with a topical steroid, such as prednisolone acetate 1% 4 times/day and cycloplegic drops (homatropine 5% 3 to 4 times/day or atropine 1% 1 time/day).

Zoster keratouveitis can become chronic or recurrent in 25% of patients up to 5 years after disease onset.[1] Sequelae of this uveitis include neurotrophic keratitis, segmental iris atrophy, glaucoma, and cataract formation. Cataracts can occur earlier in these patients and can be more complicated due to corneal scarring, decreased corneal sensation, abnormal iris/pupil posterior synechiae, and persistent intraocular inflammation.

A dreaded late clinical presentation of herpes zoster can occur in immunocompetent patients weeks to months after resolution of symptoms. Patients have rapid worsening of vision, with retinal whitening and hemorrhages termed *acute retinal necrosis*, which must be treated aggressively with systemic and intravitreal antivirals. There is also a suggestion that VZV may trigger giant cell arteritis, although additional studies are needed on this topic.[2]

The most significant long-term consequence of HZO is corneal disease, which occurs in approximately 40% of all cases.[3] Such patients often complain of decreased vision, photosensitivity, and pain. As the virus penetrates the epithelium and stroma, cumulative damage weakens the cornea, resulting in delayed epithelial healing and increased susceptibility to microtrauma. With continued progression, substantial corneal scarring can result, potentially leading to corneal thinning and perforation. In this scenario, you may need to discuss with your patient the possibility of full- or partial-thickness corneal transplantation. It is important to advise the patient that corneal sensitivity will decrease immediately after surgery, but it may slowly and partially recover with time. These patients should also be aware that vision is very difficult to predict after keratoplasty and that several months may pass before selective suture removal takes place for visual rehabilitation. Finally, these patients should know that once suture removal is completed, glasses and/or contact lenses may still be required to improve vision after transplantation and that irregular astigmatism and/or anisometropia may limit the quality of vision. Many of these transplant patients are also placed on long-term topical corticosteroid medication to help prevent the development of neovascularization, associated lipid deposition, and graft rejection that can develop months or even years after successful surgery.

Is Vaccination Helpful?

The role of vaccination in herpes zoster prevention has been established for some time, but not much is known about its specific value in precluding the development of ophthalmologic sequelae. There are currently 2 vaccines available for VZV, a zoster live vaccine (Zostavax) and a recombinant zoster vaccine (Shingrix; GlaxoSmithKline Biologicals). The zoster live vaccine contains live, attenuated varicella virus that induces protection 70% to 90% of the time. It has been shown to greatly bolster cell-mediated immunity and thereby reduce the probability of VZV reactivation. It is recommended that immunocompetent adults over the age of 50 years receive the vaccine. The recombinant zoster vaccine contains a recombinant VZV protein that induces protection 97% of the time compared with placebo. It is also recommended for use in immunocompetent adults over 50 years of age and can be given at the same time as the quadrivalent influenza vaccine.[2]

Although increasing evidence from the Herpetic Eye Disease Study shows that oral acyclovir use (400 mg twice daily) for at least 12 months substantially reduces the number of recurrences of herpes simplex ocular infection,[4,5] there is no evidence currently to support the prophylactic use of acyclovir or other antiviral medication in case of HZO. There is an ongoing multicenter study evaluating the role of prolonged suppressive antivirals in HZO, which will hopefully provide useful guidance in the clinical management of recurrent HZO in the future.

References

1. Gnann JW Jr, Whitley RJ. Herpes zoster. *N Engl J Med.* 2002;347(5):340-346.
2. Cohen EJ, Jeng BH. Herpes zoster and the Zoster Eye Disease Study (ZEDS). In: Colby K, Dana R, eds. *Foundations of Corneal Disease: Past, Present and Future.* Springer; 2020:63-72.
3. Arffa RC. Viral diseases. In: Arffa RC, Grayson M, eds. *Grayson's Diseases of the Cornea.* 4th ed. Mosby; 1997:283-337.
4. Herpetic Eye Disease Study Group. Oral acyclovir for herpes simplex virus eye disease: effect on prevention of epithelial keratitis and stromal keratitis. *Arch Ophthalmol.* 2000;118(8):1030-1036.
5. Uchoa UBC, Rezende RA, Carrasco MA, Rapuano CJ, Laibson PR, Cohen EJ. Long-term acyclovir use to prevent recurrent ocular herpes simplex virus infection. *Arch Opthalmol.* 2003;121(12):1702-1704.

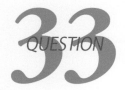

QUESTION

33

I HAVE A PATIENT WITH HERPES SIMPLEX DENDRITES. WHAT IS THE BEST PLAN TO MINIMIZE BOTH THE RECURRENCES AND POSSIBLE SCARRING?

Penny Asbell, MD, MBA;
Michael Wallace, MD; and Daniel Brocks, MD

The large, well-organized Herpetic Eye Disease Study (HEDS) continues to guide our treatment of herpes simplex virus (HSV) keratitis (Figure 33-1). It is clear from these investigations that the initial treatment of HSV epithelial keratitis with a topical antiviral agent hastens the healing process.[1,2] Since HEDS was published, several new topical antivirals have been introduced to the market, including ganciclovir ophthalmic gel 0.15% and acyclovir ointment. Ganciclovir gel has been approved by the US Food and Drug Administration (FDA) since 2009, but acyclovir ointment has not been approved by the FDA for ocular use. Studies comparing the 2 have shown similar treatment efficacy, but ganciclovir gel was better tolerated by patients. At the time of the HEDS study, trifluridine was the most commonly used topical antiviral agent for HSV keratitis, but its use has decreased since the introduction of these newer antiviral agents due to its side effects profile, notably severe ocular surface toxicity.[3] HEDS also suggested that adding an oral antiviral to topical antiviral treatment did not provide any additional benefit for treating dendritic keratitis, such as improving healing time or preventing possible additional corneal or intraocular involvement, including stromal keratitis or iridocyclitis.[1,2]

Less clear data are available regarding the use of mechanical debridement of the epithelium. A Cochrane database review revealed equivocal data as to whether adding debridement to a regimen of antiviral treatment had any benefit over topical antiviral treatment alone.[4]

The appropriate treatment to attempt to prevent recurrent herpetic eye disease requires a review of the findings of the HEDS–Acyclovir Prevention Trial. The study goal was to investigate the use of oral acyclovir 400 mg orally twice/day for 1 year vs placebo to assess the time to a recurrence of herpetic eye disease. The results showed that oral antiviral treatment reduced the rate of recurrence of herpetic eye disease by 41% in patients who had any form of HSV infection of the eye in the past year.[5] In addition, the rate of stromal keratitis was cut in half in those patients who specifically had stromal keratitis in the past year.[5]

Hardten DR, Hansen MS.
Curbside Consultation in Cornea and External Disease:
49 Clinical Questions, Second Edition (pp 185-189).
© 2022 Taylor & Francis Group.

Figure 33-1. HSV epithelial keratitis with dendritic (temporal) and geographic (inferior) lesions post–penetrating keratoplasty. (Reproduced with permission from B. Asghari, OD, BostonSight.)

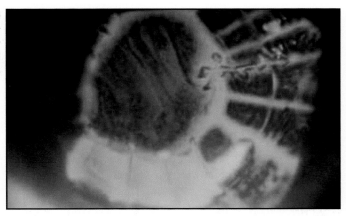

Overall, our routine care of patients with HSV epithelial keratitis includes topical or oral antivirals (oral is preferable in the presence of concurrent significant ocular surface disease), followed by a discussion with the patient regarding the usefulness of prophylaxis against recurrent disease with the use of oral antivirals. Since the HEDS study, several newer oral antivirals with greater bioavailability have been introduced, including valacyclovir and famciclovir. These agents require less frequent dosing compared with acyclovir, but they still carry the risk of renal toxicity.[3] Because most episodes of dendritic keratitis resolve without loss of vision, we generally do not suggest oral antivirals to prevent recurrences after an initial episode. In cases of recurrent stromal keratitis or if any one episode leaves residual scarring, chronic oral prophylaxis should be considered. If the patient chooses to start an antiviral, it need not be started until the current episode has resolved, as there has been no benefit found in using both topical and oral antivirals simultaneously in the treatment of a current episode of herpetic epithelial keratitis. Chronic oral antiviral usage necessitates comanagement with the primary medical physician for periodic renal function tests. Additionally, strict adherence to proper renal dosing is essential.

Management of Disciform Keratitis and Stromal Scarring

HSV disciform keratitis and stromal keratitis/scarring (Figures 33-2 and 33-3) treatment is also guided by the results of the HEDS.[6] Stromal keratitis can be divided into non-necrotizing and necrotizing. Non-necrotizing does not present with a concurrent epithelial defect, and the clinical manifestations are believed to manifest primarily from reactive, host immune-mediated stromal inflammation. Necrotizing, on the other hand, is a rare manifestation believed to be from direct viral invasion of the stroma, in addition to reactive immune stromal keratitis, and presents with an overlying epithelial defect, all of which leads to corneal ulceration.[3] The treatment of stromal keratitis was clearly shown in the HEDS to benefit from the addition of topical prednisolone phosphate 1% eye drops tapered over 10 weeks along with topical trifluridine. These patients, when compared to those who received placebo (artificial tears) and topical trifluridine only, had faster resolution of their stromal inflammation and showed no significant increase in recurrence rates. It is of vital importance to note that none of these patients had any active HSV epithelial keratitis (topical steroids are contraindicated in HSV epithelial keratitis). In addition, the use of oral acyclovir with the topical steroid/antiviral regimen was reviewed, and no significant advantage was found with adding the oral medication. Using this information, we typically treat patients with HSV stromal keratitis with the topical antiviral/steroid combination.

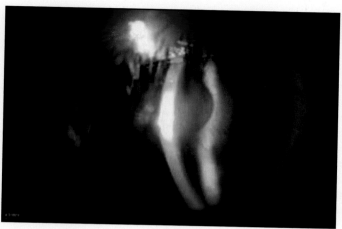

Figure 33-2. Active HSV stromal keratitis with keratic precipitates.

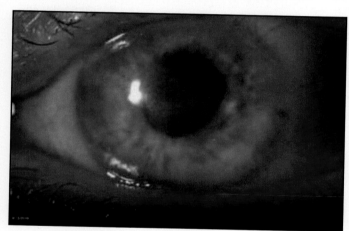

Figure 33-3. Limbal neovascularization post-HSV keratitis with residual central stromal scar. Some have advocated the use of bevacizumab topical eye drop therapy in these patients to treat neovascularization.

We generally recommend starting a combination of a topical steroid (eg, prednisolone acetate 1% or difluprednate 0.05%) about 4 times/day, combined with topical 0.15% ganciclovir gel 5 times/day. The topical steroid and ganciclovir should be slowly tapered together—for example, when the steroid is decreased to 3 times/day the ganciclovir should be similarly decreased to 4 times/day. Some patients may ultimately require a chronic, very low dose of a steroid, such as 2 to 3 times/week. Ideally, the topical antiviral should be continued until the patient is off of the steroid drops if possible. The later addition of an oral antiviral when the acute process has resolved should be discussed with the patient in an effort to decrease the risk of recurrences. Because stromal keratitis can cause corneal scarring and permanent loss of vision, prevention of recurrences is important, and the use of oral antivirals is always discussed and encouraged, unless contraindicated. The risks of oral antivirals are generally minimal and include diarrhea, nausea, and headache, but they can be more severe (ie, renal impairment). Given the likelihood of long-term use, we suggest ruling out impaired renal function prior to use as well as regular evaluation of serum kidney function tests while on the medication. Oral antivirals should be appropriately dosed according to kidney function (ie, estimated glomerular filtration rate). Avoidance is recommended if the patient is pregnant or nursing. It should be noted that the recurrence reduction effect of an oral antiviral ceases once the medication is discontinued.

New and Alternative Treatments

Research into alternative, more effective treatments is ongoing, and this research is vital due to inherent deficiencies with nucleoside analogs like acyclovir, ganciclovir, valacyclovir, and famciclovir. These deficiencies include emerging resistance to acyclovir, particularly among immunocompromised patients, and the fact that these medications do not directly inhibit viral protein synthesis. Instead, they act to prematurely terminate viral DNA synthesis. Of particular interest is the quest for an intervention that can prevent or eradicate HSV infection rather than to simply suppress the recurrent episodes that occur due to the ability of the virus to remain latent within the body. Research into novel treatment compounds, including BX795, nucleic acid aptamers, cationic peptides, and OGT 2115, is ongoing. There is also promising research in progress regarding the CRISPR/Cas9 system, a prokaryotic system for degrading the genetic material of viruses and how this system could be engineered and delivered into human cells for the eradication of even latent infections of HSV. Furthermore, monoclonal antibodies engineered to target viral glycoproteins have also been shown to be beneficial in treating HSV within animal models.[7]

Data are insufficient to come to a conclusion regarding whether diet modification plays a role in the treatment or prevention of HSV keratitis. Several animal models have shown that poor diet (malnourishment) may play an important role in the ability to heal after an HSV infection.[8] Other environmental factors were evaluated in the HEDS recurrence factor study. Specifically, patients with HSV ocular disease in the previous year were followed with a weekly questionnaire reviewing several study factors and reported whether ocular disease recurred. The study showed that no clear external factors, including psychological stress, systemic infection, ultraviolet exposure, contact lens wear, menstrual cycle, and eye injury, were associated with HSV ocular recurrence.[9] Recurrent herpes epithelial keratitis and iritis have been reported following corneal cross-linking with riboflavin and ultraviolet A for keratoconus.[10] Furthermore, recurrent HSV has also been reported after refractive laser treatment (LASIK, photorefractive keratectomy), and oral antivirals have been shown to be effective in preventing post-laser exposure HSV recurrences in an animal model.[11]

Long-Term Use of Antivirals

Although the HEDS–Acyclovir Prevention Trial showed that the use of oral acyclovir for 1 year decreased recurrence rates in patients who had previous HSV ocular disease in the preceding year, it did not answer the question of how long patients should remain taking oral antivirals. A 2003 retrospective study seemed to indicate that the use of oral acyclovir beyond 12 months continued to have efficacy in preventing ocular herpes recurrences.[12] The lack of information from a large population studied past 12 months of use must be reviewed with the patient, along with the risks, although they are fairly low for most patients on long-term oral antiviral systemic treatment. Overall, there seems to be a role for the long-term use of oral antivirals, particularly making sense in patients with a history of recurrent disease when off oral antivirals that has affected vision.

References

1. The Herpetic Eye Disease Study Group. A controlled trial of oral acyclovir for the prevention of stromal keratitis or iritis in patients with herpes simplex virus epithelial keratitis. *Arch Ophthalmol.* 1997;115(6):703-712.
2. Sudesh S, Laibson PR. The impact of the Herpetic Eye Disease Studies on the management of herpes simplex virus ocular infections. *Curr Opin Ophthalmol.* 1999;10(4):230-233.
3. Kalezic T, Mazen M, Kuklinski E, Asbell P. Herpetic eye disease study: lessons learned. *Curr Opin Ophthalmol.* 2018;29(4):340-346.
4. Wilhelmus KR. Interventions for herpes simplex virus epithelial keratitis. *Cochrane Database Syst Rev.* 2003;(3):CD002898.
5. Barron BA, Gee L, Hauck WW, et al. Herpetic Eye Disease Study. A controlled trial of oral acyclovir for herpes simplex stromal keratitis. *Ophthalmology.* 1994;101(12):1871-1882.
6. Wilhelmus KR, Gee L, Hauck WW, et al. Herpetic Eye Disease Study. A controlled trial of topical corticosteroids for herpes simplex stromal keratitis. *Ophthalmology.* 1994;101(12):1883-1895.
7. Koganti R, Yadavalli T, Shukla D. Current and emerging therapies for ocular herpes simplex virus type-1 infections. *Microorganisms.* 2019;7(10):429.
8. Benencia F, Gamba G, Benedetti R, Courreges MC, Cavalieri H, Massouh EJ. Effect of undernourishment on herpes simplex virus type 1 ocular infection in the Wistar rat model. *Int J Exp Pathol.* 2002;83(2):57-66.
9. Herpetic Eye Disease Study Group. Psychological stress and other potential triggers for recurrences of herpes simplex virus eye infections. *Arch Ophthalmol.* 2000;118(12):1617-1625.
10. Kymionis GD, Portaliou DM, Bouzoukis DI, et al. Herpetic keratitis with iritis after corneal crosslinking with riboflavin and ultraviolet A for keratoconus. *J Cataract Refract Surg.* 2007;33(11):1982-1984.
11. Asbell PA. Valacyclovir for the prevention of recurrent herpes simplex virus eye disease after excimer laser photokeratectomy. *Trans Am Ophthalmol Soc.* 2000;98:285-303.
12. Uchoa UB, Rezende RA, Carrasco MA, Rapuano CJ, Laibson PR, Cohen EJ. Long-term acyclovir use to prevent recurrent ocular herpes simplex virus infection. *Arch Ophthalmol.* 2003;121(12):1702-1704.

34
QUESTION

I Have a Patient With Diabetes Who Had Infectious Keratitis With a Bacterial Etiology, But Now After the Infection Has Cleared, I Can't Get the Epithelium to Heal. How Can I Best Manage This?

Shelby Anderson, OD and Ahmad Fahmy, OD

A recalcitrant, nonhealing epithelium is frustrating for patients and providers. The breakdown of this essential protective structure can lead to further infections, ulcers, and complications that continue to threaten the sight and comfort of the patient. It is important to trial all avenues necessary to aid in healing the epithelium in these cases, but what do you do when you have used all the preliminary therapeutic options, yet the epithelial defect persists?

Our patient is a 63-year-old White woman who had a persistent epithelial defect and epitheliopathy upon presentation to our clinic (Figure 34-1A). She had a vitrectomy for diabetic vitreous hemorrhage in the left eye 3 months prior. The patient had tried antibiotics, preservative-free lubricants, and steroids, all of which were unsuccessful in healing the corneal epithelium. Her vision was 20/300 with correction. Stage 3 neurotrophic keratitis with corneal melt was diagnosed due to absent corneal sensation throughout the cornea with cotton swab testing. We measured the epithelial defect to track progress of healing. The fellow eye was pseudophakic with mild diabetic retinopathy, best-corrected visual acuity was 20/20, and the eye had normal corneal sensation.

The options were reviewed with the patient. She was educated about the option of sewing an amniotic membrane in place, along with a permanent tarsorrhaphy, to help with healing and dryness, but the patient deferred. We then discussed the use of Oxervate (Dompé; cenegermin), a nerve growth factor that has been shown to improve corneal healing over a 2-month period of eye drop use. The patient elected to try for insurance coverage of Oxervate and was able to start treatment. Additionally, oral doxycycline and a combined nonpreserved lubricant/steroid were added to the treatment regimen to promote healing.

Hardten DR, Hansen MS.
*Curbside Consultation in Cornea and External Disease:
49 Clinical Questions, Second Edition* (pp 191-194).
© 2022 Taylor & Francis Group.

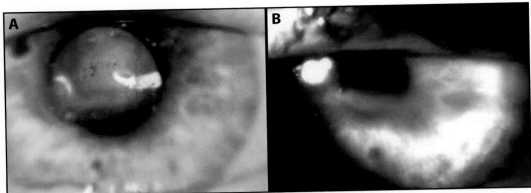

Figure 34-1. (A) The left eye of our 63-year-old woman with diabetes with a recurrent epithelial defect and severe keratopathy from topical medication toxicity. Visual acuity was 20/300 on presentation. (B) After a 2-month course of Oxervate, the epithelial defect was completely healed, and the keratopathy was resolved. Visual acuity was improved to 20/70.

Neurotrophic keratitis is a degenerative corneal condition in which there is reduced sensation of the cornea. The ophthalmic branch of the trigeminal nerve innervates the cornea, helps promote healing, and maintains the integrity and function of the corneal epithelium.[1] This condition presents from mild to severe, as defined by the Mackie classification.[2] Stage 1 includes corneal epithelial punctate staining and abnormalities with the tear film. Stage 2 is defined as a persistent epithelial defect, and stage 3 includes corneal neovascularization, ulceration with risk for perforation, corneal scar, and corneal melt.[3] Morphological changes to the subepithelial nerve plexus, including reduction in nerve density and branching, are observed in patients with neurotrophic keratitis.[4]

Degradation of the trigeminal nerve results in neurotrophic keratitis. Viral infections, such as herpetic keratitis, contact lens use, corneal dystrophies, and anesthetic abuse, can lead to initial epithelial insult, and when there is reduced innervation, it is difficult to heal the wound.[5] Brain surgery and anterior segment surgery can cause damage to the trigeminal nerve. Lesions in the brain along the course of the fifth nerve can cause impingement of the nerve. Other causes of trigeminal nerve damage can result in damage to corneal nerves, including chemical burn, ocular trauma, and even repeated/excessive use of preserved topical medications (as in glaucoma). Some systemic conditions lead to decreased corneal sensation, including multiple sclerosis and—as with our patient—diabetes.[1]

Diabetic peripheral neuropathy results in impaired sensation, foot ulceration, and amputation in 50% of patients with diabetes.[4] Small–nerve fiber injury is observed early in the disease state and can be observed in confocal microscopy studies of the corneal nerves of these patients. Corneal confocal microscopy studies have been proposed as surrogate markers for diabetic neuropathy. Decreased corneal function and lack of trophic support lead to corneal epithelial compromise in patients with neurotrophic keratitis.[4] With an estimated 34.2 million people diagnosed with diabetes mellitus in the United States and 1.5 million newly diagnosed yearly, it is critical for doctors of optometry and doctors of ophthalmology to think of neurotrophic keratitis as a possible contributor to corneal epithelial disease.[6]

Diagnosis of neurotrophic keratitis can be determined with a patient history, clinical examination, and corneal sensation testing. Patients often have a clinical history of poorly healing epithelial injury and symptoms of dryness, photophobia, or decreased vision. These patients can present with or without ocular pain. Using vital dyes in the assessment of patients suspected of neurotrophic keratitis is critical to observe epithelial irregularity, tear film insufficiency, hyperplasia, and a cloudy appearance, which is common in the early stages of neurotrophic keratitis. Staining the cornea also helps to accurately measure epithelial defects in stages 2 and 3.[3]

When neurotrophic keratitis is suspected, corneal sensation needs to be assessed, as reduced or absent corneal sensation is essential for diagnosis of this condition.[3] In the clinical research setting, quantitative sensation can be measured with an aesthesiometer. However, in clinic, a simple cotton wisp or dental floss test is performed on both eyes, and the responses are compared, providing the clinician with a quantitative measurement. An immediate blink reflex indicates normal sensation. Peripheral and central corneal sensation can be evaluated. Patients may exhibit a normal, reduced, or absent response when 4 quadrants are evaluated with the cotton wisp test.[7]

With early signs of neurotrophic keratitis (stage 1), palliative treatment can be helpful. The use of frequent lubrication with nonpreserved artificial tears is recommended, as well as appropriately discontinuing all topical medications, especially those with preservatives. In stages 2 and 3, treatment is more aggressive to help prevent progression, severe scarring, and vision loss.[8] The eyelids can help protect the cornea and promote healing through use of a tarsorrhaphy or medically induced ptosis with botulinum toxin. Additionally, a conjunctival flap or sutured amniotic membrane can be utilized. If the condition advances to corneal perforation, the cornea can be glued and may need a keratoplasty.[1]

Palliative treatment can be helpful, but disease recurrence can lead to a higher risk of visually significant subepithelial haze and a more onerous prophylactic treatment plan. Nerve growth factor is a novel option that has been shown to dramatically help patients with neurotrophic keratitis. This polypeptide stimulates neural cells to sprout and can possibly restore damaged neurons to help them function.[7] Recent studies evaluating neurotrophic persistent epithelial defects, with or without stromal thinning, have demonstrated that a 2-month course of the nerve growth factor Oxervate can resolve a nonhealing epithelial defect effectively.[8,9] During these studies, only mild adverse events were related to treatment with Oxervate, including eye pain, foreign body sensation, and tingling. In addition to resolution of corneal epithelial lesion size, other clinical studies have also demonstrated statistically significant improvements in corneal and conjunctival staining, tear break-up time, and osmolarity in patients with moderate to severe dry eye disease treated with Oxervate.[10] Oxervate is a noninvasive option that has had great success in helping these patients restore their cornea and prevent possible permanent vision loss.

After 2 months of Oxervate treatment, our patient had complete healing of the persistent epithelial defect and resolution of punctate keratopathy (Figure 34-1B). Her vision improved from 20/300 (pretreatment) to 20/70 (post treatment). Now, she is able to be fit with a rigid gas permeable contact lens to achieve improved acuity, although her vision will still be somewhat limited from diabetic macular disease. Treatment with Oxervate demonstrated an excellent benefit to risk ratio in this clinical case.

References

1. Sacchetti M, Lambiase A. Diagnosis and management of neurotrophic keratitis. *Clin Ophthalmol.* 2014;8:571-579.
2. Lambiase A, Rama P, Aloe L, Bonini S. Management of neurotrophic keratitis. *Curr Opin Ophthalmol.* 1999;10(4):270-276.
3. Dua HS, Said DG, Messmer EM, et al. Neurotrophic keratitis. *Prog Retin Eye Res.* 2018;66:107-131.
4. Tummanapalli SS, Willcox MDP, Issar T, et al. Tear film substance P: a potential biomarker for diabetic peripheral neuropathy. *Ocul Surf.* 2019;17(4):690-698.
5. Mastropasqua L, Massaro-Giordano G, Nubile M, Sacchetti M. Understanding the pathogenesis of neurotrophic keratitis: the role of the corneal nerves. *J Cell Physiol.* 2017;232(4):717-724.
6. Centers for Disease Control and Prevention. *National diabetes statistics report, 2020.* Updated February 11, 2020. Accessed October 17, 2021. https://www.cdc.gov/diabetes/library/features/diabetes-stat-report.html

7. Bonini S, Lambiase A, Rama P, Caprioglio G, Aloe L. Topical treatment with nerve growth factor for neurotrophic keratitis. *Ophthalmology.* 2000;107(7):1347-1351.
8. Bonini S, Lambiase A, Rama P, et al. Phase II randomized, double-masked, vehicle-controlled trial of recombinant human nerve growth factor for neurotrophic keratitis. *Ophthalmology.* 2018;125(9):1332-1343.
9. Pflugfelder SC, Massaro-Giordano M, Perez VL, et al. Topical recombinant human nerve growth factor (cenegermin) for neurotrophic keratopathy: a multicenter, randomized vehicle-controlled pivotal trial. *Ophthalmology.* 2020;127(1):14-16.
10. Sacchetti M, Lambiase A, Schmidl D, et al. Effect of recombinant human nerve growth factor eye drops in patients with dry eye: a phase IIa, open label, multiple-dose study. *Br J Ophthalmol.* 2020;104(1):127-135.

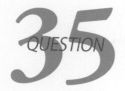
I Have a Patient With Material in the LASIK Interface at Day 1. What Do I Need to Look for to Diagnose and Manage This Problem?

Deepinder K. Dhaliwal, MD, L.Ac and Tarika Thareja, MD

The LASIK interface is a potential vulnerable space between the flap and stromal bed that can allow for the accumulation of debris, fluid, inflammatory and epithelial cells, and infectious microorganisms. While LASIK interface complications are relatively rare, a delay in recognition and treatment can lead to poor outcomes, such as flap melt, permanent corneal scarring, irregular astigmatism, and optic nerve damage. The differential diagnosis for material in the LASIK interface includes infectious keratitis, diffuse lamellar keratitis (DLK), pressure-induced stromal keratopathy (PISK), central toxic keratopathy, epithelial ingrowth, and interface debris. Although these entities may share some clinical features, particularly in the initial phases of the patient's presentation, a focused history with an emphasis on distinguishing features, such as time of presentation after surgery and the presence and severity of symptoms coupled with key clinical examination findings (such as the appearance and depth of the material), can help to hone in on the diagnosis. Ophthalmologists and eye care providers must be aware of strategies to rapidly differentiate among these conditions to allow for early recognition and prompt initiation of effective treatment.

Microbial Keratitis

Infectious keratitis after LASIK is a rare yet potentially sight-threatening complication. Early-onset infections (defined as onset within the first 2 weeks of surgery) usually start 2 to 3 days after surgery and are due to common bacterial organisms, such as staphylococcal species. In 2011, a survey by the American Society of Cataract and Refractive Surgery revealed that methicillin-resistant

Hardten DR, Hansen MS.
Curbside Consultation in Cornea and External Disease:
49 Clinical Questions, Second Edition (pp 195-199).
© 2022 Taylor & Francis Group.

Figure 35-1. Photograph of fungal keratitis post-LASIK. Note the central area of infiltration and a large, whitish endothelial mass extending into the anterior chamber from 4 o'clock to 5 o'clock. The causative organism was *Acremonium* species, and the patient ultimately required penetrating keratoplasty. (Reproduced with permission from Devin Tran, MD.)

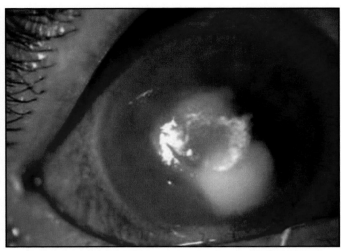

Staphylococcus aureus has emerged as the most common pathogen implicated in post-LASIK infections, mirroring the trend of increasing rates of all methicillin-resistant *Staphylococcus aureus* ocular infections.[1]

Late-onset keratitis, occurring 2 weeks to 3 months after surgery, is commonly due to opportunistic organisms, such as fungi and nontuberculous mycobacteria (NTM). Until the past decade, NTM species were the most commonly reported cause of post-LASIK infections and were implicated in several epidemics across the country related to the use of contaminated water and ice in the surgical environment.[2] However, with greater attention to sterile techniques and the routine postoperative use of fourth-generation fluoroquinolones, cases of nontuberculous mycobacterial keratitis after LASIK are now exceptionally rare.[1]

Patients with infectious keratitis are commonly symptomatic, with significant ocular pain and a variable degree of visual impairment. The infiltrate is typically focal and dense in appearance, with surrounding inflammation, and may extend anteriorly into the flap or posteriorly into the stroma, particularly in fungal infections that can penetrate Descemet's membrane (Figure 35-1). Conjunctival hyperemia and anterior chamber inflammation are often present. An epithelial defect may or may not be present, as it is not a required point of entry for the infectious organism.

Potential sources of contamination for post-LASIK infections include the patient's ocular flora, surgical equipment, fluids applied to the eye or to instruments, airborne contaminants, or inoculation from patients' hands postoperatively. Standard measures and protocols should be followed to decrease the risk of contamination from all these causes. Preoperatively, any ocular surface disease should be treated aggressively to decrease the bacterial load and optimize outcomes. Perioperative antimicrobial prophylaxis with a fourth-generation fluoroquinolone and antisepsis of the periocular area with a povidone-iodine solution is recommended, as well as careful placement of sterile drapes to completely isolate all eyelashes and meibomian gland orifices. Intraoperatively, all fluids applied to the eye and all instruments must be sterile. A separate set of instruments for each eye will eliminate the risk of cross-contamination. Finally, patients should be counseled to avoid swimming, gardening, and exposure to dirty or dusty environments for at least 2 weeks after surgery and to seek prompt attention for any warning symptoms or signs.

For both early- and late-onset infections, the mainstay of treatment is early lifting of the flap for cultures and smears, irrigating the flap interface with appropriate antibiotics, and repositioning the flap (unless necrotic). We typically use fortified vancomycin with moxifloxacin for early-onset disease and fortified amikacin with moxifloxacin for late-onset infection. Appropriate culture media include chocolate agar, blood agar, Sabouraud agar, and thioglycolate broth, with the addition of Lowenstein-Jensen medium or Middlebrook 7H9 agar for late-onset keratitis (although NTM will grow on blood agar). Smears should be sent for Gram and Giemsa stains, and special stains, such as Ziehl-Neelsen, can be considered if infection with NTM or filamentous bacteria is suspected.[1] Topical treatment with appropriate antimicrobials hourly around the clock should be initiated, as well as the prompt discontinuation of topical steroids and initiation of oral doxycycline 100 mg twice daily if corneal melting is present.

Diffuse Lamellar Keratitis

DLK is a post-LASIK complication in which white inflammatory cells enter the flap interface from the peripheral cornea, starting soon after surgery. While there are cases of delayed-onset DLK in the setting of corneal trauma, this is unusual and, in fact, if DLK is to develop, there will almost always be some evidence of it on the postoperative day 1 examination. Thus, the appearance of any new interface inflammation or infiltrate on the postoperative week 1 examination after the interface was noted to be clear previously should raise a high suspicion for infection.

Numerous risk factors for DLK have been proposed, including intraoperative epithelial defects, bacterial endotoxins from sterilization units, debris on microkeratome blades, and meibomian gland secretions.[3] In bilateral surgery, DLK typically affects both eyes, although to a varying degree, regardless of whether the surgeries were done simultaneously or sequentially.[4]

The most commonly used classification system, proposed by Eric Linebarger et al,[5] defines 4 stages of disease, based on severity and location. In stage 1, fine, flat, white granular cells are present in the interface in the flap periphery, which can sometimes be mistaken with meibomian gland secretions in the interface that will have more of an oily or refractile appearance. It is important to note that the cellular infiltration in DLK is *confined to the interface* and does not extend anteriorly into the flap or posteriorly into the stroma (in contrast to infectious keratitis). Stage 2 is the central migration of cells, resulting in the appearance of moderate, diffuse interface infiltration (Figure 35-2). Stage 3 DLK is characterized by the accumulation of more confluent and densely clumped cells in the visual axis, with clearing of the peripheral cornea. By stage 4, there is evidence of dense haze, with scarring and stromal melting. Also, in contrast to infectious keratitis post-LASIK, eyes with DLK typically appear white and quiet, and symptoms of photophobia and discomfort are usually mild. Vision is generally preserved in stages 1 and 2 and often mildly affected in stage 3.

Key principles in the management of DLK include early aggressive steroid therapy, close follow-up, and prompt surgical intervention at onset of stage 3 disease. Our treatment protocol for stage 1 disease consists of topical prednisolone acetate 1% every hour while awake and a nightly steroid ointment. Stage 2 DLK is treated with the same topical regimen with the addition of a short course of an oral corticosteroid (either a Medrol [methylprednisolone] dose pack or oral prednisone at a dose of 60 to 80 mg daily, depending on degree of inflammation and patient weight). Typically, if adequate treatment is initiated, cells in stage 1 will migrate centrally and then dissipate. The location of the cells will change, but the density will not increase. Patients are followed daily to monitor progression until the disease begins to regress. Recognition of the small percentage of cases that progress to stage 3 disease, typically between postoperative days 2 and 4, is critical and should trigger surgical intervention without delay. This entails lifting the flap to its hinge, gently irrigating the posterior surface of the flap and interface with cold balanced salt solution to eliminate the inciting toxins, and floating the flap back into position.

Figure 35-2. Photograph of late stage 2 DLK with increased density of cells in the visual axis.

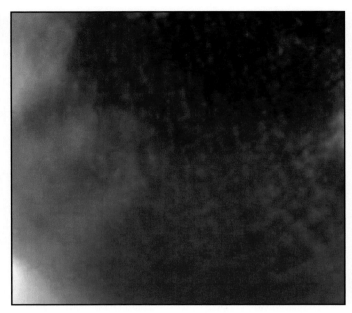

Other Etiologies

It is not uncommon to see interface debris on postoperative day 1, resulting from meibomian gland secretions, surgical sponge fibers, makeup particles, and glove talc, among others. It can be prevented by performing adequate, gentle irrigation of *both* sides of the flap and the stromal bed. Although interface debris is typically innocuous, it should be documented and observed closely to ensure that its appearance does not worsen over time, which would be indicative of an alternative diagnosis.

PISK, also referred to as *interface fluid syndrome*, is a condition in which high intraocular pressure (IOP) results in interface fluid accumulation in the setting of topical steroid use. It has been shown to develop anywhere between 1 week to years after LASIK surgery. On examination, there is evidence of diffuse interface haze, which can mimic that of DLK, and, in severe cases, there is a visible fluid cleft separating the anterior flap from the stromal bed (Figure 35-3).[6] One of the diagnostic challenges of PISK is that IOP measurements may not necessarily be elevated. Both the anatomical changes in the cornea post-refractive surgery and the shifting interface fluid can lead to underestimation of IOP when measured over the flap. A more reliable method to determine IOP is to take measurements peripheral to the flap with either a pneumotonometer or the Tono-Pen (Reichert Technologies).[7] Anterior segment optical coherence tomography can also be a very helpful diagnostic tool. PISK should be considered in presumed DLK cases that do not respond to or even worsen with steroid treatment, in the presence of significant IOP elevation, and in patients on chronic topical steroids. Management includes the discontinuation of steroids and lowering of IOP.

Central toxic keratopathy is a rare, noninflammatory condition of unknown etiology that can typically present 3 to 9 days after surgery as a central opacification of the cornea, often extending beyond the confines of the interface and typically accompanied by striae.[8] It presents acutely and does not worsen with time, but it can take months to more than 1 year to gradually clear. While no intervention is required and recovery is quite good, a persistent hyperopic shift resulting from central stromal tissue loss is not uncommon.[8]

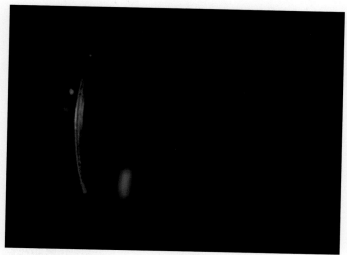

Figure 35-3. Slit-lamp photograph of PISK post-LASIK with a visible fluid cleft. (Reproduced with permission from Mahfouth A. Bamashmus and Mahmoud F. Saleh.)

References

1. Solomon R, Donnenfeld ED, Holland EJ, et al. Microbial keratitis trends following refractive surgery: results of the ASCRS infectious keratitis survey and comparisons with prior ASCRS surveys of infectious keratitis following keratorefractive procedures. *J Cataract Refract Surg.* 2011;37(7):1343-1350. doi:10.1016/j.jcrs.2011.05.006
2. Winthrop KL, Steinberg EB, Holmes G, et al. Epidemic and sporadic cases of nontuberculous mycobacterial keratitis associated with laser in situ keratomileusis. *Am J Ophthalmol.* 2003;135(2):223-224. doi:10.1016/S0002-9394(02)01955-4
3. Stulting RD, Randleman JB, Couser JM, Thompson KP. The epidemiology of diffuse lamellar keratitis. *Cornea.* 2004;23(7):680-688. doi:10.1097/01.ico.0000127477.14304.de
4. McLeod SD, Tham VMB, Phan ST, Hwang DG, Rizen M, Abbott RL. Bilateral diffuse lamellar keratitis following bilateral simultaneous versus sequential laser in situ keratomileusis. *Br J Ophthalmol.* 2003;87(9):1086-1087. doi:10.1136/bjo.87.9.1086
5. Linebarger EJ, Hardten DR, Lindstrom RL. Diffuse lamellar keratitis: diagnosis and management. *J Cataract Refract Surg.* 2000;26(7):1072-1077. doi:10.1016/S0886-3350(00)00468-5
6. Randleman JB, Shah RD. LASIK interface complications: etiology, management, and outcomes. *J Refract Surg.* 2012;28(8):575-586. doi:10.3928/1081597X-20120722-01
7. Bamashmus MA, Saleh MF. Post-LASIK interface fluid syndrome caused by steroid drops. *Saudi J Ophthalmol.* 2013;27(2):125-128. doi:10.1016/j.sjopt.2013.03.003
8. Sonmez B, Maloney RK. Central toxic keratopathy: description of a syndrome in laser refractive surgery. *Am J Ophthalmol.* 2007;143(3):420-427. doi:10.1016/j.ajo.2006.11.019

A Patient With Red, Irritated Eyes, Tearing, and Photophobia That Started Yesterday Has Mild Conjunctival Injection and 2+ Follicles of the Palpebral Conjunctiva. When the Patient Awoke, Their Eyelids Were Stuck Closed. Is This Acute Conjunctivitis?

Andrea Blitzer, MD and Marian Macsai, MD

The examination showed conjunctival injection, inflammation, and exudate (Figure 36-1). Conjunctivitis, or inflammation of the conjunctiva, is characterized by injection, dilated vessels, exudate, and often chemosis. In patients with acute conjunctivitis (less than 3 weeks), the history, age, duration of symptoms, clinical examination, type of exudate, and conjunctival scrapings help to determine the etiology.

Acute Papillary Conjunctivitis

Conjunctival papillae, a nonspecific sign of inflammation, are caused by edema and polymorphonuclear cell infiltration.[1] The hypertrophic projections of epithelium contain a central fibrovascular core on the palpebral conjunctiva. In adult patients with acute papillary conjunctivitis and mucopurulent discharge, infection by *Staphylococcus aureus*, *Haemophilus influenzae*, and streptococci are common. Methicillin-resistant *S aureus* conjunctivitis is increasing among the nursing home population and in community-acquired infections.[2] *H influenza* conjunctivitis occurs in adults chronically colonized with the bacteria, such as smokers or patients with chronic pulmonary disease.[1]

H influenza biotype III (previously called *H aegyptius*) presents with conjunctival hemorrhages, peripheral keratitis, and stromal infiltrates (Figure 36-2). In contrast, *S pneumoniae* presents with inflammatory tarsal membranes and conjunctival hemorrhages. Bacterial conjunctivitis is frequently bilateral; therefore, nasolacrimal duct obstruction, dacryocystitis, or canaliculitis should be considered in an adult with a unilateral presentation. Underlying risk factors, such as dry eye,

Hardten DR, Hansen MS.
Curbside Consultation in Cornea and External Disease:
49 Clinical Questions, Second Edition (pp 201-205).
© 2022 Taylor & Francis Group.

Figure 36-1. Acute conjunctivitis with purulent discharge on the lashes as well as diffuse conjunctival injection and edema.

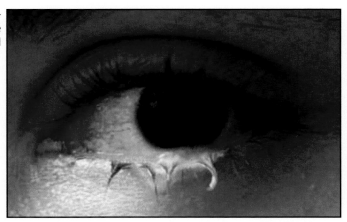

Figure 36-2. *H influenzae* biotype III (*H aegyptius*) with conjunctival hemorrhages, peripheral keratitis, and stromal infiltrates.

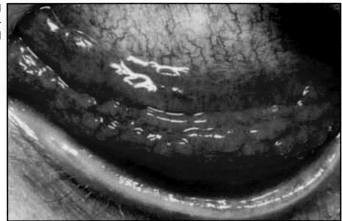

exposure due to lid abnormalities, untreated blepharitis, vitamin A deficiency, or immunosuppression, require evaluation and management after resolution of the initial episode.

In healthy adults, mild bacterial conjunctivitis may be self-limited, but using topical antibacterial drops is associated with earlier remission, occurring in 2 to 5 days in more than 60% of patients compared with placebo.[3] Our initial antibiotic choice is usually empirical, and we use polymyxin/trimethoprim drops 4 times/day for 1 week. Available as a generic, this antibiotic provides broad-spectrum coverage at a low cost to the patient, which increases compliance. Patients are instructed to follow up in 3 to 4 days if they note no improvement. In patients who are debilitated, immunocompromised, unresponsive to initial treatment, or have severe cases of purulent conjunctivitis, we perform Gram-stained smears and cultures of their conjunctiva.

In cases of acute papillary conjunctivitis with hyperpurulent discharge, *Neisseria gonorrhoeae* or *N meningitides* must be suspected.[4] Patients present with massive purulent exudation, severe chemosis, and a rapidly progressive course, often less than 24 hours. If left untreated, there may be progression to corneal ulceration, perforation, and systemic meningococcal dissemination. When gonococcal infection is a possibility, Gram stain and culture with chocolate agar media in a 4% to 8% CO_2 environment are done, and systemic therapy with daily follow-up is initiated. Frequent saline lavage can provide comfort, decrease inflammation, and prevent corneal melting. Patients without corneal ulceration are treated with 1 g of ceftriaxone given intramuscularly, whereas patients with corneal involvement re-ceive intravenous ceftriaxone (1 g every 12 hours for 3 days)

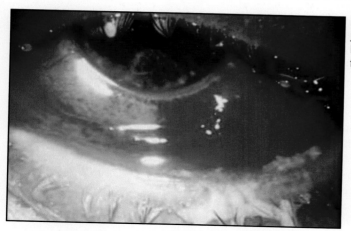

Figure 36-3. Acute follicular conjunctivitis in an adult patient, with large follicles present in the inferior fornix.

and a topical antibiotic ointment. Patients and sexual contacts are informed about the possibility of concomitant chlamydial disease. Additionally, sexual abuse is considered in children with this presentation.

In the pediatric population, the differential diagnosis for acute papillary conjunctivitis includes *S aureus, H influenza, S pneumoniae,* anaerobic bacteria (*Peptostreptococcus* species and *Peptococcus* species), and *Moraxella* species.[1] *H influenza* can occur in association with otitis media or preseptal cellulitis, which may predispose children to a fulminant meningitis. Of note, vaccination against *H influenza,* or Hib, has significantly reduced the incidence of *H influenza* conjunctivitis.

Acute Follicular Conjunctivitis

Acute follicular conjunctivitis may result from viral infections or early chlamydial inclusion conjunctivitis.[1] Follicles are aggregates of lymphocytes surrounded by mast cells and plasma in the superficial conjunctival stroma (Figure 36-3). Often, nonspecific concomitant papillae are present. Chlamydial infection from serotypes D through K is suspected in sexually active patients with unilateral acute conjunctivitis, scant discharge, and preauricular lymphadenopathy. Typically, follicles become more prominent in the second or third week of presentation. Epithelial infiltrates and micropannus involving the superior cornea may also be noted. In adult chlamydial inclusion conjunctivitis, we prescribe 1 oral dose of azithromycin 1000 mg or doxycycline 100 mg twice daily for 7 days.[2] Coinfection with gonorrhea and syphilis must be investigated, and all sexual partners must be treated.

A variety of viruses cause acute follicular conjunctivitis, including herpes simplex virus (HSV), *Paramyxoviridae,* measles, mumps, and Newcastle disease, with adenovirus being the most common.[1] Adenovirus presents as follicular conjunctivitis, epidemic keratoconjunctivitis (EKC), or pharyngeal conjunctival fever. Patients with EKC typically present with follicular conjunctivitis and preauricular lymphadenopathy, corneal subepithelial infiltrates by day 10 to 14, and blurred vision or photophobia. The highly contagious nature of this disease requires patient education to avoid transmission and possible quarantine. Patients should be reassured that EKC is self-limited. The mainstay of treatment has been aimed at symptomatic relief with the use of artificial tears, topical antihistamines, or cold compresses.[2] If a conjunctival membrane forms, debridement can be performed for patient comfort. Early clinical trials have demonstrated the efficacy of a combination of povidone-iodine (0.4% to 1.0%) and dexamethasone (0.1%) eye drops used 4 times daily to accelerate symptom resolution and adenoviral eradication.[5-7] This combination has also been shown to decrease the development of subepithelial infiltrates.[6] Topical corticosteroids should be used cautiously. Steroids provide initial symptomatic relief, but monotherapy with dexamethasone was associated with a slower rate of viral eradication and an increased risk of subepithelial infiltrates.[6] Subepithelial infiltrates with resultant visual degradation are more severe and difficult to eradicate after steroid treatment. Thus, treatment with topical corticosteroids alone is not recommended.

Pharyngeal conjunctival fever presents acutely with follicular conjunctivitis, fever, pharyngitis, and submandibular lymphadenopathy. In contrast to EKC, pharyngeal conjunctival fever rarely involves the cornea or forms membranes.

Primary HSV causes an acute follicular conjunctivitis with serous discharge and preauricular lymphadenopathy that is often associated with a vesicular lesion on the lid margin, fever, and upper respiratory symptoms.[1] Approximately 50% of patients have concomitant corneal epithelial punctate staining or dendrites. Treatment of HSV conjunctivitis includes use of topical trifluridine 1% solution 8 times/day, oral acyclovir 200 to 400 mg 5 times/day, oral valacyclovir (500 mg 2 or 3 times/day), or famciclovir (250 mg twice/day) for the prevention of corneal infection.[2]

Acute Membranous Conjunctivitis

The etiology of acute membranous or pseudomembranous conjunctivitis may be elusive and requires that cultures be obtained.[1] Common causes include EKC, HSV, beta-hemolytic streptococci, S aureus, and rarely C diphtheria.

As discussed, being able to classify the type of conjunctivitis is essential in determining the etiology, directing the necessary laboratory workup, and tailoring therapy.

Giant Papillary Conjunctivitis

Unlike the other types of conjunctivitis mentioned here, giant papillary conjunctivitis (GPC) is not caused by an infection. Instead, it is directly correlated to the presence of a foreign body that is in contact with the palpebral conjunctiva. Patients with GPC present with ocular irritation, redness, and itching. Examination reveals papillae on the upper palpebral conjunctiva that are larger than 0.3 mm. GPC is classically associated with contact lenses, and it is most commonly seen in patients who exchange their contact lenses infrequently or are allergic to their contact lens solution. GPC can also be caused by chronic microtrauma from exposed sutures or ocular prostheses. The pathophysiology of GPC involves both mechanical irritation and immune-mediated inflammation.[8] Untreated GPC can lead to contact lens intolerance and, in extreme cases, cause damage to the cornea, as the giant papillae abrade the corneal surface with each blink.

The primary treatment for GPC is to remove the aggravating entity. Contact lens wearers should go on a contact lens holiday, and any exposed sutures should be removed, replaced, or rotated so that the suture knot is buried. In patients with an allergic component, topical antihistamines may improve symptoms. Steroids can be considered in refractory cases.[9] Contact lens wearers can reduce their risk of GPC by changing their contact lenses and cases frequently, using nonpreserved contact lens solution, limiting the number of hours per day that they wear contact lenses, and ensuring that they have a good fit of their lenses.

References

1. Krachmer JH, Mannis MJ, Holland EJ. *Cornea: Fundamentals, Diagnosis and Management*. Vol 1, 2nd ed. Mosby; 2005.
2. American Academy of Ophthalmology Cornea/External Disease Panel, Preferred Practice Patterns Committee. *Conjunctivitis*. American Academy of Ophthalmology; 2008.
3. Sheikh A, Hurwitz B. Antibiotics versus placebo for acute bacterial conjunctivitis. *Cochrane Database Syst Rev.* 2006;19(2):CD001211.
4. Ullman S, Roussel TJ, Forster RK. Gonococcal keratoconjunctivitis. *Surv Ophthalmol.* 1987;32(3):199-208.
5. Pinto RDP, Lira RPC, Abe RY, et al. Dexamethasone/povidone eye drops versus artificial tears for treatment of presumed viral conjunctivitis: a randomized clinical trial. *Curr Eye Res.* 2015;40(9):870-877.
6. Kovalyuk N, Kaiserman I, Mimouni M, et al. Treatment of adenoviral keratocon-junctivitis with a combination of povidone-iodine 1.0% and dexamethasone 0.1% drops: a clinical prospective controlled randomized study. *Acta Ophthalmol.* 2017;95(8):e686-e692.
7. Pepose JS, Ahuja A, Liu W, Narvekar A, Haque R. Randomized, controlled, phase 2 trial of povidone-iodine/dexa-methasone ophthalmic suspension for treat-ment of adenoviral conjunctivitis. *Am J Ophthalmol.* 2018;194:7-15.
8. Elhers WH, Donshik PC. Giant papillary conjunctivitis. *Curr Opin Allergy Clin Immunol.* 2008;8(5):445-449.
9. Bartlett JD, Howes JF, Ghormley NR, Amos JF, Laibovitz R, Horwitz B. Safety and efficacy of loteprednol etabonate for treatment of papillae in contact lens-associated giant papillary conjunctivitis. *Curr Eye Res.* 1993;12(4):313-21.

SECTION V

CORNEAL REFRACTIVE

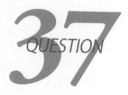

My Patient Underwent LASIK Previously and Now Is Interested in Cataract Surgery. What Is the Most Appropriate Formula for IOL Calculations? Would They Be a Good Candidate for a Multifocal IOL? What About After Corneal Cross-Linking?

Brent Kramer, MD and Mitch Ibach, OD

Advancements in cataract surgery and intraocular lenses (IOLs) have led to improved refractive outcomes, which in turn has led to higher patient expectations. The same patient population that invested in their vision to achieve spectacle independence with laser vision correction (LVC) surgery earlier in life may now desire to invest again to re-achieve spectacle independence—this time for both distance and near. Cataract surgery in patients with previous corneal refractive surgery is an ever-evolving subject, as there continues to be improvements with the initial laser surgery, IOL formulas, and IOL technology. Herein are a few considerations when you find this patient in your chair, asking about their options.

Patient Selection

It is important that these patients considering premium IOLs undergo the same rigorous evaluation to ensure they have not developed any underlying pathology since their initial LVC surgery. Treating any underlying surface disease, such as dry eye or anterior basement membrane dystrophy, should remain a high priority. While topography is essential for all patients considering a premium IOL, an extra consideration for this patient population is to ensure that there is no underlying ectatic process and that their ablation is well centered. Assessing the amount of higher-order aberrations is also key.

While improvements in IOL formulas have been made, it is a far from perfect process in LVC patients. With current technology and methods, one can expect that only 60% to 70% of their patients will fall within 0.5 diopters of their target.[1] A postoperative plan for refractive misses

Hardten DR, Hansen MS.
Curbside Consultation in Cornea and External Disease:
49 Clinical Questions, Second Edition (pp 209-215).
© 2022 Taylor & Francis Group.

needs to be clearly laid out for each individual patient. Assessing the residual stromal bed depth is critical to ensure that a patient is a candidate for a laser refractive touch-up. If this is not an option, ametropia can be managed only by spectacle correction or a lens exchange. If that is not a reasonable plan for the patient or surgeon, diffractive multifocal IOLs should be avoided.

The initial indication for refractive surgery should also be considered. Patients with mild myopic ablations typically tolerate multifocal IOLs more so than patients with hyperopic ablations or a high amount of either ablative pattern.[2,3] Monovision with monofocal IOLs is a low-risk alternative for patients who tolerated this as their initial LVC target.

Patient Counseling

Setting reasonable expectations through patient counseling is one of the most important steps of standard cataract surgery with a monofocal IOL, and it is even truer for the LVC patient who is investing in a premium IOL. A patient who enjoyed years of spectacle independence on postoperative day 1 after LASIK may be approaching this surgery with that exact expectation as well. Explain to the patient that this may be a multistep process that requires secondary steps, such as a YAG capsulotomy or laser touch-up, and that, rarely, despite a rigorous selection process, intolerable glare and halo may require an IOL exchange.

IOL Formulas

THE PROBLEM

The difficulty with IOL calculations for eyes with previous LASIK/photorefractive keratectomy (PRK) exists for 3 main reasons:

1. Index of refraction error: Keratometers and topographers measure the radius of curvature of the anterior cornea and then use a standard index of refraction (1.3375 in the Gullstrand eye, which is NOT uniformly used by all devices) to calculate its power in diopters. When eyes undergo LASIK/PRK, the anterior surface of the cornea changes, while the posterior surface largely remains the same, rendering the standard index of refraction invalid and the measured corneal power inaccurate[4] (Figure 37-1).

2. Radius error (also known as *instrument error*): Most devices produce a "Sim K," which is commonly used in IOL power calculations, by taking paracentral corneal measurements and extrapolating the central power. In cases of small and/or decentered ablations, this will be inaccurate.[5]

3. Effective lens position error: A majority of third-generation and later formulas utilize the measured corneal power to determine the effective lens position. Underestimation occurs in myopic ablations and overestimation occurs in hyperopic ablations.

If no consideration is taken, myopic ablations would result in a hyperopic surprise, and hyperopic ablations would result in a myopic surprise.

A FEW SOLUTIONS

Since Holladay's initial publication on the matter in 1989, there have been 30+ proposed formulas for post-LVC patients.[1,6] While no gold standard has been established, a few methods have stood out from the others as follows:

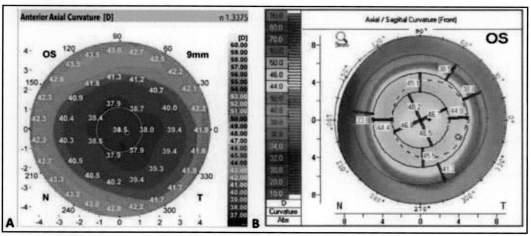

Figure 37-1. Post-ablative topography. (A) GALILEI G4 (Ziemer Ophthalmic Systems) demonstrating central cornea flattening after a myopic ablation. (B) Pentacam (OCULUS) demonstrating central corneal steepening after a hyperopic ablation.

- Barrett True-K: Regardless of historical data availability, the Barrett True-K has been proven to be the most accurate formula for both myopic and hyperopic ablations, and it is typically what we use.[7-9] The Barrett True-K Toric formula is also available for patients with a significant amount of corneal astigmatism. With rollout of version 2.0 of these formulas, Dr. Barrett has allowed users to enter the posterior corneal power (opposed to using his standard regression formula). While data have yet to be published, preliminary results are promising.[10] Both formulas are freely available on the Asia Pacific Association of Cataract & Refractive Surgeons website.

- American Society of Cataract and Refractive Surgery Post-Refractive Calculator (Figure 37-2): Drs. Hill, Wang, and Koch have helped to develop a calculator that allows users to enter data once and obtain results from a few of the most accurate formulas (individual and averaged together). Some of these formulas have been shown to be more accurate than others, but a downfall is when there are outliers, which can leave surgeons wondering.[8]

- Intraoperative Aberrometry (Figure 37-3): The Optiwave Refractive Analysis System (Alcon Laboratories Inc) is a key tool to have in the toolbox and can be used as a confirmatory measurement for the most difficult cases. Limited literature have shown promising results when compared with some of the most accurate formulas.[11-13]

Not listed here are many other methods that have been shown to be reliable. It is critical to stay up to date on the most current literature, as this is a rapidly evolving area that will continue to improve.

IOL Selection

There have been numerous studies that have shown the safety and efficacy of diffractive multifocal IOLs in patients with previous myopic[3,8,14-17] and hyperopic[2,9,18,19] ablations. As mentioned previously, patient selection and patient counseling is key. While no standard cutoff has been established, higher ablations lead to more corneal higher-order aberrations, which in turn leads to more bothersome dysphotopsias for the patient. When selecting the IOL, it is important to

A

IOL Calculator for Eyes with Prior Myopic LASIK/PRK
(Your data will not be saved. Please print a copy for your record.)

Please enter all data available and press "Calculate"

Doctor Name Brent Kramer	Patient Name Prev Myope	Patient ID 2020
Eye OD	IOL Model ZC800	Target Ref (D) 0

Pre-LASIK/PRK Data:

Refraction*	Sph(D)	Cyl(D)*	Vertex (If empty, 12.5 mm is used)
Keratometry	K1(D)	K2(D)	

Post-LASIK/PRK Data:

Refraction*§	Sph(D) -0.50	Cyl(D)* +1.25	Vertex(If empty, 12.5 mm will be used) 12.5
Topography	EyeSys EffRP	Tomey ACCP Nidek#ACP/APP	Galilei TCP2 41.36
Atlas Zone value	Atlas 9000 4mm zone		Pentacam TNP_Apex_4.0 mm Zone
Atlas Ring Values	0mm	1mm	2mm 3mm
OCT (RTVue or Avanti XR)	Net Corneal Power	Posterior Corneal Power	Central Corneal Thickness

Optical/Ultrasound Biometric Data:

Ks	K1(D) 42.25	K2(D) 43.28	Device Keratometric ● ○ ○ Index (n) 1.3375 1.332 Other
	AL(mm) 24.35	ACD(mm) 3.35	Lens Thick (mm) 4.61 WTW (mm) 11.7
Lens Constants**	A-const(SRK/T) 119.3	SF(Holladay1) 2.02	
	Haigis a0 (If empty, converted value is used) -1.023	Haigis a1 (If empty, 0.4 is used) +0.174	Haigis a2 (If empty, 0.1 is used) +0.286

*if entering "Sph(D)", you must enter a value for "Cyl(D)", even if it is zero.
§Most recent stable refraction prior to development of a cataract.
Magellan ACP or OPD-Scan III APP 3-mm manual value (personal communication Stephen D. Klyce, PhD).
**Enter any constants available; others will be calculated from those entered. If ultrasonic AL is entered, be sure to use your ultrasound lens constants. It is preferable to use optimized a0, a1, and a2 Haigis constants.

Calculate	Reset Form

IOL calculation formulas used: Double-K Holladay 1[1], Shammas-PL[2], Haigis-L[3], OCT-based[4], & Barrett True K[5]

B

Using ΔMR		Using no prior data	
[1]Adjusted EffRP	--	[2]Wang-Koch-Maloney	--
[2]Adjusted Atlas 9000 (4mm zone)	--	[2]Shammas	20.97 D
[1]Adjusted Atlas Ring Values	--	[3]Haigis-L	--
Masket Formula	--	[1]Galilei	19.51 D
Modified-Masket	--	[2]Potvin-Hill Pentacam	--
[1]Adjusted ACCP/ACP/APP	--	[4]OCT	--
[5]Barrett True K	--	[5]Barrett True K No History	20.78 D

Average IOL Power (All Available Formulas):   20.42 D

Min: 19.51 D

Max: 20.97 D

Figure 37-2. The online American Society of Cataract and Refractive Surgery post-refractive IOL calculator for previous myopic patients. Hyperopic and RK options are also available. (A) The data entry page can be populated based on the technology you have available to you. Be sure to enter the correct A-constants for your IOL/Biometry. (B) The results section displays the IOL power recommended to achieve the desired refractive target. More formulas populate as more data are entered and details for each formula can be seen by clicking on their name. (Source: Accessed online August 2019; ASCRS.org.)

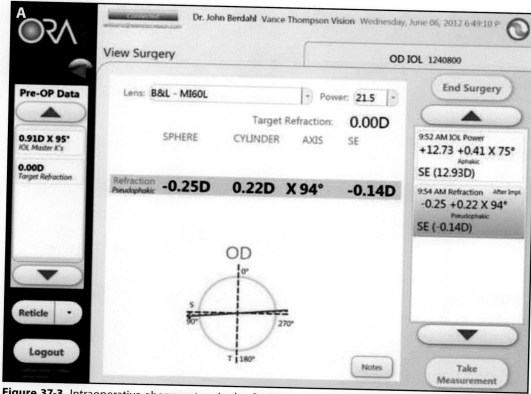

Figure 37-3. Intraoperative aberrometry via the Optiwave Refractive Analysis System showing both (B) aphakic and (A) pseudophakic measurements. (Reproduced with permission from Alcon Laboratories Inc.) *(continued)*

remember that myopic ablations induce positive spherical aberrations and therefore, in theory, benefit from an aspheric IOL, while the opposite is true for hyperopic ablations, which induce negative spherical aberrations and benefit from spherical IOLs.

GOING FORWARD

The Light Adjustable Lens (RxSight Inc) has a lot to offer patients with previous refractive surgery. All the difficulties of IOL power calculation are minimized, with the surgeon being able to dial in any postoperative refraction and ultimately minimize this refractive error with ultraviolet light polymerization of the lens "inside the eye." This allows the surgeon to "just get close," and then come back and adjust with ultraviolet light. This will be of particular benefit for patients who are not candidates for or do not desire postoperative LASIK/PRK.

Corneal Cross-Linking

Since its US Food and Drug Administration-approval in 2016, more post cross-linking (CXL) patients are presenting for cataract surgery. The biggest consideration that needs to be taken for these patients is whether or not the cornea is still changing. While CXL is an effective treatment for halting the progression of corneal ectasia, the average patient will also experience a residual flattening and decrease in their irregular astigmatism. It is ideal to wait 6 to 12 months to ensure

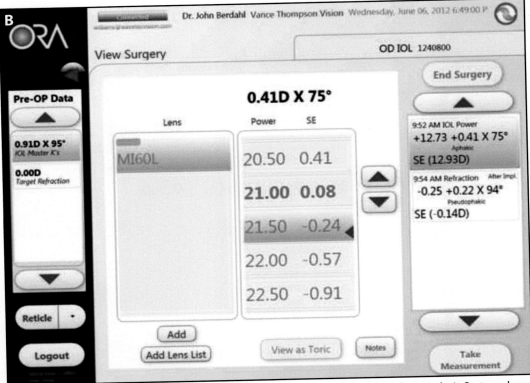

Figure 37-3 (continued). Intraoperative aberrometry via the Optiwave Refractive Analysis System showing both (B) aphakic and (A) pseudophakic measurements. (Reproduced with permission from Alcon Laboratories Inc.)

the shape of the cornea has stabilized. However, if CXL has just been performed or is planned to be performed after cataract surgery (a discussion beyond the scope of this question), one should aim slightly myopic in anticipation of a hyperopic shift. Also note that in some cases, the cornea continues to flatten, even after 12 months.

References

1. Savini G, Hoffer KJ. Intraocular lens power calculation in eyes with previous corneal refractive surgery. *Eye Vis (Lond).* 2018;5:18.
2. Alfonso JF, Fernández-Vega L, Ortí S, Ferrer-Blasco T, Montés-Micó R. Refractive and visual results after implantation of the AcrySof ReSTOR IOL in high and low hyperopic eyes. *Eur J Ophthalmol.* 2009;19(5):748-753.
3. Vrijman V, van der Linden JW, van der Meulen IJE, Mourits MP, Lapid-Gortzak R. Multifocal intraocular lens implantation after previous corneal refractive laser surgery for myopia. *J Cataract Refract Surg.* 2017;43(7):909-914.
4. Wang L, Mahmoud AM, Anderson BL, Koch DD, Roberts CJ. Total corneal power estimation: ray tracing method versus Gaussian optics formula. *Invest Ophthalmol Vis Sci.* 2011;52(3):1716-1722.
5. Savini G, Carbonelli M, Barboni P, Hoffer KJ. Clinical relevance of radius of curvature error in corneal power measurements after excimer laser surgery. *J Cataract Refract Surg.* 2010;36(1):82-86.
6. Holladay JT. Consultations in refractive surgery. *Refract Corneal Surg.* 1989;5:203.
7. Abulafia A, Hill WE, Koch DD, Wang L, Barrett GD. Accuracy of the Barrett True-K formula for intraocular lens power prediction after laser in situ keratomileusis or photorefractive keratectomy for myopia. *J Cataract Refract Surg.* 2016;42(3):363-369.

8. Vrijman V, Abulafia A, van der Linden JW, van der Meulen IJE, Mourits MP, Lapid-Gortzak R. Evaluation of different IOL calculation formulas of the ASCRS calculator in eyes after corneal refractive laser surgery for myopia with multifocal IOL implantation. *J Refract Surg.* 2019;35(1):54-59.

9. Vrijman V, Abulafia A, van der Linden JW, van der Meulen IJE, Mourits MP, Lapid-Gortzak R. ASCRS calculator formula accuracy in multifocal intraocular lens implantation in hyperopic corneal refractive laser surgery eyes. *J Cataract Refract Surg.* 2019;45(5):582-586.

10. Barrett G. Getting it right when the cornea has been adjusted. Session SYM-107. Presented at: ASCRS 2019 Annual Meeting; May 3-7, 2019; San Diego, CA.

11. Ianchulev T, Hoffer KJ, Yoo SH, et al. Intraoperative refractive biometry for predicting intraocular lens power calculation after prior myopic refractive surgery. *Ophthalmology.* 2014;121(1):56-60.

12. Fram NR, Masket S, Wang L. Comparison of intraoperative aberrometry, OCT-based IOL formula, Haigis-L, and Masket formulae for IOL power calculation after laser vision correction. *Ophthalmology.* 2015;122(6):1096-1101.

13. Fisher B, Potvin R. Clinical outcomes with distance-dominant multifocal and monofocal intraocular lenses in post-LASIK cataract surgery planned using an intraoperative aberrometer. *Clin Exp Ophthalmol.* 2018;46(6):630-636.

14. Alfonso JF, Madrid-Costa D, Poo-López A, Montés-Micó R. Visual quality after diffractive intraocular lens implantation in eyes with previous myopic laser in situ keratomileusis. *J Cataract Refract Surg.* 2008;34(11):1848-1854.

15. Fernández-Vega L, Madrid-Costa D, Alfonso JF, Montés-Micó R, Poo-López A. Optical and visual performance of diffractive intraocular lens implantation after myopic laser in situ keratomileusis. *J Cataract Refract Surg.* 2009;35(5):825-832.

16. Ferreira TB, Pinheiro J, Zabala L, Ribeiro FJ. Comparative analysis of clinical outcomes of a monofocal and an extended-range-of-vision intraocular lens in eyes with previous myopic laser in situ keratomileusis. *J Cataract Refract Surg.* 2018;44(2):149-155.

17. Palomino-Bautista C, Carmona-González D, Sánchez-Jean R, et al. Refractive predictability and visual outcomes of an extended range of vision intraocular lens in eyes with previous myopic laser in situ keratomileusis. *Eur J Ophthalmol.* 2019;29(6):593-599.

18. Alfonso JF, Fernández-Vega L, Baamonde B, Madrid-Costa D, Montés-Micó R. Visual quality after diffractive intraocular lens implantation in eyes with previous hyperopic laser in situ keratomileusis. *J Cataract Refract Surg.* 2011;37(6):1090-1096.

19. Vrijman V, van der Linden JW, van der Meulen IJE, Mourits MP, Lapid-Gortzak R. Multifocal intraocular lens implantation after previous hyperopic corneal refractive laser surgery. *J Cataract Refract Surg.* 2018;44(4):466-470.

38 QUESTION

I HAVE A PATIENT WITH A PHAKIC IOL THAT NOW HAS A CATARACT. WHAT SPECIAL METHODS DO I NEED TO USE TO MANAGE THIS PATIENT?

Nikolas Raufi, MD and Terry Kim, MD

Phakic intraocular lenses (pIOLs) are divided into 3 classes: anterior chamber or angle fixated (AC), iris fixated (IF), and sulcus fixated or posterior chamber (PC). In the United States, they include the Verisyse (Johnson & Johnson Vision; IF-pIOL) and Visian (Staar Surgical; PC-pIOL) lenses. The AC-pIOLs have not been US Food and Drug Administration–approved and will not be discussed in detail. Despite their advantages over keratorefractive surgery and clear lens exchange, pIOLs are susceptible to complications that are mostly dependent on their placement and design.

Cataract

Cataract is an uncommon complication of these lenses, necessitating explantation in 0.86% (AC-pIOL), 0.58% (IF-pIOL), and 3.42% (PC-pIOL) of cases.[1] The most common types of cataract in AC and IF lenses is the nuclear sclerotic cataract. In contrast, about 91% of cataracts in PC-pIOLs are of the anterior subcapsular variety, usually secondary to surgical trauma and pIOL-crystalline lens touch.[1] Other contributory factors include changes in the blood–aqueous barrier, inflammation, myopia, age, and lens material biocompatibility.[1] Most nonfoldable AC- and IF-pIOLs are made of polymethyl methcrylate, a very biocompatible material, and the newer collamer PC-pIOLs (eg, Visian) are made of extremely flexible collagen, which is believed to be even less cataractogenic.

Hardten DR, Hansen MS.
*Curbside Consultation in Cornea and External Disease:
49 Clinical Questions, Second Edition* (pp 217-219).
© 2022 Taylor & Francis Group.

Figure 38-1. Diffuse illumination slit-lamp photograph of the Verisyse lens. Posteriorly, an anterior subcapsular cataract is evident, as well as pigment deposition on the anterior lens capsule.

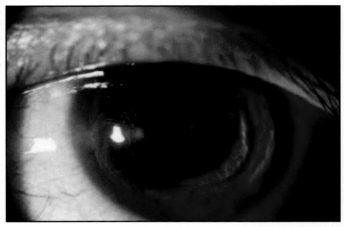

The 2 most important factors to consider in reducing risk of anterior subcapsular cataract formation include surgical technique and appropriate lens vaulting. Surgical experience is paramount, as any inadvertent crystalline lens contact, and even overuse of viscoelastic, can promote nonprogressive or slowly progressive cataracts.[2] Average lens vault is 0.8 mm for IF-pIOLs and 0.15 mm for PC-pIOLs.[3]

Surgery

Preoperatively, it is imperative to discuss with patients the possibility of cataract formation because they will immediately lose accommodative ability after removal of the crystalline lens. Many cataracts that develop are not visually significant; however, when they are, the examination will reveal a ring or circular opacity corresponding to the area of pIOL-crystalline lens touch (Figure 38-1). Typically, biometry data will exist from before the original surgery, and these data can be used for calculating the power of the new IOL. However, when not available, most modern optical coherence biometers have a "phakic" mode that provides good accuracy and reliability, especially for the Visian PC-pIOL. If this is not available, Hoffer[4,5] has provided a correction of ultrasound axial length measurements. Nonetheless, if available, we recommend employing the use of intraoperative aberrometry after pIOL extraction to confirm the IOL power choice. We recommend generally leaving these patients slightly myopic rather than aiming for plano.

Due to their rigid 5.0- or 6.0-mm polymethyl methcrylate optic, IF-pIOLs must be removed out of a 6-mm incision, ideally via a scleral tunnel to reduce surgically induced astigmatism (Figure 38-2A). We recommend using 2 side ports for these lenses, 1 at each enclavation site to assist in lens manipulation. Using lens forceps through the main incision, the lens can be grasped while a Sinskey hook disinserts each claw from the iris (Figure 38-2B). After IF-pIOL removal (Figure 38-2C), the crystalline lens can be removed through a separate 2.2-mm clear corneal incision.

The technique for removing PC-pIOLs is more straightforward, as the same corneal incision can be used for this procedure. After injecting a dispersive ophthalmic viscosurgical device over and under the pIOL, a Koch spatula (or similar blunt instrument) through properly positioned paracentesis incisions can be used to lift and free the haptics from behind the iris. If the corneal incision size is smaller (ie, 2.2 to 2.4 mm), we then recommend grasping the lens with MST forceps (MicroSurgical Technology) through a paracentesis incision while cutting the lens in half along its long axis with MST scissors through the temporal clear corneal incision. This maneuver

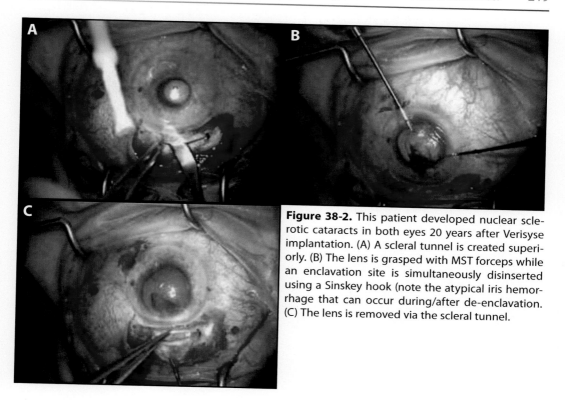

Figure 38-2. This patient developed nuclear sclerotic cataracts in both eyes 20 years after Verisyse implantation. (A) A scleral tunnel is created superiorly. (B) The lens is grasped with MST forceps while an enclavation site is simultaneously disinserted using a Sinskey hook (note the atypical iris hemorrhage that can occur during/after de-enclavation. (C) The lens is removed via the scleral tunnel.

aids in removal because, despite its flexibility, the lens is prone to fragmentation when pulled through a small corneal incision. If the corneal incision is larger, the Visian PC-pIOL can simply be removed by grasping it (without cutting it) with a forceps and removing it from the anterior chamber. With the main incision already created, the crystalline lens can then be removed in the usual fashion.

It is important to note that most patients with pIOLs are highly myopic, which originally precluded them from undergoing LASIK/photorefractive keratectomy. Highly myopic patients tend to develop cataracts earlier than emmetropic patients, even without a history of ocular surgery. They typically have deep anterior chambers and floppy lens capsules, as well as a higher risk for postoperative intraocular pressure spikes and retinal detachment (especially if their posterior vitreous is not detached from the retina). However, in our experience, most patients do very well after surgery, and visual outcomes are comparable to traditional cataract surgery.

References

1. Chen LJ, Chang YJ, Kuo JC, Rajagopal R, Azar DT. Metaanalysis of cataract development after phakic intraocular lens surgery. *J Cataract Refract Surg.* 2008;34(7):1181-1200.
2. Kohnen T, Kook D, Morral M, Güell JL. Phakic intraocular lenses: part 2: results and complications. *J Cataract Refract Surg.* 2010;36(12):2168-2194.
3. Gonvers M, Bornet C, Othenin-Girard P. Implantable contact lens for moderate to high myopia; relationship of vaulting to cataract formation. *J Cataract Refract Surg.* 2003;29(5):918-924.
4. Hoffer KJ. Ultrasound axial length measurement in biphakic eyes. *J Cataract Refract Surg.* 2003;29(5):961-965.
5. Hoffer KJ. Addendum to ultrasound axial length measurement in biphakic eyes: factors for Alcon L12500-L14000 anterior chamber phakic IOLs. *J Cataract Refract Surg.* 2007;33(4):751-752.

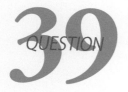

How Do I Manage a Patient Who Rubbed Their Eye Just After LASIK? What Could Go Wrong?

Majid Moshirfar, MD; James R. Barnes, BS;
Grant C. Hopping, MD; and Yasmyne C. Ronquillo, MD, MSc, JD

Shortly after LASIK surgery, patients may be tempted to rub their eyes. LASIK can affect the eyes of some patients due to the incision, abrasion of the cornea, and inflammatory factors released from cells at the surgical site. Symptoms can include irritation from inflammation, itchy eyes, and dry eyes. Quick diagnosis and management of these symptoms are crucial in preventing the complications that can occur due to post-LASIK eye rubbing.

After LASIK surgery, patients should be consulted to avoid rubbing their eyes to avoid potential complications, such as flap dislocation and flap striae. Flap dislocation involves dislodgement of the surgical flap from its proper position and is usually visually significant. On the other hand, flap striae occurs when the cornea is reshaped and the flap is repositioned. Corrugations can form on the surgical flap due to the cornea's new shape. Striae may or may not be visually significant. Methods to diagnose and treat these conditions are outlined in this question.

Flap Dislocation

Flap dislocation is a rare but serious complication involving dehiscence of the surgical flap after LASIK. Clinical signs and symptoms of flap dislocations vary, based on the timing, location, and severity of the dislocation. Flap dislocations generally cause visual symptoms, but clinical judgment should be used in cases of mild dislocations where the patient reports no symptoms. If the patient is asymptomatic and maintains appropriate visual acuity, no treatment is needed, but careful observation and documentation should be performed.

Dislocations to the periphery of the field of vision cause fewer visual symptoms than those near the center of the visual field. Another potential complication of flap dislocation is epithelial

Hardten DR, Hansen MS.
*Curbside Consultation in Cornea and External Disease:
49 Clinical Questions, Second Edition* (pp 221-226).
© 2022 Taylor & Francis Group.

Figure 39-1. Flap dislocation of the inferior portion of the surgical flap.

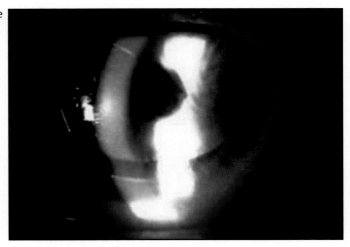

ingrowth, which may cause flap elevation, affecting vision and flap melt in rare cases. Other complications of flap dislocation include infection, irregular astigmatism, and hyperopia.[1]

The early diagnosis and treatment of flap dislocation are vital to help the patient avoid complications. Flap dislocations should be examined using slit-lamp biomicroscopy, looking for partial or full dehiscence of the flap along the surgical cut (Figure 39-1). Flap dislocations should be examined for flap striae, infection, and epithelial ingrowth. Timing, severity, and sequelae of the dislocation are important factors in determining the treatment plan (Figure 39-2).

EARLY INTERVENTION

Flap dislocations within the first 24 to 72 hours are often due to poor adhesion of the surgical flap. These acute dislocations can occur due to myriad reasons, including inadvertent eye rubbing, excessive dryness (which may be exacerbated by topical anesthetics), or adhesion to the upper eyelid. Flap dislocations that are treated within the first 5 days can be treated by irrigation with an isotonic or hypotonic solution, refloating, and repositioning of the flap. Irrigation with an isotonic or hypotonic solution can cause swelling of the flap, making it easier to reposition. After the flap has been refloated, it should be examined for any re-epithelialization that should subsequently be removed from the stromal face and the underside of the surgical flap. Then, the flap can be repositioned using gentle strokes with microsponges to massage the flap into its proper orientation, ensuring a symmetrical flap border. Some clinicians find it useful to use tools, such as the Johnston LASIK applanator (Katena), to aid in the smoothing of the flap. Sutures are generally not needed to hold the flap in place.

After the flap is repositioned, we strongly recommend applying a bandage contact lens and keeping the patient in the clinic for several hours to monitor for flap slippage and proper position of the bandage lens. Having the patient lie in a supine position for 5 minutes with their eyes closed can encourage the flap to remain in a stable position. A topical antibiotic and steroid should be administered to prevent infection and reduce inflammation. The bandage contact lens can be removed after 48 hours. Follow-up should be done to monitor for possible diffuse lamellar keratitis, epithelial ingrowth, and redislocation.[2]

LATE INTERVENTION

In certain clinical scenarios, a patient with an acute flap dislocation may not be seen for several weeks or months. These patients require a slightly different management plan compared with patients who are treated immediately after the dislocation.

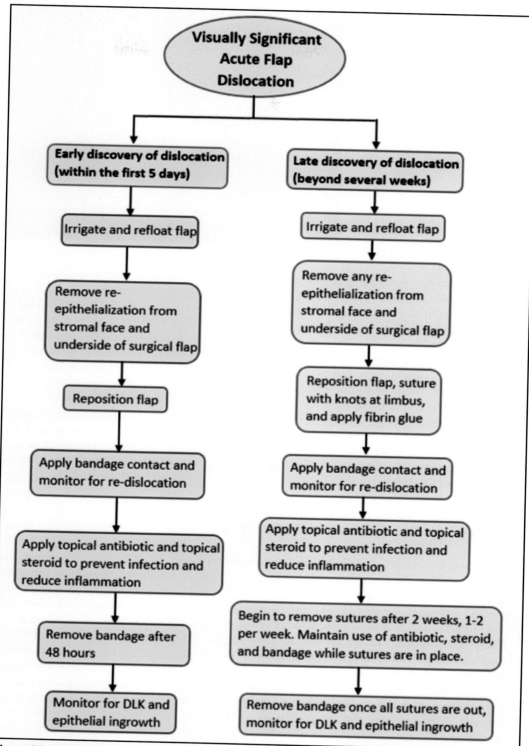

Figure 39-2. Management of visually significant acute flap dislocation post-LASIK.

Figure 39-3. Flap striae observed under the slit lamp.

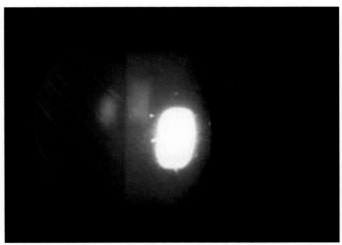

Severe dislocations involving near-complete or full dehiscence of the flap often require surgical intervention, including suturing of the flap. Immediate treatment is necessary in the case of an epithelial ingrowth to prevent impaired vision, astigmatism, or flap melt.[3] Late management of an acute flap dislocation involves irrigating and refloating the flap, followed by examining for and removing any re-epithelialization from the stromal face and the underside of the surgical flap. The flap can then be repositioned using surgical sponges. After the flap is repositioned, multiple radially oriented 10-0 nylon interrupted sutures are placed to fix the flap in place. We do not recommend burying the knots but instead rotating them toward the limbus to limit stress on the flap.[4] Fibrin glue is also placed along the flap to prevent recurrence of flap dislocation and epithelial ingrowth.[5] A bandage contact lens should be applied and the patient kept in clinic for several hours to monitor for redislocation. Stepwise removal of the sutures should begin 2 weeks postoperatively, and use of a topical antibiotic and topical steroid should continue while sutures are present. The bandage contact lens should be removed when all sutures are out, and the patient should continue to be monitored for diffuse lamellar keratitis, epithelial ingrowth, and redislocation.

Flap Striae

Flap striae are classified as macro- and microstriae and can also form due to postoperative rubbing of the eyes. The mechanical pressure on the surgical flap caused by rubbing can cause folding and rolling of the flap. Macrostriae are large, full-thickness folds that are usually visually obstructive and require treatment. Microstriae may sometimes cause visual symptoms depending on their location and thickness; those that are symptomatic require treatment.

Macrostriae and microstriae are best detected during slit-lamp examination (Figure 39-3). Macrostriae are generally easy to observe, but microstriae may require staining to be detected. Sodium fluorescein may aid in the visualization of microstriae, causing them to appear as negatively stained lines. This finding is due to the absence of tear film over the protruding microstriae.[6] Visual significance of microstriae can be reported by the patient. If the patient is asymptomatic, then careful documentation and observation are sufficient. In more difficult cases, another way to determine the visual significance of microstriae is to take advantage of the similarities between the striae and the cylindrical grooves of a Maddox rod (US Neurologicals LLC). Microstriae that are clinically significant will act like a Maddox rod by producing streaks of light perpendicular to the striae.[7]

Early recognition and treatment of flap striae lead to better visual outcomes and reduced likelihood of the patient experiencing fixed folds. As with flap dislocations, management of striae varies depending on the severity and time of recognition.

EARLY INTERVENTION

Visually significant striae that are diagnosed within the first 24 to 48 hours can be flattened with microsponges under the slit lamp by applying gentle pressure to the fold.[8,9] If symptoms persist, then striae can be treated by hydrating and sponging the flap under the slit lamp. If the striae do not resolve, ironing the flap can be an effective treatment. Ironing of flap striae involves using heated spatulas to flatten the striae. The newly flat striae are then held in place with warm water and warm instrument massage for 5 to 10 minutes. Ironing is an effective treatment for persistent striae and may help to prevent recurrence for 6 months postoperatively.[10] If the striae continue to remain symptomatic, then the flap can be repositioned by irrigation with an isotonic or hypotonic solution, refloating, and replacing with surgical sponges.[11] Some striae may require only rehydration and irrigation to disappear.[12] If symptomatic flap striae do not resolve with these measures, then more aggressive treatment may be required. Please follow the steps for "late discovery of striae" to treat persistent symptomatic striae (Figure 39-4.)

LATE INTERVENTION

Persistent striae that are diagnosed weeks or months after LASIK or those that do not respond to initial treatment need to be treated with a more permanent solution. The surgical flap should be irrigated and refloated. The stromal face and both sides of the surgical flap should then be thoroughly inspected for epithelial ingrowth. Any re-epithelialization should be removed, and the epithelium overlying the LASIK flap may need to be completely debrided. After the removal of the epithelium, the flap should be stretched, repositioned, and sutured in place. Suturing is a common method of treatment that can eliminate striae and prevent recurrence by mechanically stretching the surgical flap.[13] Potential complications include the formation of new striae in the opposite direction due to overstretching and irregular astigmatism. If symptomatic flap striae persist, phototherapeutic keratectomy can be used to treat the patient. Phototherapeutic keratectomy is the standard treatment for refractive striae and is performed by debriding the epithelium and ablating the striae with an excimer laser, rendering it smooth.[13] Flap amputation can be used as a last resort in rare cases of striae refractory to the treatments outlined herein.[14]

References

1. Henderson BA, Yoo SH. *Curbside Consultation in Refractive and Lens-Based Surgery: 49 Clinical Questions*. SLACK Incorporated; 2014.
2. Aldave AJ, Hollander DA, Abbott RL. Late-onset traumatic flap dislocation and diffuse lamellar inflammation after laser in situ keratomileusis. *Cornea*. 2002;21(6):604-607.
3. Azar DT, Kock DD. *LASIK: Fundamentals, Surgical Techniques, and Complications*. Marcel Dekker Inc; 2003.
4. Moshirfar M, Anderson E, Taylor N, Hsu M. Management of a traumatic flap dislocation seven years after LASIK. *Case Rep Ophthalmol Med*. 2011;2011:514780. doi:10.1155/2011/514780
5. Anderson NJ, Hardten DR. Fibrin glue for the prevention of epithelial ingrowth after laser in situ keratomileusis. *J Cataract Refract Surg*. 2003;29(7):1425-1429.
6. Steinert RF. Early flap striae. In: *Difficult and Complicated Cases in Refractive Surgery*. Springer Berlin Heidelberg; 2015:175-176. doi:10.1007/978-3-642-55238-0_38
7. Choi CJ, Melki SA. Maddox rod effect to confirm the visual significance of laser in situ keratomileusis flap striae. *J Cataract Refract Surg*. 2011;37(10):1748-1750. doi:10.1016/j.jcrs.2011.08.001
8. Jackson DW, Hamill MB, Koch DD. Laser in situ keratomileusis flap suturing to treat recalcitrant flap striae. *J Cataract Refract Surg*. 2003;29(2):264-269.

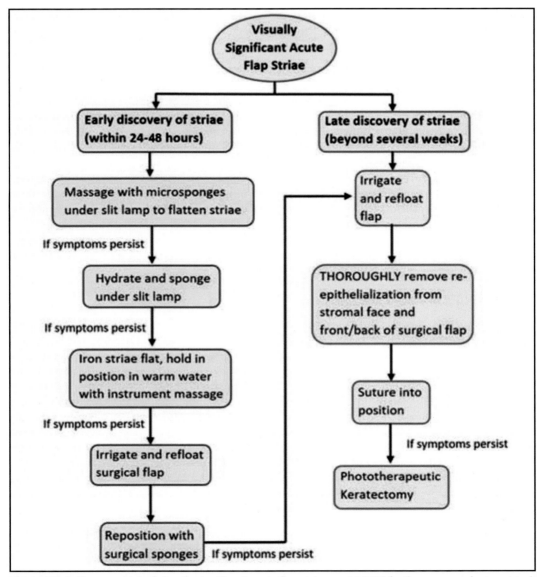

Figure 39-4. Management of visually significant acute flap striae post-LASIK (both macro- and microstriae).

9. Moshirfar M. Flap striae after LASIK. *EyeWiki*. Published 2015. Updated July 31, 2020. Accessed October 19, 2021. https://eyewiki.aao.org/Flap_Striae_After_LASIK

10. Donnenfeld ED, Perry HD, Doshi SJ, Biser SA, Solomon R. Hyperthermic treatment of post-LASIK corneal striae. *J Cataract Refract Surg*. 2004;30(3):620-625. doi:10.1016/j.jcrs.2003.08.019

11. Lam DS, Leung AT, Wu JT, et al. Management of severe flap wrinkling or dislodgment after laser in situ keratomileusis. *J Cataract Refract Surg*. 1999;25(11):1441-1447.

12. Muñoz G, Alió JL, Pérez-Santonja JJ, Attia WH. Successful treatment of severe wrinkled corneal flap after laser in situ keratomileusis with deionized water. *Am J Ophthalmol*. 2000;129(1):91-92.

13. Steinert RF, Ashrafzadeh A, Hersh PS. Results of phototherapeutic keratectomy in the management of flap striae after LASIK. *Ophthalmology*. 2004;111(4):740-746. doi:10.1016/j.ophtha.2003.06.015

14. Chhadva P, Cabot F, Galor A, Karp CL, Yoo SH. Long-term outcomes of flap amputation after LASIK. *J Refract Surg*. 2016;32(2):136-137. doi:10.3928/1081597X-20151229-01

40

MY PATIENT RECENTLY HAD LASIK, BUT I NOTICED NEW EPITHELIAL CELLS IN THE FLAP INTERFACE. WHEN DO I LIFT THE FLAP TO TREAT EPITHELIAL INGROWTH AND WHAT IS THE BEST METHOD?

Zachary Zavodni, MD

Thankfully, epithelial ingrowth after primary LASIK surgery is a rare event, especially in the era of femtosecond laser flaps—occurring in less than 1% of cases.[1] When it does occur, it is typically in the far periphery of the flap and is of no visual or clinical consequence. Nonetheless, these patients warrant close monitoring because if epithelial ingrowth extends radially beyond the flap edge, it can induce irregular astigmatism and result in decreased vision.

Unquestionably, the biggest risk factor for epithelial ingrowth is a LASIK retreatment in which the flap is lifted.[2] In these cases, epithelial defects are common and an irregular epithelial edge is created while lifting the flap. The rate of ingrowth in these cases ranges from 7% to 31%.[3] Risk factors for developing ingrowth in primary LASIK patients include anterior basement membrane dystrophy, epithelial defect during surgery, and vertical gas breakthrough. As alluded to earlier, the rate of ingrowth seems to be lower with femtosecond laser–created flaps, presumably because the vertical geometry of the flap edge creates a barrier to epithelial growth.[4,5]

Epithelial ingrowth can present with various clinical patterns. Early (or mild) ingrowth is asymptomatic and typically presents as a faint, peripheral interface opacity, with a whitish-gray demarcation line. As more epithelial cells migrate into the interface, ingrowth will become thicker, and more discrete forming nests, or pearls, of cells will cluster together. Late, or advanced, ingrowth will develop a more homogenous dense whitish appearance, with associated flap edge distortion and overlying flap necrosis.

Advanced cases of ingrowth require immediate debridement, but these scenarios are thankfully very rare. More often than not, refractive surgeons must decide when to intervene if ingrowth is mild to intermediate in nature. Indications for ingrowth flap-lift removal include:

Hardten DR, Hansen MS.
*Curbside Consultation in Cornea and External Disease:
49 Clinical Questions, Second Edition* (pp 227-229).
© 2022 Taylor & Francis Group.

- Ingrowth that is clearly expanding in size and extending beyond 2 mm from the flap edge
- Ingrowth that has grown thick enough or radially enough to induce irregular astigmatism, resulting in decreased vision. Typically, in these cases, the epithelium will clearly track from a flap edge, but sometimes there may be an island of central ingrowth not seemingly connected to a flap edge.
- Ingrowth that is affecting the health of the cornea (ie, flap necrosis, with or without an epithelial defect)

There are several methods for the removal of epithelial cell ingrowth. Fundamentally, the technique involves lifting the LASIK flap with reflection and subsequently debriding cells from the posterior flap surface and the stromal bed. Surgeons should be familiar with several surgical pearls when performing ingrowth removal, including the following:

- If ingrowth is only in 1 quadrant, then the surgeon should lift only that section, minimizing the area for possible subsequent recurrence.
- Initially entering the flap interface with a 30-gauge needle at the slit lamp can be very helpful. It is easier to lift the flap edge at the slit lamp than under a diffuse operating microscope light. The sharp edge of the needle also creates a cleaner entry into the interface space and makes it less likely to create an irregular epithelial defect at the site of entry.
- Debride cells from both the underside of the flap and stromal side with both a bladed spatula and Weck-Cel (BVI Medical) sponges.
- Once the flap has been replaced, irrigate aggressively in the interface to wash out any epithelial cells.

Typically, these measures will lead to successful ingrowth removal without recurrence. There remains ongoing debate regarding the importance of removing peripheral epithelium beyond the flap edges. The conceptual idea is that with a larger epithelial defect, the flap may have more time to adhere before epithelium grows over the flap interface. Consequently, epithelium may be less likely to grow underneath the flap. Although some surgeons support this technique, there is not significant published data to support that recurrence rates are necessarily lower with this approach. If there is recurrence of significant ingrowth after initial removal, and the procedure must be repeated, then supplementary operative measures should be taken to seal down the flap edges. Both sutures and fibrin glue have been used in this setting with good results.[6-8]

Finally, it is important to note that ingrowth can also be treated with neodymium:yttrium aluminum garnet (Nd:YAG) laser.[9] This approach is typically used for cases of focal central islands of epithelial cells in the visual axis. The YAG laser energy creates cavitation bubbles that can kill epithelial cells. Although effective, this technique frequently requires several applications of laser energy for full eradication.

References

1. Kamburoglu G, Ertan A. Epithelial ingrowth after femtosecond laser-assisted in situ keratomileusis. *Cornea*. 2008;27(10):1122-1125.
2. Caster AI, Friess DW, Schwendeman FJ. Incidence of epithelial ingrowth in primary and retreatment laser in situ keratomileusis. *J Cataract Refract Surg*. 2010;36(1):97-101.
3. Moshirfar M, Jehangir N, Fenzl CR, McCaughey M. LASIK enhancement: clinical and surgical management. *J Refract Surg*. 2017;33(2):116-127.
4. Letko E, Price MO, Price FW Jr. Influence of original flap creation method on incidence of epithelial ingrowth after LASIK retreatment. *J Refract Surg*. 2009;25(11):1039-1041.
5. Henry CR, Canto AP, Galor A, Vaddavalli PK, Culberson WW, Yoo SH. Epithelial ingrowth after LASIK: clinical characteristics, risk factors, and visual outcomes in patients requiring flap lift. *J Refract Surg*. 2012;28(7):488-492.

6. Anderson NJ, Hardten DR. Fibrin glue for the prevention of epithelial ingrowth after laser in situ keratomileusis. *J Cataract Refract Surg.* 2003;29(7):1425-1429.

7. Rapuano CJ. Management of epithelial ingrowth after laser in situ keratomileusis on a tertiary care cornea service. *Cornea.* 2010;29(3):307-313.

8. Narváez J, Chakrabarty A, Chang K. Treatment of epithelial ingrowth after LASIK enhancement with a combined technique of mechanical debridement, flap suturing, and fibrin glue application. *Cornea.* 2006;25(9):1115-1117.

9. Lindfield D, Ansari G, Poole T. Nd:YAG laser treatment for epithelial ingrowth after laser refractive surgery. *Ophthalmic Surg Lasers Imaging.* 2012;43(3):247-249.

SECTION VI

TRAUMA

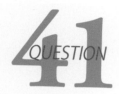

A PIECE OF GLASS FLEW INTO MY PATIENT'S EYE. THE EXAM SHOWS CENTRAL CORNEAL PERFORATION < 1 MM IN DIAMETER. THE ANTERIOR CHAMBER IS SHALLOW BUT FORMED. HOW SHOULD I CLOSE THIS WOUND?

Roberto Pineda, MD and Ramon Joaquim Hallal Jr, MD

This patient has suffered a perforating corneal injury from a projectile. A careful history is mandatory but often is difficult if the patient was chemically impaired at the time of injury or if the patient is a child. In such cases, it is prudent to obtain imaging studies of the eye and orbit. If suspicion of a foreign body is low or more advanced imaging modalities are not available, plain film radiography may be all that is required. However, nonmetallic foreign bodies, such as glass, are not easily seen on plain radiographs and may be missed. Computed tomography (CT) is now the standard diagnostic test for imaging the traumatized eye and orbit and is available in most hospitals. Current-generation CT machines can detect nonmetallic radiolucent foreign bodies 1 mm in size. A CT scan of the eye and orbit is suggested, with both axial and coronal sections (1-mm sections). Magnetic resonance imaging may detect and localize a small nonmetallic foreign body, such as glass, with an image quality superior to that provided by CT for soft tissues and nonmagnetic intraocular foreign bodies, but this study takes longer, is less available, and is more expensive. The etiology of the foreign body is paramount. Glass is an inert material—different from iron or copper—which should be removed as soon as possible due to inherent toxicity.

In addition to the slit-lamp examination, the pupil should be dilated so that the fundus can be examined. Careful examination of the periocular tissue is also warranted to rule out other sites of penetration from foreign body material. Seidel testing of the corneal wound is necessary to help determine the best options for closing it (Figures 41-1A and B). Prophylactic antibiotics (oral or intravenous) are mandated in all cases of ocular perforation.

Hardten DR, Hansen MS.
*Curbside Consultation in Cornea and External Disease:
49 Clinical Questions, Second Edition* (pp 233-235).
© 2022 Taylor & Francis Group.

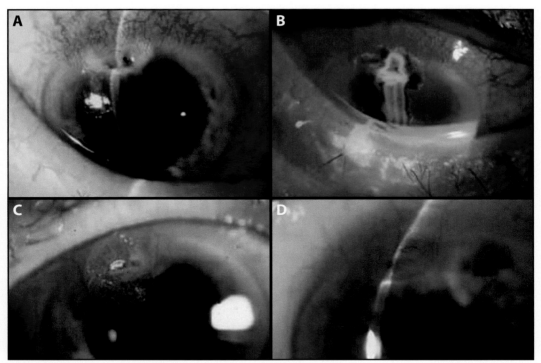

Figure 41-1. (A) Peripheral corneal ulceration with perforation. (B) Positive Seidel test corneal ulceration. (C) Corneal perforation 1 month after application of glue. (D) Area of perforation after removal of glue with wound healing. (Reproduced with permission from Jonathan Primack, MD.)

Treatment

Depending on the Seidel testing results, different approaches can be employed to close the 1-mm perforation. If the wound is self-sealing and relatively clean with little debris, placement of an extended-wear therapeutic soft contact lens and aqueous suppression (topical beta-blocker or alpha-agonist) may be adequate for wound closure, allowing the anterior chamber to reform. An eye shield or glasses should be worn to avoid inadvertent touching of the cornea. The contact lens is usually left in place for several weeks, with use of topical antibiotics and a mild steroid. This approach is particularly beneficial when the perforation involves the visual axis as in this case because unlike glue, it does not interfere with vision. Avoiding closure of the wound with sutures eliminates additional scarring and astigmatism. However, many times, the perforation is not self-sealing and surgical closure of the wound is required.

The use of tissue adhesives is an effective means of addressing small corneal perforations and has been used for defects of up to 2 mm. The application of cyanoacrylate glue is a simple in-office or minor surgery procedure used to close this type of defect.[1] Another benefit from glue is the bacteriostatic and bactericidal properties against gram-positive and gram-negative microorganisms.[2]

Several brands of medical grade isobutyl 2-cyanoacrylate glue have been used, such as Dermabond (Ethicon). Commercial glues, such as Super Glue (Super Glue Corp), are methyl 2-cyanoacrylate adhesives and should be avoided because they result in secondary irritation due to formaldehyde released into the tear film during polymer breakdown.[3] Median glue retention is 58 days, according to a recent study from Massachusetts Eye and Ear.[4]

For this patient, it is easiest to glue the perforation under a microscope while they are lying down. However, adhesive application may be possible at the slit lamp as well. Topical anesthesia and a lid speculum are employed. Formal prepping of the eye is usually not necessary. First, epithelium around the perforation needs to be removed (1 to 2 mm) so that the glue can adhere. Application of glue over the epithelium will result in loss of the polymerized glue plug within a few days of application as the corneal epithelium sloughs off. Although not mentioned in this scenario, if iris is plugging the wound, consider filtered air or light use of a viscoelastic to displace the iris before applying the glue. Next, attempt to dry the stromal bed as much as possible before the application of glue. It is very important to avoid excess glue around the site, as it irritates the eye, often resulting in early expulsion of glue, and limits examination of the treated area.

Application of the glue may be performed in many ways, including directly to the cornea, through the use of a microapplicator (with glue) or microtip (27- or 30-gauge needle), or via a blunt side of a cellulose spear or plastic disc (2 to 3 mm) attached to a wooden applicator for 30 seconds (polymerization is enhanced by the presence of hydroxide anions, which are abundant in aqueous and water; Figures 41-1C and D).

If glue is not available or cannot effectively seal the corneal perforation, suturing the perforation is always an option. With a central corneal perforation, consider 11-0 nylon sutures to minimize scarring, using as few sutures as possible. Use of 10-0 nylon is acceptable if 11-0 nylon sutures are not available. If the wound continues to leak, consider the addition of glue and/or a therapeutic contact lens.

In cases where gluing is not possible, a rotational autograft has been described as an alternative option. Several case reports have been published with good outcomes that avoid the risk of rejection and are less dependent on corticosteroids compared with corneal allograft transplantation.[5] To this point, a rotational autograft should be an option only in countries where access to corneal tissue is limited or unavailable. In countries with an adequate supply of donor corneas, one should consider an emergent penetrating keratoplasty if other modalities fail or are not available.

Finally, with irregular central corneal perforations that do not close with a few simple sutures, or if there are issues with cyanoacrylate glue and long-term contact lenses, several layers of amniotic membrane can be used to close a small corneal perforation. This can be combined with the use of a fibrin-thrombin tissue adhesive such as Tisseel (Baxter) to avoid sutures and, therefore, scarring.

Our current in-hospital management for healthy adult open globes includes vancomycin 1 g every 12 hours and ceftazidime 1 g every 8 hours intravenously for 48 hours as well as 1 week of oral antibiotics.

References

1. Vote BJ, Elder MJ. Cyanoacrylate glue for corneal perforations: a description of a surgical technique and a review of the literature. *Clin Exp Ophthalmol.* 2000;28(6):437-442.
2. Chen WL, Lin CT, Hsieh CY, Tu IH, Chen WY, Hu FR. Comparison of the bacteriostatic effects, corneal cytotoxicity, and the ability to seal corneal incisions among three different tissue adhesives. *Cornea.* 2007;26(10):1228-1234.
3. Chan SM, Boisjoly H. Advances in the use of adhesives in ophthalmology. *Curr Opin Ophthalmol.* 2004;15(4):305-310.
4. Yin J, Singh RB, Al Karmi R, Yung A, Yu M, Dana R. Outcomes of cyanoacrylate tissue adhesive application in corneal thinning and perforation. *Cornea.* 2019;38(6):668-673.
5. Gunes A, Kansu Bozkurt T, Unlu C, Sezgin Akcay BI, Bayramlar H. Ipsilateral rotational autokeratoplasty for the management of traumatic corneal scar. *Case Rep Ophthalmol Med.* 2012;2012:853584.

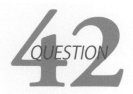

My Patient Was Splashed With Cement in Both Eyes. They Have Red, Irritated Eyes and Blurry Vision. The Exam Shows Debris on the Conjunctiva and Under the Lids, Diffuse SPK in the Right Eye, and a Central Corneal Epithelial Defect in the Left Eye. What Should I Watch for?

Bennie H. Jeng, MD

The spectrum of chemical burns to the eye is very broad, ranging from mild epithelial disruption to severe ocular and intraocular damage. While acid burns can cause severe destruction of the ocular surface, alkali burns can be even more destructive because saponification of cell membranes can lead to rapid penetration of the alkali through the cornea and sclera into the eye, causing destruction of intraocular contents. Although the prognosis of the injured eye depends on the extent of the injury, it also depends on the rapidity and modalities of treatment. Thus, all chemical burns to the eye, no matter how seemingly minor, must be treated immediately, as the extent of ocular surface damage can be severe depending on the chemical involved.

For this particular patient, if irrigation of the eyes has not yet been performed on arrival to the office, immediate irrigation of both eyes must be done, even before visual acuity is checked. Manual irrigation with saline or lactated Ringer's solution using a bottle or through intravenous tubing directly into the eyes as well as the upper and lower fornices should be performed. If a Morgan lens (MorTan Inc) setup is available, it can be used after the initial manual irrigation; otherwise, manual irrigation should be continued. Either way, copious irrigation should be done for at least 30 minutes. Topical proparacaine drops can be useful during this process. After this irrigation is performed, one should wait a few minutes to allow equilibration, and then the pH should be tested. During the equilibration period, visual acuities can be checked and a quick slit-lamp examination can be performed to assess the ocular surface and anterior segment structures. Irrigation should then be continued until a neutral pH of 7.0 is reached.

When the pH has been normalized, re-examination at the slit lamp should be performed, and cotton-tipped applicators or jeweler forceps should be used to remove the cement debris from the ocular surface. Special care should be taken to check in the inferior fornices and under the

Hardten DR, Hansen MS.
*Curbside Consultation in Cornea and External Disease:
49 Clinical Questions, Second Edition* (pp 237-240).
© 2022 Taylor & Francis Group.

Figure 42-1. Cement particles lodged in the upper fornix of a man who suffered an alkali burn to the eye with cement. Failure to identify and remove these particles will result in a reservoir for continued alkali release onto the ocular surface. (Reproduced with permission from Richard L. Abbott, MD.)

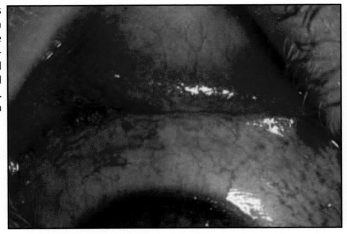

Figure 42-2. Diffuse epithelial disruption of the inferior two-thirds of the cornea after an acute alkali burn to the eye from cement. (Reproduced with permission from Richard L. Abbott, MD.)

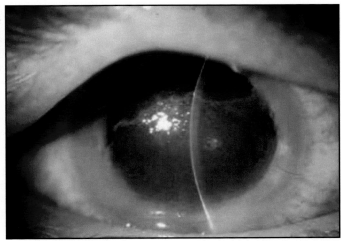

upper eyelid in the superior fornices (Figure 42-1). Double eversion of the upper eyelids must be performed to ensure that there is no debris in the upper fornices. It is imperative to ensure that no debris remains, as any leftover debris will continue to serve as a reservoir of alkali in the form of lime, which will continue to cause damage. Any areas of frank necrosis of the ocular surface should also be noted, and necrotic material should be debrided to remove any residual caustic material and to promote better epithelialization. After all of the debris and necrosis is removed, irrigation with a few more liters of normal saline should be performed to wash out any residual alkali. When the pH is confirmed to be normalized, irrigation can be stopped and the eyes should be re-examined once again. The epithelial defects on both the corneas and the conjunctiva should be noted (Figure 42-2), and the intraocular pressures should be checked because alkali burns can frequently cause raised intraocular pressures. The presence of intraocular inflammation should be noted, and a special assessment of the limbus should be undertaken to grade the damage based on the Roper-Hall modification of the Hughes classification[1] or the Dua classification.[2]

Early Medical Management

The outcome of the injury now rests on the initial medical management. Contrary to the conservative practices that are frequently employed, the use of an intensive regimen of corticosteroid eye drops is essential to a favorable outcome, and, in fact, the benefit of corticosteroid-induced reduction in inflammation from prolonged use of corticosteroids is not associated with significant corneal stromal melting.[3] Thus, in this case, I would favor the use of prednisolone acetate 1% drops every 2 hours in both eyes. Along with this, I would cover with a broad-spectrum antibiotic drop, such as a fourth-generation fluoroquinolone 4 times daily. I would also add a cycloplegic agent such as scopolamine 0.25% 4 times daily or atropine 1% twice daily—do not use phenylephrine because of its vasoconstrictive properties. Furthermore, I would consider using either oral vitamin C 1 g 4 times daily (do not forget to remind the patient to drink a lot of water) or oral doxycycline 100 mg twice daily (or both) to prevent stromal melting.[4] Sodium citrate 10% drops can also be used for this purpose, but it is difficult to obtain and, in this case, is probably not necessary. If the intraocular pressure is elevated, oral acetazolamide 250 mg 4 times daily or 500 mg twice daily can be used or a topical beta-blocker should be given. Frequent use of preservative-free artificial tears should be encouraged on an hourly basis and, if necessary, an oral analgesic can be prescribed.

Amniotic Membrane Grafting for Severe Burns

Unless a Roper-Hall grade IV burn is noted, surgical intervention is typically not necessary at this time. However, with severe burns, and more recently even in moderate burns, amniotic membrane grafting has become a popular modality for the early treatment of ocular burns.[5] Amniotic membrane possesses nutrients and growth factors that can help suppress inflammation and promote epithelialization. In addition, it can be useful in helping to protect the fragile, damaged ocular surface. Sometimes, the placement of an amniotic membrane is done in conjunction with the placement of a temporary tarsorrhaphy. A sutureless, temporary, amniotic membrane patch is also available commercially, and this may prove to be an efficient and efficacious treatment modality during the acute phase of ocular chemical burns.[5] Other biologics, such as autologous serum or platelet-rich plasma, have also demonstrated some positive effects in such settings where an amniotic membrane might be used.

Ongoing Medical Management

During the first week after injury, medical therapy should be continued, and the patient should be seen daily until the epithelium (cornea and conjunctiva) is healed. It is common to overlook conjunctival defects, which could end up melting and necrosing. Any new areas of necrosis should be treated with debridement, and topical collagenase inhibitors, such as acetylcysteine 10%, can be used 4 times daily. If perforation is a threat, then a corneal or scleral patch graft (depending on the location of the necrosis) may be warranted. During this time, the intraocular pressure should be monitored and treated, and any conjunctival adhesions seen in the fornices (Figure 42-3) can be lysed with a cotton-tipped applicator.

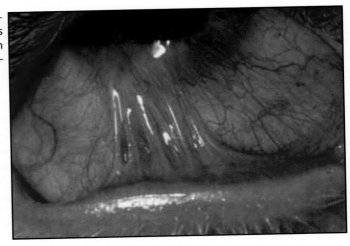

Figure 42-3. Symblepharon formation in the lower fornix several weeks after an alkali burn to the eye with cement. (Reproduced with permission from Richard L. Abbott, MD.)

After the first week, the topical corticosteroid drops should be tapered to 4 times daily and, if the epithelium is not healed, consideration should be made to intervene with a bandage contact lens. Aggressive lubrication should also be continued. Alternatively, pressure patching with an antibiotic/corticosteroid combination ointment in the eye is an option. If this is unsuccessful, an amniotic membrane graft, with or without a temporary tarsorrhaphy, may be warranted at this time. Ultimately, chronic dry eyes and limbal stem cell deficiency can be sequelae of chemical burns that may require long-term or even lifelong care. That being said, aggressive and prompt initial management of such cases will give the patient the best chance for a more favorable outcome.

References

1. Roper-Hall MJ. Thermal and chemical burns. *Trans Ophthalmol Soc UK*. 1965;85:631-653.
2. Dua HS, King AJ, Joseph A. A new classification of ocular surface burns. *Br J Ophthalmol*. 2001;85(11):1379-1383.
3. Brodovsky SC, McCarty CA, Snibson G, et al. Management of alkali burns: an 11-year retrospective review. *Ophthalmology*. 2000;107(10):1829-1835.
4. Wagoner MD. Chemical injuries of the eye: current concepts in pathophysiology and therapy. *Surv Ophthalmol*. 1997;41(4):275-313.
5. Kheirkhah A, Johnson DA, Paranjpe DR, Raju VK, Casas V, Tseng SCG. Temporary sutureless amniotic membrane patch for acute alkaline burns. *Arch Ophthalmol*. 2008;126(8):1059-1066.

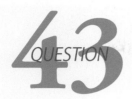

WHAT CAN I OFFER A PATIENT WHO SUSTAINED EYE TRAUMA AND LOSS OF IRIS TISSUE?

Walter T. Parker, MD

Iris trauma can be a daunting challenge at first glance, but finding a way to remedy the problem can be quite rewarding for both the patient and physician. In many cases, a surgical or clinical remedy that has been in use for years will be the easiest and most effective. However, advances in surgical techniques and technologies have given the clinician more options than we have ever had to address this issue.

Diagnosis

The importance of individualizing the treatment to the patient's particular complaints is crucial to the result that we all desire—a happy patient. A detailed history and physical examination should help reveal subtle aspects that might help lead to a more personalized approach to the patient. In many cases involving trauma, the iris defects are obvious. However, a subtle defect in the iris could result in monocular diplopia or multiplopia. Additionally, comorbid conditions like corneal, retinal, or glaucomatous damage that commonly exist in patients with previous trauma will help to direct overall treatment. Sometimes, patients with seemingly small defects will have more complaints than others, with larger and more obvious abnormalities due to differences in choroidal pigment. Importantly, mydriasis without tissue loss from associated trauma allows for ambient light to hit an optic edge in some cases, causing significant glare and photophobia. The psychosocial impact of iris trauma and defects is underappreciated, leaving many patients with depression and anxiety related to their disease.[1]

Hardten DR, Hansen MS.
*Curbside Consultation in Cornea and External Disease:
49 Clinical Questions, Second Edition* (pp 241-246).
© 2022 Taylor & Francis Group.

Figure 43-1. Preoperative superior iris defect.

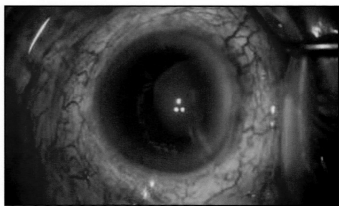

Treatment

CONTACT LENSES

This approach is uniquely suited for the patient who is absolutely averse to surgery at all costs. "Aniridic contacts" use an opaque periphery to block out the incoming light with a diaphragm. However, due to decreased oxygen transmissibility and thickness, many patients report that they are too uncomfortable to wear them. Also, the diaphragm blocks light from the corneal plane instead of the nodal point, causing ambient light to contribute to photic symptoms, particularly in pseudophakes, and visual field defects in others.

CORNEAL TATTOOS

In select patients, corneal tattoos have been successful and remain a way to avoid intraocular surgery in a previously traumatized eye, and some studies report only minimal adverse effects. Femtosecond lasers have been used to create a pocket for deposition of the tattoo pigment. However, it is important to note that this is a permanent treatment and may prevent examination of other parts of the eye, which is particularly important in traumatic patients who often have existing comorbidities. A recent study by Alio et al[2] reviewed 234 patients, where 49% experienced at least some light sensitivity. Others experienced visual field defects and problems with magnetic resonance imaging testing.[2-4]

IRIS SUTURING

Directly suturing the iris should be implemented in patients where there is enough iris tissue to adequately close the existing defect. In a peripheral defect with only a small sector missing, a McCannel suture technique can be used.[5] If the defect is more central but still involving a few clock hours (Figure 43-1), then a Siepser knot or its variants can be employed (Figures 43-2A and 43-3).[6,7] In cases of iridodialysis (Figure 43-4), then a 9-0 or 10-0 PROLENE suture (J&J Medical Devices) on a double-armed needle can be used to suture the iris to the scleral wall (Figures 43-5 and 43-6). However, even a hang-back technique can result in pupillary distortion. Other instances of no iris tissue loss but symptomatic pupillary mydriasis can be cured with an iris cerclage technique.[8] It will be important to note whether the previous iris trauma caused subtle iris transillumination defects (especially in a light-colored iris), where even an excellent cosmetic closure will still leave the patient with symptomatic glare and passage of ambient light.

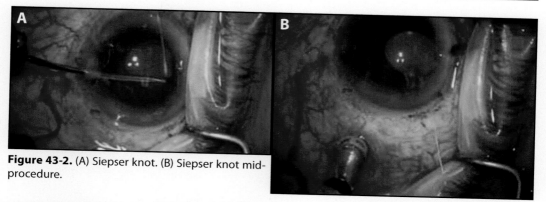

Figure 43-2. (A) Siepser knot. (B) Siepser knot mid-procedure.

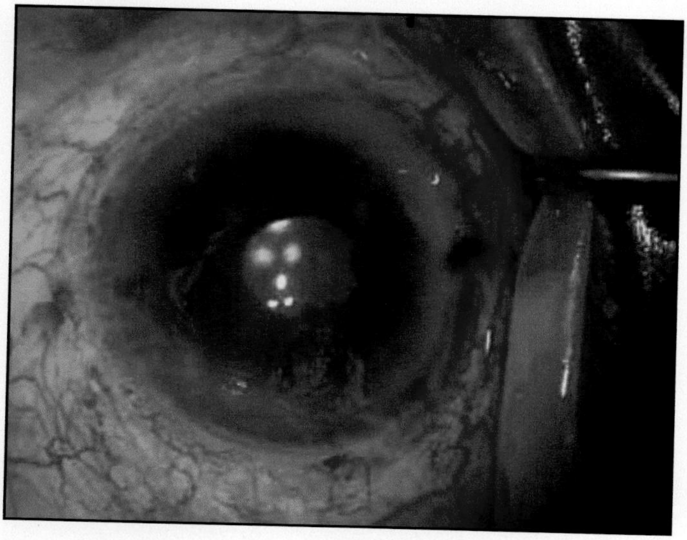

Figure 43-3. Status/post–Siepser knot.

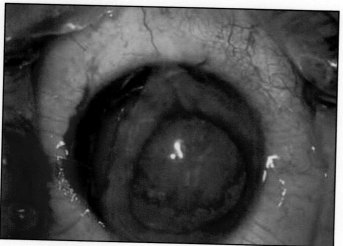

Figure 43-4. Preoperative iridodialysis.

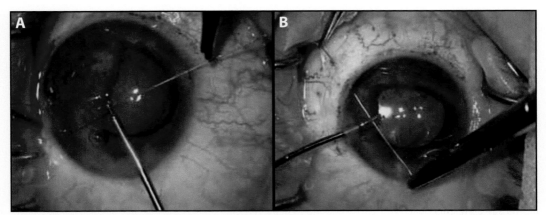

Figure 43-5. (A) Iridodialysis repair 1. (B) Iridodialysis repair 2.

Figure 43-6. Status/post–iridodialysis repair.

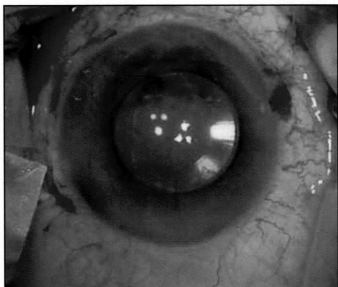

IRIS PROSTHESIS

In cases where there is not enough iris tissue for suturing, a concomitant cataract, or significant transillumination defects, then an iris prosthesis is a useful option. In 2018, the US Food and Drug Administration (FDA) approved the CustomFlex Artificial Iris (HumanOptics AG). This foldable, silicone intraocular iris prosthesis is currently both FDA approved and available in the United States.[9,10] The prosthesis is customized to the patient by sending a hard copy photo of the fellow eye or a photo of the desired iris color in patients with bilateral iris defects. This prosthesis has the advantage of requiring only a small incision for implantation of 2.5 mm to 3.2 mm in most cases, and it comes in a foldable fiber (for suturing) and fiber-free option. It can be suture fixated, with or without an intraocular lens, placed in the capsular bag with an endocapsular tension ring, with or without an intraocular lens, or, in some cases, passively in the sulcus. However, cost should be a significant consideration for these patients due to the customization required for each individual (Figures 43-7 through 43-9).[11-15]

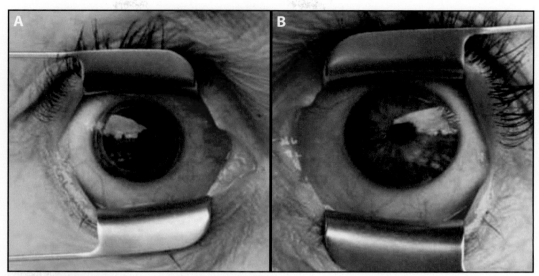

Figure 43-7. Preoperative HumanOptics prosthesis.

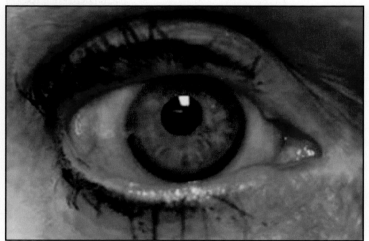

Figure 43-8. Postoperative HumanOptics prosthesis.

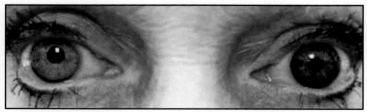

Figure 43-9. Postoperative HumanOptics prosthesis with fellow eye.

For the sake of a global perspective, other options are available outside of the United States. The 3 main categories of iris prostheses are combined iris prosthesis-intraocular lens, rigid endocapsular iris prostheses, and foldable iris prostheses. Morcher GmbH and Ophtec both manufacture the prosthesis-intraocular lens and rigid endocapsular models. These models are made of polymethyl methacrylate and can be quite large and difficult to manipulate in the eye. They also come in less natural colors of light blue, light green, or medium brown (Ophtec) or black (Morcher).[16-18] Reper-NN Ltd also makes a hydrophobic acrylic model that comes in a wider variety of embedded colors and can be placed as a foldable model in the capsular bag or with 5-point fixation loops in the sulcus, either passively or with suture fixation.[19]

An entirely separate category of cosmetic iris prostheses are designed for patients with no ocular abnormalities and for patients only with the desire to change eye color. It is important to note that the cosmetic iris prosthesis models like BrightOcular (Stellar Devices) are not recommended because of their associated severe complications when the device is placed above native iris. There have been reports of irreversible vision loss, severe iris damage, glaucoma, uveitis, and corneal decompensation. We are unaware of any studies showing their safety.[20-22]

References

1. Snyder ME, Han DC. Prosthetic iris device implantation. In: Randleman B, Ahmed I, eds. *Intraocular Lens Surgery: Selection, Complications, and Complex Cases*. Thieme; 2016: Chapter 26.
2. Alio JL, Al-Shymali O, Amesty MA, Rodriguez AE. Keratopigmentation with micronised mineral pigments: complications and outcomes in a series of 234 eyes. *Br J Ophthalmol*. 2018;102(6):742-747.
3. Alio JL, Rodriguez AE, El Bahrawy M, Angelov A, Zein G. Keratopigmentation to change the apparent color of the human eye: a novel indication for corneal tattooing. *Cornea*. 2016;35(4):431-437.
4. Alio JL, Rodriguez AE, Toffaha BT, El Aswad A. Femtosecond-assisted keratopigmentation double tunnel technique in the management of a case of Urrets-Zavalia syndrome. *Cornea*. 2012;31(9):1071-1074.
5. McCannel MA. A retrievable suture idea for anterior uveal problems. *Ophthalmic Surg*. 1976;7(2):98-103.
6. Siepser SB. The closed chamber slipping suture technique for iris repair. *Ann Ophthalmol*. 1994;26(3):71-72.
7. Osher RH, Snyder ME, Cionni RJ. Modification of the Siepser slip-knot technique. *J Cataract Refract Surg*. 2005;31(6):1098-1100.
8. Rosenthal KJ. Iris defects and complications. In: Fishkind WJ, ed. *Phacoemulsification and Intraocular Lens Implantation: Mastering Techniques and Complications in Cataract Surgery*. 2nd ed. Thieme; 2017; 263-274.
9. HumanOptics A. *CustomFlex Artificial Iris: Professional Use Information*. July 28, 2019. Accessed October 20, 2021. https://www.accessdata.fda.gov/cdrh_docs/pdf17/P170039d.pdf
10. FDA approves first artificial iris [News release]. *U.S. Food & Drug Administration*. May 30, 2018. Updated May 31, 2018. Accessed October 20, 2021. https://www.fda.gov/newsevents/newsroom/pressannouncements/ucm609291.htm
11. Srinivasan S, Ting DSJ, Snyder ME, Prasad S, Koch HR. Prosthetic iris devices. *Can J Ophthalmol*. 2014;49(1):6-17.
12. Ayliffe W, Groth SL, Sponsel WE. Small-incision insertion of artificial iris prostheses. *J Cataract Refract Surg*. 2012;38(2):362-367.
13. Rana M, Savant V, Prydal JI. A new customized artificial iris diaphragm for treatment of traumatic aniridia. *Cont Lens Anterior Eye*. 2013;36(2):93-94.
14. Mayer CS, Reznicek L, Hoffmann AE. Pupillary reconstruction and outcome after artificial iris implantation. *Ophthalmology*. 2016;123(5):1011-1018.
15. Mayer C, Tandogan T, Hoffmann AE, Khoramnia R. Artificial iris implantation in various iris defects and lens conditions. *J Cataract Refract Surg*. 2017;43(6):724-731.
16. Mavrikakis I, Mavrikakis E, Syam PP, et al. Surgical management of iris defects with prosthetic iris devices. *Eye (Lond)*. 2005;19(2):205-209.
17. Burk SE, Da Mata AP, Snyder ME, Cionni RJ, Cohen JS, Osher RH. Prosthetic iris implantation for congenital, traumatic, or functional iris deficiencies. *J Cataract Refract Surg*. 2001;27(11):1732-1740.
18. Aslam SA, Wong SC, Ficker LA, MacLaren RE. Implantation of the black diaphragm intraocular lens in congenital and traumatic aniridia. *Ophthalmology*. 2008;115(10):1705-1712.
19. Pozdeyeva NA, Pashtayev NP, Lukin VP, Batkov YN. Artificial iris-lens diaphragm in reconstructive surgery for aniridia and aphakia. *J Cataract Refract Surg*. 2005;31(9):1750-1759.
20. Mansour AM, Ahmed II, Eadie B, et al. Iritis, glaucoma and corneal decompensation associated with BrightOcular cosmetic iris implant. *Br J Ophthalmol*. 2016;100(8):1098-1101.
21. Chaurasia S. Devastating complication of cosmetic iris implants. *Indian J Ophthalmol*. 2017;65(8):771-772.
22. Kelly A, Kaufman SC. Corneal endothelial cell loss and iritis associated with a new cosmetic iris implant. *JAMA Ophthalmol*. 2015;133(6):723-724.

SECTION VII

POSTOPERATIVE

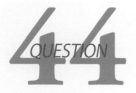

A Patient Who Had Been Doing Well After DMEK Presents With New Corneal Edema. What Should I Do?

Yuri McKee, MD, MS

By definition, a patient who had initial graft clearing followed by subsequent edema has secondary corneal graft failure. The differential diagnosis of secondary graft failure after Descemet's membrane endothelial keratoplasty (DMEK) includes graft rejection, viral infection, graft dislocation, medication-induced graft failure, and late graft failure. While none of these scenarios is common, the time-sensitive diagnoses are those of corneal graft rejection and viral endotheliitis, as endothelial damage is ongoing during these processes.

Diagnostic Considerations

The corneal evaluation of a patient with new-onset corneal edema after a previous functioning DMEK should quantify the area and density of the edema. If edema is diffusely noted across the area of the graft, then graft failure or rejection should be considered (Figure 44-1). If a focal area of edema exists overlying an area of graft detachment, then late graft failure or rejection may be less likely (Figure 44-2). In focal secondary edema, a history of blunt trauma may be elicited. Another reason for a focal DMEK detachment could be a physical repulsion of the graft by an irregularity in the posterior corneal stroma from old corneal wounds or a tight suture (Figure 44-3). Anterior segment optical coherence tomography may help to confirm the etiology of a partial graft detachment if the corneal edema is dense enough to preclude the view of the graft. Specular microscopy is useful in these cases to ensure that the areas of attached graft still have viable endothelial cells.

Certain medications are also known to affect endothelial function. Feng et al[1] described a case of memantine-associated endothelial dysfunction and subsequent DMEK failure. Once memantine was discontinued, the subsequent DMEK grafts were successful.

Hardten DR, Hansen MS.
Curbside Consultation in Cornea and External Disease:
49 Clinical Questions, Second Edition (pp 249-252).
© 2022 Taylor & Francis Group.

Figure 44-1. Large areas of DMEK detachment in a failed graft.

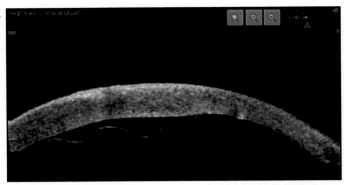

Figure 44-2. A focal area of graft detachment caused by accidental blunt trauma 4 weeks after surgery. Anterior segment optical coherence tomography easily demonstrates the focal graft detachment.

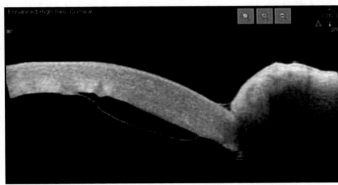

Figure 44-3. Focal repulsion of a DMEK graft at the graft–host junction of a previous penetrating keratoplasty.

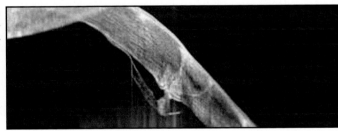

In cases of DMEK graft rejection, there may or may not be corneal edema. The typical rejection line with trailing corneal edema may not be seen. The patient may be completely asymptomatic or present with decreased vision, redness, photophobia, discomfort, anterior chamber cell or flare, and keratic precipitates (KPs). Graft KPs in DMEK rejection are typically diffuse (Figure 44-4), and the eye is generally much less inflamed compared with graft rejection in a penetrating keratoplasty. Because the signs and symptoms of DMEK graft rejection are so much less intense than the classic signs of penetrating keratoplasty graft rejection, the condition may be initially missed. Careful examination for even the slightest anterior chamber cell or KP on the graft should be undertaken. Graft edema is typically a late finding in DMEK graft rejection.

Fortunately, the rate of DMEK graft rejection is far less than other corneal graft modalities. Anshu et al[2] initially reported a DMEK graft rejection rate of less than 1%. Price et al[3-5] have further described very low rejection rates, even with less potent topical steroids. They also reported that cessation of topical steroids for rejection prophylaxis can raise long-term rejection rates from 1% to 3% to 3% to 6%.[3-5] Therefore, it is advisable to keep DMEK patients on at least once-daily low-potency steroids such as fluorometholone or loteprednol.

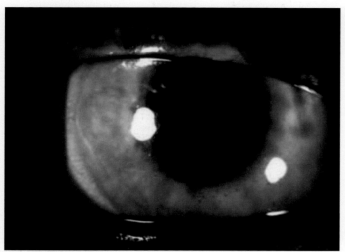

Figure 44-4. Diffuse KP within the confines of the DMEK graft without corneal edema.

A critical consideration in DMEK graft rejection that does not improve with topical steroid application is the possibility of herpetic or cytomegalovirus infection or reactivation. Tan and Tan[6] reported a retrospective review of 4 cases of cytomegalovirus endotheliitis. It was noted that the signs of cytomegalovirus can closely mimic signs of graft rejection; however, graft rejection will not have KP outside of the confines of the graft, whereas viral endotheliitis is not always restricted only to transplanted cells. A high index of suspicion and aqueous polymerase chain reaction testing are critical in establishing the proper diagnosis. Topical and oral ganciclovir yielded eventual success in all cases in their case series.

Treatment

The treatment of graft rejection in DMEK is similar to immune rejection in other corneal transplant types. The frequent use of topical steroids for several weeks tends to rapidly diminish the signs and symptoms. Graft loss is rare if rejection is diagnosed and treated promptly. Nonresolving graft rejection, initial intraocular pressure elevation at diagnosis, or significant uveitis should raise suspicion of viral endotheliitis. When a rejection episode is resolved, it may be advisable to either increase the potency or the frequency of the steroid prophylaxis above the level at which the immune rejection occurred. Complete DMEK failure after rejection episodes has been reported at very low rates in the peer-reviewed literature.[2,7]

If rejection or infection is either not suspected or has completely resolved, the surgeon may consider pneumatic assistance for graft detachments larger than 30% of the graft. In cases of localized graft detachment or an overall tenuous graft attachment, the surgeon may attempt an injection of air or nonexpansile gas into the anterior chamber if a patent inferior iridotomy is present. The patient would then require supine positioning to allow for graft–host apposition. A graft that fails to reattach after 2 or 3 air injection cycles may require replacement. Graft rejection may not cause graft dislocation. The time required for the body to mount an immune response against graft antigens is typically long enough for the DMEK graft to have created adhesions to the host cornea that may maintain graft adhesion, even after graft failure and the onset of edema.

Conclusion

Secondary graft failure after DMEK is generally rare. Graft rejection and viral infection are considerations of utmost importance in this condition. Appropriate antiviral or antirejection medications are critical to prevent further damage to the endothelial cells. Even more unusual conditions are partial graft detachment from physical forces or complete late graft failure. An appropriate clinical examination, diagnostic modalities, and prompt treatment may save the graft and spare the patient from unnecessary surgery. Referral to a corneal specialist with DMEK experience is suggested if any doubt exists as to the cause of secondary graft edema or the proper treatment regimen.

References

1. Feng MT, Price FW Jr, McKee Y, Price MO. Memantine-associated corneal endothelial dysfunction. *JAMA Ophthalmol*. 2015;133(10):1218-1220.
2. Anshu A, Price MO, Price FW Jr. Risk of corneal transplant rejection significantly reduced with Descemet's membrane endothelial keratoplasty. *Ophthalmology*. 2012;119(3):536-540.
3. Price MO, Feng MT, Scanameo A, Price FW Jr. Loteprednol etabonate 0.5% gel vs. prednisolone acetate 1% solution after Descemet membrane endothelial keratoplasty: prospective randomized trial. *Cornea*. 2015;34(8):853-858.
4. Price MO, Price FW Jr, Kruse FE, Bachmann BO, Tourtas T. Randomized comparison of topical prednisolone acetate 1% versus fluorometholone 0.1% in the first year after Descemet membrane endothelial keratoplasty. *Cornea*. 2014;33(9):880-886.
5. Price MO, Scanameo A, Feng MT, Price FW Jr. Descemet's membrane endothelial keratoplasty: risk of immunologic rejection episodes after discontinuing topical corticosteroids. *Ophthalmology*. 2016;123(6):1232-1236.
6. Tan TE, Tan DTH. Cytomegalovirus corneal endotheliitis after Descemet membrane endothelial keratoplasty. *Cornea*. 2019;38(4):413-418.
7. Price DA, Kelley M, Price FW Jr, Price MO. Five-year graft survival of Descemet membrane endothelial keratoplasty (EK) versus Descemet stripping EK and the effect of donor sex matching. *Ophthalmology*. 2018;125(10):1508-1514.
8. Ham L, Dapena I, Liarakos VS, et al. Midterm results of Descemet membrane endothelial keratoplasty: 4 to 7 years clinical outcome. *Am J Ophthalmol*. 2016;171:113-121.
9. Hos D, Tuac O, Schaub F, et al. Incidence and clinical course of immune reactions after Descemet membrane endothelial keratoplasty: retrospective analysis of 1000 consecutive eyes. *Ophthalmology*. 2017;124(4):512-518.
10. Monnereau C, Bruinsma M, Ham L, et al. Endothelial cell changes as an indicator for upcoming allograft rejection following Descemet membrane endothelial keratoplasty. *Am J Ophthalmol*. 2014;158(3):485-495.
11. Price MO, Feng MT, McKee Y, Price FW Jr. Repeat Descemet membrane endothelial keratoplasty: secondary grafts with early intervention are comparable with fellow-eye primary grafts. *Ophthalmology*. 2015;122(8):1639-1644.

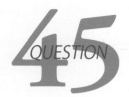

How Should I Manage an Intraocular Pressure Spike of 43 mm Hg in a Patient With DMEK Who Is Taking 1 Drop of Pred Forte 1% Daily?

Laura Voicu, MD and Krishna Surapaneni, MD

Elevated intraocular pressure (IOP) after corneal transplantation is a common problem due to the long-term use of steroid eye drops to prevent graft rejection. High steroid responses (IOP > 21 mm Hg) may occur in more than 15% of transplant patients. The incidence IOP elevation in Descemet's membrane endothelial keratoplasty (DMEK) is 6.5% to 12.1%, most frequently due to steroid response.[1] Descemet's stripping endothelial keratoplasty (DSEK) has a higher reported incidence of IOP elevation of 17% to 43%,[1,2] which may support considering a DMEK procedure over DSEK when appropriate in patients who are at risk for developing IOP elevation postoperatively.

Minimizing the Likelihood of Elevated Pressures

It is important to identify patients preoperatively who are at increased risk for developing IOP elevation postoperatively. Risk factors include preexisting glaucoma, bullous keratopathy, history of steroid response, damage to outflow mechanisms, and angle closure due to peripheral anterior synechiae.[1] Careful preoperative examination with gonioscopy is important to identify patients at increased risk of elevated IOP, which, after DMEK, is most often due to steroid use,[1] but it may also include inflammation and/or damage to the trabecular meshwork. Additionally, herpetic disease may be reactivated in the setting of corneal transplantation and can be associated with a trabeculitis.[3] Before any cornea transplant, especially in patients with preexisting glaucoma, it is prudent to optimize the IOP. In the case of a known steroid responder, careful optimization

Hardten DR, Hansen MS.
*Curbside Consultation in Cornea and External Disease:
49 Clinical Questions, Second Edition* (pp 253-256).
© 2022 Taylor & Francis Group.

of IOP before surgery and a low threshold to optimize medical management early in the post-transplant time period may reduce the likelihood of an IOP spike in the postoperative period.[1,2]

Given the need for an air or gas bubble to promote graft adherence postoperatively, patients may develop a mechanical angle-closure glaucoma in the immediate postoperative period, but this has not been shown to lead to a higher risk of developing peripheral anterior synechiae that would increase the long-term risk of glaucoma.[1] This can be managed and/or avoided by decreasing the bubble size at the end of surgery, dilating the pupil, or by performing an inferior iridotomy peri-operatively. A study that compared the use of sulfur hexachloride and air in DMEK surgery did not show a difference in the rate of elevated IOP in the immediate postoperative period.[4]

DMEK in eyes with previous trabeculectomy or glaucoma drainage devices have been shown to have good postoperative outcomes, and DMEK may be preferable compared to DSEK in patients who are at high risk for developing steroid response postoperatively, due to the ability to taper steroid doses faster in these eyes.[5,6]

IOP Management

Most likely, a patient with IOP elevation after DMEK is a steroid responder, and our preferred initial treatment would be monotherapy using a topical, nonselective, beta-adrenergic blocker; an adrenergic agonist; or a prostaglandin analog.[7] Other causes of late postoperative IOP elevations, including damage to the trabecular meshwork, persistent inflammation, or preexisting glaucoma, have to be considered as well.

If the medication is effective and there are no side effects, the regimen can be continued. Often, an IOP decrease of at least 20% from baseline is defined as an effective initial treatment in glaucoma management. However, the goal depends on the baseline IOP and optic nerve status—if the IOP is extremely high, such as 43 mm Hg, multiple medications may be necessary to reach an acceptable IOP.

If the first-choice drug is not effective or if side effects occur, then therapy is switched within the first-choice drug group. If the drug is effective but the target IOP is not reached, a switch between monotherapies is an option. However, if the first drug has decreased IOP sufficiently but the target IOP is not reached, combining drugs from the first-choice group is a good next step.

The newer medication netarsudil may become an excellent early treatment option for use in post-DMEK eyes. Netarsudil, a Rho-associated protein kinase (ROCK) inhibitor, may have effects on endothelial cell migration that could potentially be beneficial in post-transplant eyes. ROCK inhibitors may play a part in increasing cell adhesion and proliferation, and this may allow for preservation of corneal endothelium and the slowing of apoptosis.[8] This new class of glaucoma medication adds to our toolbox in treating these patients, although its role is still evolving. Additional research will be needed to identify the best use of these newer medications in post-transplant eyes with elevated IOP.

Nonselective adrenergic agents, parasympathomimetic, and topical and systemic carbonic anhydrase inhibitors are considered a lesser preferred second-choice group. Treatment of high IOP with carbonic anhydrase inhibitors may have an adverse effect on corneal endothelial cells by attenuating the bicarbonate efflux and subsequent loss of stroma dehydration. Dorzolamide has been reported to lead to increased corneal thickness, but the effect on corneal cell morphology and corneal cell density is unknown. However, carbonic anhydrase inhibitor therapy may have a stronger effect on corneal thickness in patients with preexisting corneal endothelium problems (such as those due to Fuchs' endothelial dystrophy or following penetrating keratoplasty), which has also been suggested in the literature.[9,10] Even though the effect of carbonic anhydrase inhibitors on corneal endothelium is not fully elucidated, it would be prudent to be careful with these agents in patients with a compromised corneal endothelium. Concomitant oral therapy might even enhance the negative effects of topical carbonic anhydrase on corneal endothelium.

To avoid steroid response, an effective topical steroid with the least chance to increase IOP should be chosen. The ability of topical steroids to induce IOP elevation depends on the dosage, treatment duration, drug formulation (hydrophilic phosphate form or lipophilic alcohol or acetate form), and the anti-inflammatory potency of the steroid. Dexamethasone and prednisolone are highly potent steroids and cause steroid responses more often than less potent steroids. Fluorometholone and loteprednol are less potent steroids that are effective in controlling ocular inflammation but lead to substantially less IOP elevation. This is possibly due to local steroid metabolism in the cornea and subsequent reduced penetration into the aqueous humor. In a prospective, randomized study conducted comparing the use of loteprednol vs prednisolone acetate 1% after DMEK by Price et al,[5] loteprednol was as effective in preventing immunologic graft rejection and significantly less likely to cause IOP elevation.

Tapering the frequency of steroid drops can be effective in managing a steroid response. In the case that elevated IOP persists despite lowering the corticosteroid dose and initiating antiglaucomatous drugs, the use of systemic immunosuppressive drugs (eg, cyclosporine, mycophenolate mofetil) could be considered in patients with high risk for immune graft rejection. Stopping topical steroids in the setting of elevated IOP is a consideration. However, Price et al[5] found that topical steroids 1 year after DMEK transplantation may be protective against graft rejection and that 6% of patients who discontinued steroids after this time period experienced graft rejection. Those authors also found in this prospective trial that 0% of patients who had reduced topical steroid use to once daily after the first year had experienced graft rejection, and hence lowering steroid frequency should be considered.[11]

If IOP is refractory to medical treatment, interventions such as selective laser trabeculoplasty, trabeculectomy, XEN implant (Allergan Inc), angle surgery, or a glaucoma shunt can be considered. The management of glaucoma should be commensurate with the status of the optic nerve as well as whether there is any evidence of glaucomatous optic neuropathy. There is currently no specific consensus on glaucoma surgical management after endothelial keratoplasty. Surgical outcomes may be more favorable in patients who have had previous endothelial keratoplasty vs penetrating keratoplasty.[12] Placement of any kind of glaucoma filter should be carefully considered to avoid endothelial contact, as this may result in corneal decompensation.

IOP Measurement After DMEK

The interpretation of IOP in the post-transplant eye is challenging because corneal irregularity and increased corneal thickness influence the validity of applanation measurements. It has been postulated that a 10% change in central corneal thickness will result in a 3.4 mm Hg change of IOP.[13] After endothelial keratoplasty, the corneal thickness increases during and after the postoperative period. Goldmann tonometer (Haag-Streit Diagnostics) is calibrated for a corneal thickness of 520 µm; therefore, Goldmann tonometry is less accurate in corneas with a thickness out of the normal range. Nomograms to correct for the falsely increased IOP in thick corneas are not commonly used because their accuracy is questionable. It has been suggested that dynamic contour tonometry (DCT; PASCAL, Swiss Microtechnology) measures IOP independent from curvature and corneal thickness. Although there is less research published in post-DMEK eyes, a recent study comparing IOP after DSEK with 3 measurement techniques (Goldmann tonometry, DCT, and pneumotonometry), found that Goldmann tonometry measured lower IOP levels (4 mm Hg lower on average) compared with DCT and pneumotonometry.[14] In addition, no correlation was found between IOP and corneal thickness. Because the DSEK graft is not attached to the limbus, these findings suggested that the grafted part of the cornea does not contribute to the biomechanical effects on IOP measurement (Figure 45-1). It is also possible that the viscous properties of the post-DSEK cornea have changed because of the resolution of previous corneal edema, which could

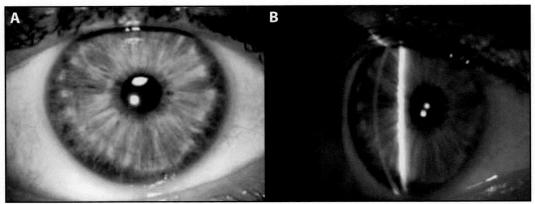

Figure 45-1. (A) Eye with DMEK showing a clear, nicely centered posterior lamellar disc. (B) Eye with DMEK showing the posterior lamellar disc that is not attached to the limbus; therefore, it has no biomechanical effect on measuring IOP.

be responsible for the lower IOP measured by Goldmann tonometry.[2] One study of IOP measurement techniques in post-DMEK eyes observed broad variability between different techniques and suggested that consistently using one IOP measurement technique to follow IOP changes would be beneficial in these eyes.[15]

References

1. Maier AKB, Wolf T, Gundlach E, et al. Intraocular pressure elevation and post-DMEK glaucoma following Descemet membrane endothelial keratoplasty. *Graefes Arch Clin Exp Ophthalmol*. 2014;252(12):1947-1954.
2. Naveiras M, Dirisamer M, Parker J, et al. Causes of glaucoma after Descemet membrane endothelial keratoplasty. *Am J Ophthalmol*. 2012;153(5):958-966.e1.
3. Asi F, Milioti G, Seitz B. Descemet membrane endothelial keratoplasty for corneal decompensation caused by herpes simplex virus endotheliitis. *J Cataract Refract Surg*. 2018;44(1):106-108.
4. Einan-Lifshitz A, Sorkin N, Boutin T, et al. Comparison of sulfur hexafluoride (SF6) and air tamponade in noniridectomized Descemet membrane endothelial keratoplasty. *Cornea*. 2018;37(3):273-276.
5. Price MO, Feng MT, Scanameo A, Price FW Jr. Loteprednol etabonate 0.5% gel vs. prednisolone acetate 1% solution after Descemet membrane endothelial keratoplasty: prospective randomized trial. *Cornea*. 2015;34(8):853-858.
6. Aravena C, Yu F, Deng SX. Outcomes of Descemet membrane endothelial keratoplasty in patients with previous glaucoma surgery. *Cornea*. 2017;36(3):284-289.
7. Webers CAB, Beckers HJM, Nuijts RMMA, Schouten JSAG. Pharmacological management of primary open-angle glaucoma: second-line options and beyond. *Drugs Aging*. 2008;25(9):729-759.
8. Moshirfar M, Parker L, Birdsong OC, et al. Use of Rho kinase inhibitors in ophthalmology: a review of the literature. *Med Hypothesis Discov Innov Ophthalmol*. 2018;7(3):101-111.
9. Konowal A, Morrison JC, Brown SV, et al. Irreversible corneal decompensation in patients treated with topical dorzolamide. *Am J Ophthalmol*. 1999;127(4):403-406.
10. Wirtitsch MG, Findl O, Heinzl H, Drexler W. Effect of dorzolamide hydrochloride on central corneal thickness in humans with cornea guttata. *Arch Ophthalmol*. 2007;125(10):1345-1350.
11. Price MO, Scanameo A, Feng MT, Price FW Jr. Descemet's membrane endothelial keratoplasty: risk of immunologic rejection episodes after discontinuing topical corticosteroids. *Ophthalmology*. 2016;123(6):1232-1236.
12. Kornmann HL, Gedde SJ. Glaucoma management after corneal transplantation surgeries. *Curr Opin Ophthalmol*. 2016;27(2):132-139.
13. Price MO, Price FW Jr. Descemet's stripping with endothelial keratoplasty: comparative outcomes with microkeratome-dissected and manually dissected donor tissue. *Ophthalmology*. 2006;113(11):1936-1942.
14. Vajaranant TS, Price MO, Price FW, Wilensky JT, Edward DP. Intraocular pressure measurements following Descemet stripping endothelial keratoplasty. *Am J Ophthalmol*. 2008;145(5):780-786.
15. Maier AK, Gundlach E, Pahlitzsch M, et al. Intraocular pressure measurements after Descemet membrane endothelial keratoplasty. *J Glaucoma*. 2017;26(3):258-265.

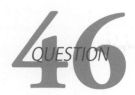
A Patient Is 5 Months After Corneal Transplant for a Corneal Scar and Now Has a New Epithelial Defect That Is Part on the Graft and Part on the Host Cornea. How Should I Manage This Patient?

Gary Legault, MD

A decrease in the rate of penetrating keratoplasty is likely due to the advancement of contact lens technology, corneal cross-linking, and earlier diagnosis of corneal pathology.[1] Despite this trend, we still need to prepare to manage postoperative complications from a penetrating keratoplasty. The first step is managing patient expectations prior to surgery. Often, patients think a penetrating keratoplasty is similar to LASIK, and they will be able to see immediately after surgery. Preoperative education about slow recovery, numerous follow-up examinations, a lifetime of steroid eye drops, and risk of postoperative complications is paramount for successful outcomes. An epithelial defect is one of the postoperative complications that risks a graft failure.

What Caused the Epithelial Defect?

The differential for an epithelial defect is broad, and eliciting an accurate patient history aids in making the diagnosis. Knowing the indication for the patient's corneal transplant often provides a clue because history often repeats itself. An infectious etiology, such as herpes simplex virus (HSV) keratitis, should remain high in the differential, especially if the patient had a corneal transplant due to a corneal scar from an infection. Multiple studies have shown higher rates of epithelial defects in patients with a history of HSV or adenovirus compared with patients without a viral infection.[2-3] Mechanical trauma, such as a fingernail scratch or foreign body, can be determined from the patient's history and examination. Additionally, decreased tear production from a vitamin A deficiency or Sjogren's syndrome can predispose a patient to an epithelial defect.

Hardten DR, Hansen MS.
Curbside Consultation in Cornea and External Disease:
49 Clinical Questions, Second Edition (pp 257-259).
© 2022 Taylor & Francis Group.

Other possibilities to consider are limbal stem cell deficiency from chemical burns, a neurotrophic trigeminal nerve from HSV, varicella zoster virus, diabetes, exposure keratopathy, or even topical anesthetic abuse.[4]

How to Treat the Epithelial Defect

Determining the etiology of the epithelial defect can help guide the treatment plan. If there is any possibility that the defect could be HSV, I have a low threshold for starting oral acyclovir or valacyclovir. While the epithelial defect persists, I add a prophylactic antibiotic eye drop, such as Polytrim (polymyxin B/trimethoprim), 4 times daily to avoid a bacterial infection. I always start with aggressive lubrication with ointment and preservative artificial tears at least every hour. To avoid rejection, I keep patients on lifelong steroid eye drops and do not stop the drops for an epithelial defect. Because the patient is only 5 months post-surgery, sutures are typically still in place. I will remove any loose or broken sutures. Finally, if there are no contraindications, I will start doxycycline 100 mg twice daily. Oral tetracycline (250 mg 4 times daily) and doxycycline (20 to 100 mg twice daily) have each demonstrated benefits in patients with persistent epithelial defects.[5]

What if the Epithelial Defect Persists?

If there is little or no improvement of the epithelial defect after 3 days, I will add a bandage contact lens. A Kontur lens (Kontur Kontact Lens Co Inc) is preferable because it typically fits better in patients after penetrating keratoplasty than a standard soft contact lens. If the epithelial defect persists after 1 week of contact lens use, I will add amniotic membrane such as a PROKERA Slim (Bio-Tissue Inc). Amniotic membrane can accelerate the recovery of the cornea epithelium.[6] At the same time, I place an order for autologous serum tears. Autologous serum tears can be challenging to acquire for patients, but, anecdotally, I have seen restoration of the epithelium within days of starting the tears. A recent report from the American Academy of Ophthalmology identified no published controlled studies to support the use of serum tears, even though 4 papers showed a benefit for patients with persistent epithelial defects.[7] If there is still no resolution, I will perform a temporary tarsorrhaphy. Sometimes, I may have already placed a tarsorrhaphy in noncompliant patients, patients with exposure keratopathy, or when a PROKERA amniotic membrane constantly comes out of the fornix. A last resort is the use of a Prosthetic Replacement of the Ocular Surface Ecosystem (PROSE; Boston Sight).[8] Cenergermin is another option if there is a neurotrophic component. It has shown positive results when used 6 times daily for 8 weeks in the US Food and Drug Administration trials.[9]

How Can the Risk of Recurrence Be Minimized?

Minimizing the recurrence of an epithelial defect can vary depending on the etiology. All patients should continue artificial tears to improve the ocular surface. In exposure keratopathy, I refer the patient for a consultation with an oculoplastics specialist to consider a procedure to tighten the eyelids. For patients with HSV, I recommend oral acyclovir 400 mg twice daily for prophylaxis for at least 1 year. For all patients, I continue daily steroid eye drops to prevent an immunologic graft rejection while closely monitoring for any signs of glaucoma.

Conclusion

A penetrating keratoplasty requires numerous follow-up examinations and a long recovery period. Prompt recognition and treatment of postoperative complications is necessary to optimize visual outcomes.

References

1. Wagoner MD, Ba-Abbad R, Al-Mohaimeed M, et al. Postoperative complications after primary adult optical penetrating keratoplasty: prevalence and impact on graft survival. *Cornea.* 2009;28(4):385-394.
2. Beyer CF, Byrd TJ, Hill JM, Kaufman HE. Herpes simplex virus and persistent epithelial defects after penetrating keratoplasty. *Am J Opthalmol.* 1990;109(1):95-96.
3. Ricci F, Missiroli F, Ciotti M, Perno CF, Cerulli L. Persistent epithelial defects after penetrating keratoplasty caused by adenoviral infectious keratitis. *New Microbiol.* 2010;33(2):171-174.
4. Dahlgren MA, Dhaliwal A, Huang AJW. Persistent epithelial defects. In: Albert DM, Miller JW, eds. *Albert & Jakobiec's Principles and Practice of Ophthalmology.* Elsevier; 2008:749-759.
5. Cykiert RC. Systemic tetracycline therapy for epithelial defects. *Ophthalmology.* 1987;94(7):894-895.
6. Cehng AMS, Tseng SCG. Self-retained amniotic membrane combined with antiviral therapy for herpetic epithelial keratitis. *Cornea.* 2017;36(11):1383-1386.
7. Shtein RM, Shen JF, Kuo AN, Hammersmith KM, Li JY, Weikert MP. Autologous serum-based eye drops for treatment of ocular surface disease: a report by the American Academy of Ophthalmology. *Ophthalmology.* 2020;127(1):128-133.
8. Lim P, Ridges R, Jacobs DS, Rosenthal P. Treatment of persistent corneal epithelial defect with overnight wear of a prosthetic device for the ocular surface. *Am J Ophthalmol.* 2013;156(6):1095-1101.
9. Sheha H, Tighe S, Hashem O, Hayashida Y. Update on cenegermin eye drops in the treatment of neurotrophic keratitis. *Clin Ophthalmol.* 2019;13:1973-1980.

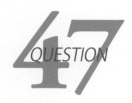

QUESTION

47

What Should I Do for a Patient Who Presents With 6.0 Diopters of Astigmatism After Undergoing Penetrating Keratoplasty 24 Months Ago?

Elaine Zhou, MD and Zaina Al-Mohtaseb, MD

The goal of a penetrating keratoplasty (PK) is to provide patients with optimal vision postoperatively. Despite having a clear graft, remnant refractive error (especially astigmatism) may limit vision. A high degree of postoperative astigmatism is a common dilemma that requires careful consideration.

In the initial postoperative period, post-PK astigmatism may be managed conservatively with spectacles and rigid gas permeable or scleral contact lenses. Selective topography-guided suture removal may begin 3 months postoperatively if interrupted sutures are used. In selective suture removal, corneal topography should be correlated to the patient's manifest refraction to confirm the steep axis before removal of tight sutures corresponding to the steep axis. We dislike removing more than 2 or 3 sutures at a time, given the risk of rejection and potential for major changes in astigmatism after removal.

After complete suture removal, 15% to 31% of patients still have residual astigmatism greater than 5.0 diopters (D).[1] In fact, average post-PK astigmatism is 4.0 to 6.0 D.[2]

The timing of surgical correction of residual refractive error and astigmatism is the most important consideration. The graft–host junction generally reaches maximal healing (although there will always be a weak point) by 1 year and corneal topography is stable 2 to 3 months after complete suture removal. If all sutures have been removed, astigmatism that is present 24 months post-PK will likely not improve with time. The following interventions may be considered to correct post-PK astigmatism.

Hardten DR, Hansen MS.
Curbside Consultation in Cornea and External Disease:
49 Clinical Questions, Second Edition (pp 261-264).
© 2022 Taylor & Francis Group.

Contact Lens

The least invasive intervention that will most quickly achieve an optimal visual outcome is contact lenses, especially in patients who have additional spherical error, high degrees of anisometropia, or aphakia. Traditional rigid gas permeable lenses are most commonly used.[3] However, many patients may be intolerant to rigid gas permeable lenses due to poor ocular surface, large degree of corneal irregularity, or discomfort. In these patients, scleral contact lenses should be tried. Newer designs of scleral lenses, including Boston Sight's Prosthetic Replacement of the Ocular Surface Ecosystem (PROSE) and EYEPRINT Prosthetics, can be custom-made, custom fit to the patient's eye, and made to contour over irregular surfaces, such as glaucoma blebs.[4] These contact lens fittings often require multiple visits and specialized training. A close relationship with an optometrist who specializes in contact lens fittings would likely lead to more successful outcomes.

Relaxing Incisions

The basic principle of relaxing incisions is to create partial-depth arcuate incisions that flatten at the meridian of the incision and steepen 90 degrees away. These quick procedures can be performed at the slit lamp, minor procedure room, or operating room. Patients generally stabilize within 6 to 8 weeks. The incision can be performed in the host or in the graft. Arcuate incisions within the graft (termed *astigmatic keratotomy*) are more effective because the graft–host junction may block the effects of the incision if placed outside of the graft.

Older nomograms for congenital astigmatism generally do not apply to post-PK patients. However, several newer nomograms, including the Hanna nomogram, Nordan nomogram, and Saint-Clair nomogram are validated for post-PK eyes.

Relaxing incisions can be performed manually or can be laser-assisted. Femtosecond laser-assisted arcuate keratotomy has been shown to have lower rates of wound dehiscence, epithelial down growth, infection and perforation.[5] We prefer not to perform an astigmatic keratotomy that is longer than 50 degrees, given the risk of irregular astigmatism and patient discomfort.

Laser Refractive Surgery

LASIK and photorefractive keratectomy (PRK) are also effective options for improving post-PK astigmatism, especially if a spherical correction is needed as well. However, these options are limited by corneal thickness, stromal bed size, and status of the ocular surface. Greater astigmatic corrections may be obtained with PRK because the lack of flap allows for greater availability of corneal stroma. Often, the goal of laser refractive surgery in cases of large refractive error or large astigmatism (> 6.0 D) is to attenuate refractive error or anisometropia and to make contact lenses or spectacles more tolerable.[6]

LASIK and PRK both have their own advantages. LASIK has a faster healing and visual rehabilitation time, minimal regression, and low risk for stromal haze. PRK eliminates the risk for flap complications, but it has a risk of stromal haze, especially with higher amounts of correction. The use of mitomycin-C has decreased the incidence of stromal haze.

Traditionally, laser refractive surgery has been limited by irregular astigmatism post-PK. Advances in custom ablation, including topography-guided and wavefront-guided ablations, have allowed for treatment of irregular astigmatism. Topography-guided ablation creates laser ablation patterns by comparing the topography of the patient's anterior corneal surface to a perfect sphere.

This technology has been shown to reduce corneal irregularities and astigmatism, but it may still not improve uncorrected visual acuity.[7] It is important to discuss with the patient that the goal for this refractive surgery may be to improve best-corrected vision, but the patient may still be contact lens or spectacle dependent.

Toric Intraocular Lenses

In patients with regular, symmetric astigmatism and a visually significant cataract after PK, toric intraocular lenses (IOL) may provide a potential solution. Combining implantation of a toric IOL with intraoperative use of aberrometry devices (such as the Optiwave Refractive Analysis; Alcon) may improve refractive predictability. However, the highest power toric IOL currently available corrects only up to +4.5 D of astigmatism at the corneal plane. In patients with higher amounts of astigmatism, spectacles or additional procedures may be needed to correct residual astigmatism.

In patients with clear lenses with no cataract, phakic IOLs may also be an option. However, a patient must be counseled about the increased risk of endothelial cell loss, immunologic rejection, and earlier formation of cataract.[8]

Additionally, the physician must remember that correcting for corneal astigmatism with an IOL makes the future use of hard contact lenses or scleral contact lenses difficult because a contact lens will eliminate corneal astigmatism, and the toric IOL cylinder will be left uncorrected. In patients who are dependent on contact lenses for corneal surface irregularity or poor ocular surface disease, a toric IOL may not be a good option. The best candidates are patients with regular astigmatism and those who wear spectacles that correct for that astigmatism and were happy prior to formation of cataract.

Historical Options

Wedge resection for high astigmatism (> 10.0 D), in which a thin slice of cornea is excised at the flat meridian, has fallen out of favor because of the unpredictability of outcomes and relative ease of other procedures.[9] Intrastromal corneal ring segments are also an option; however, they are limited by the need for corneal thickness and risk for infection and extrusion.

Conclusion

Patient satisfaction with their postoperative vision is highly dependent on expectations. Prior to surgery, discussing the likely need for further refractive correction after PK is essential. The goal of the procedures discussed is often to improve best-corrected visual acuity and to possibly decrease dependence on spectacles or contact lenses. It is important to understand the options available for astigmatic correction, tailor treatment plans for your specific patient, and be able to preemptively counsel patients on the appropriate options.

References

1. Feizi S, Zare M. Current approaches for management of postpenetrating keratoplasty astigmatism. *J Ophthalmol.* 2011;2011:708736.
2. Skeens HM. Management of postkeratoplasty astigmatism. In: Krachmer JH, Mannis MJ, Holland EJ, eds. *Cornea: Fundamentals, Diagnosis, and Management.* 3rd ed. Elsevier; 2011:1397-1408.
3. Wietharn BE, Driebe WT Jr. Fitting contact lenses for visual rehabilitation after penetrating keratoplasty. *Eye Contact Lens.* 2004;30(1):31-33.
4. Lee JC, Chiu GB, Bach D, Bababeygy SR, Irvine J, Heur M. Functional and visual improvement with prosthetic replacement of the ocular surface ecosystem scleral lenses for irregular corneas. *Cornea.* 2013;32(12):1540-1543.
5. Hoffart L, Proust H, Matonti F, Conrath J, Ridings. Correction of postkeratoplasty astigmatism by femtosecond laser compared with mechanized astigmatic keratotomy. *Am J Ophthalmol.* 2009;147(5):779-787 e1.
6. Kovoor TA, Mohamed E, Cavanagh HD, Bowman RW. Outcomes of LASIK and PRK in previous penetrating corneal transplant recipients. *Eye Contact Lens.* 2009;35(5):242-245.
7. Kwitko S, Cabal FP, de Araujo BS, Jung YP. Topography-guided ablation for the treatment of irregular astigmatism. *J EuCornea.* 2019;2:20-23.
8. Wade M, Steinert RF, Garg S, Farid M, Gaster R. Results of toric intraocular lenses for post-penetrating keratoplasty astigmatism. *Ophthalmology.* 2014;121(3):771-777.
9. Ezra DG, Hay-Smith G, Mearza A, Falcon MG. Corneal wedge excision in the treatment of high astigmatism after penetrating keratoplasty. *Cornea.* 2007;26(7):819-825.

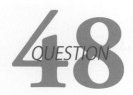

I HAVE A PATIENT WITH POOR VISION AFTER DMEK. WHAT WENT WRONG, AND HOW DO I GET BETTER VISION FOR THEM?

Bryan S. Lee, MD, JD

Descemet membrane endothelial keratoplasty (DMEK) has significantly improved the treatment of endothelial disease. It offers several advantages over its predecessor, Descemet stripping automated endothelial keratoplasty (DSAEK). Because the tissue being transplanted is thinner, there is a lower risk of rejection.[1] Accordingly, patients may use a less intense regimen to prevent rejection and have a high likelihood of success discontinuing steroids completely.[2,3]

Additionally, DMEK offers better postoperative vision than prior forms of endothelial keratoplasty. Presumably, this results from the anatomic replacement that DMEK offers, which avoids creation of a stromal–stromal interface. Even in comparison to ultrathin DSAEK, DMEK offers significantly better best-corrected visual acuity—about 1.5 lines better in one recent randomized trial.[4]

As surgeons have gained more experience with DMEK and as eye banks have performed more steps to prepare the tissue, the number of DMEK procedures has continued to increase each year.

Problems Related to the DMEK

During the immediate postoperative period, the presence of a large air bubble will obstruct the patient's vision. If 20% sulfur hexafluoride was used, the bubble can persist for several days. Once the bubble clears the visual axis, the visual acuity is usually good within a few days. If not, one possibility is an inverted graft. However, this complication has become less common because the eye bank can place a mark, usually an "S" or "F," at the surgeon's request to mark graft orientation (Figure 48-1). Other techniques used intraoperatively to reduce the risk of flipped tissue include intraoperative optical coherence tomography (OCT) or visual techniques such as the Moutsouris sign.[5]

Hardten DR, Hansen MS.
*Curbside Consultation in Cornea and External Disease:
49 Clinical Questions, Second Edition* (pp 265-268).
© 2022 Taylor & Francis Group.

Figure 48-1. A mark, such as the "S" pictured here, simplifies the process of determining graft orientation intraoperatively.

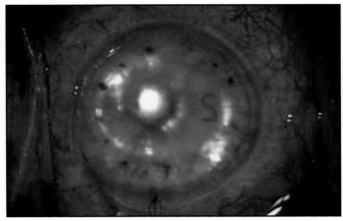

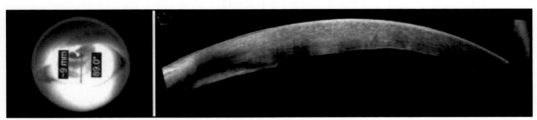

Figure 48-2. This anterior segment OCT demonstrates a small inferior graft detachment, which is the most common type to occur after DMEK. Because the area involved was small and the central graft was well attached, the DMEK was observed and adhered completely without any additional intervention.

Minimizing graft trauma and utilizing efficient techniques to decrease graft manipulation may not play as critical a role as assumed if the unfolding is done reasonably expeditiously.[6] Using a glass injector instead of plastic may cause less endothelial damage.[7] Having the eye bank preload the tissue may cause more endothelial cell loss compared with prestripping alone,[8] but the surgeon's loading of a prestripped tissue will certainly cause additional cell loss.

Poor or incomplete attachment will sometimes require rebubbling or perhaps even graft replacement. A graft that had significant endothelial loss from the surgery will take longer to clear the cornea, if it does at all. Anterior segment OCT may be helpful in identifying areas of detachment and anatomic factors that may be harming graft adhesion, such as posterior stromal irregularity, retained Descemet's membrane, or graft–host mismatch from tight sutures.

As a general rule, if 70% of the graft is attached, the likelihood is that the DMEK will remain attached (Figure 48-2). However, if more than 30% is detached, the detachment affects the visual axis, or the detachment is worsening while being observed, rebubbling can be done at the slit lamp.[9] If the view through the cornea is limited by postoperative edema, OCT can help to make the determination of what percentage is attached.

Posterior Segment Pathology

As with any intraocular surgery, postoperative cystoid macular edema (CME) can explain poor vision, especially in patients with an epiretinal membrane or diabetic retinopathy. If the patient is not seeing well after the graft has cleared, then a dilated fundus examination and potentially macular OCT are warranted. Studies have reported the incidence of post-DMEK CME to be between 7% and 15.6%. One study of 77 Asian eyes found a statistically significant increased risk of CME with greater iris damage, larger air volume, rebubbling, and performing staged DMEK (after phacoemulsification).[10] However, a larger study did not find a relationship between staging of the phacoemulsification and CME, and another did not find any clear risk factors for CME.[11,12]

Retinal or optic nerve pathology may have been difficult to visualize preoperatively because of the corneal disease. Examples include diseases such as epiretinal membrane, age-related macular degeneration, diabetic retinopathy, glaucoma, or optic nerve atrophy.

Additional Media Opacities

Although performing phakic DMEK is rare, it sometimes makes sense if the lens is essentially clear or if the patient is young and would benefit from preserving accommodation. A patient with very poor quality biometry because of corneal disease could potentially decide to perform the DMEK first, followed by repeat biometry. After DMEK, cataract progression is highly likely from the intraocular gas and postoperative steroids. Follow-up visits should include continued evaluation of the lens.

Once the patient is pseudophakic, posterior capsular opacification is another possible explanation for poor post-DMEK vision. If the intraocular lens (IOL) material is hydrophilic acrylic, then intraocular gas, including air and 20% sulfur hexafluoride, has been shown to cause IOL opacification from calcification.[13] A patient undergoing combination phacoemulsification-DMEK should not have a hydrophilic acrylic IOL implant. The surgeon should discuss the possibility of opacification preoperatively if a pseudophakic patient with a hydrophilic acrylic IOL is having DMEK.

Longer Term

For the cornea to clear, the endothelial cells must migrate from the DMEK to the surrounding cornea.[14,15] This migration may not happen symmetrically, resulting in variable refraction for months to beyond 1 year.[16] Those authors reported that endothelial cells preferentially migrated from the radial cut edges of a quarter DMEK graft rather than from the outer edge.

Although DMEK resolves edema and reduces the visual effect of guttae, it does not resolve anterior corneal disease. Several reports have shown improvement from phototherapeutic keratectomy (PTK) after DSAEK in patients with anterior basement membrane dystrophy or anterior stromal disease.[17,18] Additionally, PTK can be performed in combination with a refractive treatment with fairly good predictability.[19] Most likely, the same results would apply to PTK after DMEK, although studies would be needed to establish this.

References

1. Anshu A, Price MO, Price FW Jr. Risk of cornea transplant rejection significantly reduced with Descemet's membrane endothelial keratoplasty. *Ophthalmology*. 2012;119(3):536-540.
2. Price MO, Price FW Jr, Kruse FE, Bachmann BO, Tourtas T. Randomized comparison of topical prednisolone acetate 1% versus fluorometholone 0.1% in the first year after Descemet membrane endothelial keratoplasty. *Cornea*. 2014;33:880-886.
3. Price MO, Feng MT, Scanameo A, Price FW Jr. Loteprednol etabonate 0.5% gel vs. prednisolone acetate 1% solution after Descemet membrane endothelial keratoplasty: prospective randomized trial. *Cornea*. 2015;34(8):853-858.

4. Chamberlain W, Lin CC, Austin A, et al. Descemet endothelial thickness comparison trial: a randomized trial comparing ultrathin Descemet stripping automated endothelial keratoplasty with Descemet membrane endothelial keratoplasty. *Ophthalmology.* 2019;126(1):19-26.
5. Dapena I, Moutsouris K, Droutsas K, Ham L, van Dijk K, Melles GRJ. Standardized "no-touch" technique for Descemet membrane endothelial keratoplasty. *Arch Ophthalmol.* 2011;129(1):88-94.
6. Sales CS, Terry MA, Veldman PB, Mayko ZM, Straiko MD. Relationship between tissue unscrolling time and endothelial cell loss. *Cornea.* 2016;35(4):471-476.
7. Rickmann A, Wahl S, Katsen-Globa A, Szurman P. Safety analysis and results of a borosilicate glass cartridge for no-touch graft loading and injection in Descemet membrane endothelial keratoplasty. *Int Ophthalmol.* 2019;39(10):2295-2301.
8. Tran KD, Dye PK, Odell K, et al. Evaluation and quality assessment of prestripped, preloaded Descemet membrane endothelial keratoplasty grafts. *Cornea.* 2017;36(4):484-490.
9. Yeh RY, Quilendrino R, Musa FU, Liarakos VS, Dapena I, Melles GRJ. Predictive value of optical coherence tomography in graft attachment after Descemet's endothelial keratoplasty. *Ophthalmology.* 2013;120(2):240-245.
10. Inoda S, Hayashi T, Takahashi H, et al. Risk factors for cystoid macular edema after Descemet membrane endothelial keratoplasty. *Cornea.* 2019;38(7):820-824.
11. Flanary WE, Vislisel JM, Wagoner MD, et al. Incidence of cystoid macular edema after Descemet membrane endothelial keratoplasty as a staged and solitary procedure. *Cornea.* 2016;35(8):1040-1044.
12. Kocaba V, Mouchel R, Fleury J, et al. Incidence of cystoid macular edema after Descemet membrane endothelial keratoplasty. *Cornea.* 2018;37(3):277-282.
13. Werner L, Wilbanks G, Ollerton A, Michelson J. Localized calcification of hydrophilic acrylic intraocular lenses in association with intracameral injection of gas. *J Cataract Refract Surg.* 2012;38(4):720-721.
14. Jacobi C, Zhivov A, Korbmacher J, et al. Evidence of endothelial cell migration after Descemet membrane endothelial keratoplasty. *Am J Ophthalmol.* 2011;152(4):537-542.e2.
15. Hos D, Heindl LM, Bucher F, Cursiefen C. Evidence of donor corneal endothelial cell migration from immune reactions occurring after Descemet membrane endothelial keratoplasty. *Cornea.* 2014;33(4):331-334.
16. Miron A, Spinozzi D, Bruinsma M, et al. Asymmetrical endothelial cell migration from in vitro quarter-Descemet membrane endothelial keratoplasty grafts. *Acta Ophthalmol.* 2018;96(8):828-833.
17. Hongyok T, Kim A, Jun AS, Ladas JG, Chuck RS. Phototherapeutic keratectomy with mitomycin C after Descemet stripping automated endothelial keratoplasty. *Br J Ophthalmol.* 2010;94(3):377-378.
18. Awdeh RM, Abbey AM, Vroman DT, et al. Phototherapeutic keratectomy for the treatment of subepithelial fibrosis and anterior corneal scarring after Descemet stripping automated endothelial keratoplasty. *Cornea.* 2018;31(7):761-763.
19. Lee BS, Hardten DR. Visual and subjective outcomes of phototherapeutic keratectomy after Descemet's stripping endothelial keratoplasty. *Clin Ophthalmol.* 2014;8:1011-1015.

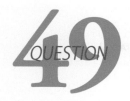

QUESTION 49

I Have a Patient Who Had Prior Verisyse IOL Implantation 20 Years Ago, and They Now Present With Posterior Synechiae, Moderate Cataract, a Shallow Anterior Chamber, and New Corneal Edema. How Should I Best Help This Patient With Their Vision?

Daniel Terveen, MD;
Vance Thompson, MD; and John Berdahl, MD

Background on Phakic Intraocular Lenses

The first phakic intraocular lenses (pIOLs) were introduced by Strampelli in 1953 and designed for placement in the anterior chamber, supported by the angle structures.[1] These IOLs were fraught with severe complications, including angle fibrosis and glaucoma, endothelial decompensation, and pupillary abnormalities. A large number required explantation, and pIOLs were largely abandoned for the next 35 years.[2] In 1998, the Artisan IOL (Ophtec BV) was introduced, featuring a 5- to 6-mm optic, 8.5-mm overall length, 0.87-mm vault to the anterior iris, and available in powers –5.0 to –20.0 diopters. In 2004, this lens gained US Food and Drug Administration (FDA) approval under the name Verisyse Phakic IOL (Abbott Medical Optics Inc).[3,4] Fyodorov introduced the first phakic posterior chamber IOL in 1986.[5] The only lens of this type available in the United States is the Visian implantable collamer lens (STAAR Surgical Co). This lens has a foldable 4.9- to 5.8-mm optic and can be placed through a 3.0-mm clear corneal incision. It is made from a collamer material composed of hydroxyethyl methacrylate and porcine collagen and can be used to treat myopia ranging from –3.0 to –20.0 diopters.[5]

Several randomized controlled trials have evaluated the effectiveness of pIOL placement compared with photoablative procedures.[6,7] These studies found that the 2 methodologies were equally effective at treating refractive error and myopia, but pIOL placement had better contrast sensitivity, higher patient satisfaction, and a lower risk of loss of best-corrected visual acuity at 1 year (0% vs 12%, P = .001).[8]

Hardten DR, Hansen MS.
*Curbside Consultation in Cornea and External Disease:
49 Clinical Questions, Second Edition* (pp 269-272).
© 2022 Taylor & Francis Group.

Table 49-1

Contraindications for pIOLs Based on FDA Data

Contraindications	Visian ICL	Verisyse pIOL
Anterior chamber depth (mm)	< 3.0	< 3.2
Anterior chamber angle	Less than grade II on gonioscopy	Any angle abnormalities
Pregnant or nursing	Contraindicated	Contraindicated
Endothelial density	Age-dependent minimum (range, 1900 to 3875 cells/mm^2)	Age-dependent minimum (range, 2000 to 3550 cells/mm^2)
Iris changes	None	Abnormal iris, such as peaked pupil

Source: US Food and Drug Administration. Accessed October 24, 2021. https://www.accessdata.fda.gov/scripts/cdrh/devicesatfda/index.cfm and https://www.accessdata.fda.gov/scripts/cdrh/devicesatfda/index.cfm

Complications From Phakic IOLs

Thorough preoperative evaluation is important in reducing the risk of complications from pIOLs (Table 49-1). The FDA pivotal trial for the Verisyse and Visian IOLs found several complications with both lenses (Table 49-2). Subsequent studies have evaluated the complications and found similar rates of cataract formation and endothelial cell loss with long-term follow-up. These complications may require IOL explantation. A Spanish study of 240 explanted pIOLs found that the average time for explantation of the iris-claw type lens was 9.36 ± 6.75 years and 4.49 ± 4.25 years for the posterior chamber pIOL.[9] Cataract formation was the cause of explantation in 45.83% of iris claw type and 65.28% in posterior chamber IOLs. Endothelial cell loss was the cause in 8.33% of iris claw type and 1.39% in posterior chamber IOLs.[9]

Monitoring of pIOLs

Following the initial placement of pIOLs, the patient should typically be seen at 1 day, 1 week, 1 month, 2 months, 6 months, and 1 year after surgery and then yearly thereafter. Postoperative examinations should include keratometry, intraocular pressure (IOP) monitoring, and endothelial cell density monitoring at 6 months and yearly thereafter. It is important to monitor yearly for progressive shallowing of the anterior chamber from cataract formation, which can lead to endothelial cell loss as described previously.[10]

Table 49-2

Complications Reported in the FDA Submission

Model	Eyes	Glare/ Halos	Hyphema	Mean ECD Loss	Cataract	Iritis	IOP Elevation
Verisyse	662	18.2%	0.2%	4.75% at 3 years	5.2%	0.5%	0%
Visian	526	9.7% worse 12.0% better	0%	12.8% at 5 years	ASC 0.4%; NS 1.0%	0%	0.4%

ECD = endothelial cell density.

Adapted from the Basic and Clinical Science Course. *Refractive Surgery.* American Academy of Ophthalmology; 2008.

Surgical Technique for This Patient

This patient requires pIOL explantation as well as cataract extraction and possible endothelial keratoplasty. The surgeon should first consider the impact of the endothelial cell loss and resulting corneal edema on the visual complaints. Preoperative endothelial cell count, pachymetry, and densitometry obtained from the Pentacam (OCULUS) can help to guide the surgeon in determining the proportion of visual decline due to corneal changes. If it is determined to be visually significant, endothelial transplantation can be performed at the time of cataract surgery or in a staged procedure.

The Verisyse lens requires a 6.2-mm incision for removal of a 6.0-mm diameter optic and a 5.2-mm incision for a 5.0-mm optic. A self-sealing scleral tunnel is made superiorly, and 2 paracenteses are made on each side of the scleral tunnel, keeping in mind future cataract surgery. Cohesive viscoelastic is placed into the anterior chamber, and the IOL is disenclaved from the iris and carefully removed from the superior incision. The surgeon can now decide whether to perform cataract extraction and endothelial transplantation through the superior incision or after suturing the superior incision to create a new temporal clear-cornea incision for phacoemulsification/ endothelial keratoplasty. If using the superior incision, 2 or 3 interrupted sutures can be placed in the scleral tunnel to reduce the size to better fit the phacoemulsification handpiece. The surgery then proceeds as a normal Descemet's membrane endothelial keratoplasty/Descemet's stripping automated keratoplasty triple procedure, with synechiolysis and management of a small pupil. Alternatively the surgeon can secure the superior scleral tunnel and perform a standard Descemet's membrane endothelial keratoplasty triple from the temporal approach. A larger gas fill is recommended, as the superior incision can cause some gas to escape from the anterior chamber. IOL calculation can be obtained in the traditional manner. The IOP should be closely monitored in the postoperative period, as high myopes with synechia are at high risk for an IOP spike.

Conclusion

With proper yearly monitoring, pIOLs are a great option for vision correction in patients who are contact lens intolerant or who have difficulty with high spectacle correction. Yearly monitoring can prevent additional complications, as described in this case, and these IOLs can provide high-quality spectacle-independent vision until the patient is a candidate for cataract surgery.

References

1. Chen LJ, Chang YJ, Kuo JC, Rajagopal R, Azar DT. Metaanalysis of cataract development after phakic intraocular lens surgery. *J Cataract Refract Surg*. 2008;34(7):1181-1200.
2. Praeger DL, Momose A, Muroff LL. Thirty-six month follow-up of a contemporary phakic intraocular lens for the surgical correction of myopia. *Ann Ophthalmol*. 1991;23(1):6-10.
3. Fechner PU, Strobel J, Wichmann W. Correction of myopia by implantation of a concave Worst-iris claw lens into phakic eyes. *Refract Corneal Surg*. 1991;7(4):286-298.
4. Alexander L, John M, Cobb L, Noblitt R, Barowsky RT. U.S. clinical investigation of the Artisan myopia lens for the correction of high myopia in phakic eyes: report of the results of phases 1 and 2, and interim phase 3. *Optometry*. 2000;71(10):630-642.
5. Jimenez-Alfaro I, Benitez del Castillo JM, Garcia-Feijoo J, Gil de Berenabe JG, Serrano de La Iglesia JM. Safety of posterior chamber phakic intraocular lenses for the correction of high myopia: anterior segment changes after posterior chamber phakic intraocular lens implantation. *Ophthalmology*. 2001;108(1):90-99.
6. El Danasoury MA, El Maghraby A, Gamali TO. Comparison of iris-fixed Artisan lens implantation with excimer laser in situ keratomileusis in correcting myopia between −9.00 and −19.50 diopters: a randomized study. *Ophthalmology*. 2002;109(5):955-964.
7. Schallhorn S, Tanzer D, Sanders DR, Sanders ML. Randomized prospective comparison of Visian toric implantable collamer lens and conventional photorefractive keratectomy for moderate to high myopic astigmatism. *J Refract Surg*. 2007;23(9):853-867.
8. Barsam A, Allan BD. Excimer laser refractive surgery versus phakic intraocular lenses for the correction of moderate to high myopia. *Cochrane Database Syst Rev*. 2014;6:CD007679.
9. Alió JL, Toffaha BT, Peña-Garcia P, Sádaba LM, Barraquer RI. Phakic intraocular lens explantation: causes in 240 cases. *J Refract Surg*. 2015;31(1):30-35.
10. Huang D, Schallhorn SC, Sugar A, et al. Phakic intraocular lens implantation for the correction of myopia. *Ophthalmology*. 2009;116(11):2244-2258.

FINANCIAL DISCLOSURES

Dr. Natalie A. Afshari reported no financial or proprietary interest in the materials presented herein.

Dr. Zaina Al-Mohtaseb reported no financial or proprietary interest in the materials presented herein.

Dr. Brian D. Alder reported no financial or proprietary interest in the materials presented herein.

Dr. Shelby Anderson has not disclosed any relevant financial relationships.

Dr. Penny Asbell reported no financial or proprietary interest in the materials presented herein.

Dr. Brandon Baartman reported no financial or proprietary interest in the materials presented herein.

James R. Barnes reported no financial or proprietary interest in the materials presented herein.

Dr. Melissa Barnett reported no financial or proprietary interest in the materials presented herein.

Dr. John Berdahl reported no financial or proprietary interest in the materials presented herein.

Dr. Benjamin B. Bert reported no financial or proprietary interest in the materials presented herein.

Dr. Andrea Blitzer reported no financial or proprietary interest in the materials presented herein.

Dr. Daniel Brocks reported no financial or proprietary interest in the materials presented herein.

Dr. Jessica Chow reported no financial or proprietary interest in the materials presented herein.

Dr. Reza Dana reported being an equity holder in Aramis Biosciences and a consultant for Novartis, Kala, Kowa.

Dr. Derek W. DelMonte reported no financial or proprietary interest in the materials presented herein.

Dr. Deepinder K. Dhaliwal reported no financial or proprietary interest in the materials presented herein.

Dr. Ali R. Djalilian reported no financial or proprietary interest in the materials presented herein.

Dr. Ahmad Fahmy reported no financial or proprietary interest in the materials presented herein.

Dr. Brad H. Feldman reported no financial or proprietary interest in the materials presented herein.

Dr. C. Stephen Foster reported no financial or proprietary interest in the materials presented herein.

Dr. Martin L. Fox reported no financial or proprietary interest in the materials presented herein.

Dr. Frederick (Rick) W. Fraunfelder reported no financial or proprietary interest in the materials presented herein.

Dr. Prashant Garg has not disclosed any relevant financial relationships.

Dr. Mark S. Gorovoy reported no financial or proprietary interest in the materials presented herein.

Dr. Preeya K. Gupta reported no financial or proprietary interest in the materials presented herein.

Dr. Ramon Joaquim Hallal Jr reported no financial or proprietary interest in the materials presented herein.

Dr. Sadeer B. Hannush has not disclosed any relevant financial relationships.

Dr. Mark S. Hansen has not disclosed any relevant financial relationships.

Dr. David R. Hardten reported financial interest in Minnesota Eye Consultants, Unifeye Vision Partners, Dompe, ESI, Glaukos, HumanOptics, Johnson & Johnson, MicroOptx, OSD, and Sightpath.

Dr. Grant C. Hopping reported no financial or proprietary interest in the materials presented herein.

Dr. Mitch Ibach reported no financial or proprietary interest in the materials presented herein.

Dr. Bennie H. Jeng reported no financial or proprietary interest in the materials presented herein.

Dr. Kyle Jones reported no financial or proprietary interest in the materials presented herein.

Dr. *Sumitra S. Khandelwal* reported no financial or proprietary interest in the materials presented herein.

Dr. *Terry Kim* reported no financial or proprietary interest in the materials presented herein.

Dr. *Thomas Kohnen* has not disclosed any relevant financial relationships.

Dr. *Brent Kramer* reported no financial or proprietary interest in the materials presented herein.

Dr. *Bryan S. Lee* reported no financial or proprietary interest in the materials presented herein.

Dr. *Gary Legault* reported no financial or proprietary interest in the materials presented herein.

Dr. *Erik Letko* has not disclosed any relevant financial relationships.

Dr. *Wendy Liu* reported no financial or proprietary interest in the materials presented herein.

Dr. *Marian Macsai* has not disclosed any relevant financial relationships.

Dr. *Yuri McKee* reported no financial or proprietary interest in the materials presented herein.

Dr. *Jill S. Melicher* reported no financial or proprietary interest in the materials presented herein.

Dr. *Mark S. Milner* has not disclosed any relevant financial relationships.

Dr. *Majid Moshirfar* reported no financial or proprietary interest in the materials presented herein.

Dr. *Muanploy Niparugs* reported no financial or proprietary interest in the materials presented herein.

Dr. *Manachai Nonpassopon* reported no financial or proprietary interest in the materials presented herein.

Dr. *Walter T. Parker* reported no financial or proprietary interest in the materials presented herein.

Dr. *Samuel Passi* has not disclosed any relevant financial relationships.

Dr. *Stephen C. Pflugfelder* has not disclosed any relevant financial relationships.

Dr. *Roberto Pineda* reported receiving royalties from Elsevier.

Dr. *Christopher J. Rapuano* reported no financial or proprietary interest in the materials presented herein.

Dr. *Nikolas Raufi* reported no financial or proprietary interest in the materials presented herein.

Dr. *Sherman W. Reeves* reported no financial or proprietary interest in the materials presented herein.

Dr. Yasmyne C. Ronquillo reported no financial or proprietary interest in the materials presented herein.

Dr. Cullen D. Ryburn reported no financial or proprietary interest in the materials presented herein.

Dr. Konstantinos D. Sarantopoulos reported no financial or proprietary interest in the materials presented herein.

Dr. Celine E. Satija reported no financial or proprietary interest in the materials presented herein.

Dr. Mohamed Abou Shousha reported no financial or proprietary interest in the materials presented herein.

Dr. Krishna Surapaneni reported no financial or proprietary interest in the materials presented herein.

Dr. Daniel Terveen reported no financial or proprietary interest in the materials presented herein.

Dr. Tarika Thareja reported no financial or proprietary interest in the materials presented herein.

Dr. Vance Thompson reported financial relationships with Ophtec, Johnson and Johnson, Alcon, and Staar.

Dr. Kevin R. Tozer reported no financial or proprietary interest in the materials presented herein.

Dr. Elmer Y. Tu has not disclosed any relevant financial relationships.

Dr. Nandini Venkateswaran reported no financial or proprietary interest in the materials presented herein.

Dr. David D. Verdier reported no financial or proprietary interest in the materials presented herein.

Dr. Jesse M. Vislisel reported no financial or proprietary interest in the materials presented herein.

Dr. Laura Voicu reported no financial or proprietary interest in the materials presented herein.

Dr. Michael Wallace reported no financial or proprietary interest in the materials presented herein.

Dr. Yvonne Wang reported no financial or proprietary interest in the materials presented herein.

Dr. Steven E. Wilson reported no financial or proprietary interest in the materials presented herein.

Dr. Sonia H. Yoo reported no financial or proprietary interest in the materials presented herein.

Dr. Zachary Zavodni reported no financial or proprietary interest in the materials presented herein.

Dr. Elaine Zhou reported no financial or proprietary interest in the materials presented herein.

Printed in the United States
by Baker & Taylor Publisher Services